heal your brain

heal your brain

How the New Neuropsychiatry Can Help You Go from Better to Well

David J. Hellerstein, MD

The Johns Hopkins University Press

BALTIMORE

Disclaimer: This book is not intended to give medical advice and is not a substitute for your personal physician. Do not modify your treatment or prescription dosage without first consulting your physician. While I give specific information about drugs and dosages used in individual cases presented in this book, this is not a substitute for consultation with your own physician. Be sure to follow the treatment regimen he or she recommends for you, and do not attempt to make changes on your own!

© 2011 The Johns Hopkins University Press
All rights reserved. Published 2011
Printed in the United States of America on acid-free paper
9 8 7 6 5 4 3 2 1

The Johns Hopkins University Press
2715 North Charles Street
Baltimore, Maryland 21218-4363
www.press.jhu.edu

Library of Congress Cataloging-in-Publication Data

Hellerstein, David.
  Heal your brain : how the new neuropsychiatry can help you go from better to well / David J. Hellerstein.
      p. cm.
Includes bibliographical references and index.
ISBN-13: 978-0-8018-9883-9 (hardcover : alk. paper)
ISBN-10: 0-8018-9883-8 (hardcover : alk. paper)
  1. Neuropsychiatry—Popular works. I. Title.
RC343.H315 2011
616.8—dc22   2010022279

A catalog record for this book is available from the British Library.

Special discounts are available for bulk purchases of this book. For more information, please contact Special Sales at 410-516-6936 or specialsales@press.jhu.edu.

The Johns Hopkins University Press uses environmentally friendly book materials, including recycled text paper that is composed of at least 30 percent post-consumer waste, whenever possible. All of our book papers are acid-free, and our jackets and covers are printed on paper with recycled content.

Contents

Introduction

THIS BOOK IS ABOUT what I do every day—every day that I see patients, that is. About two or three afternoons a week, I leave my office at the New York State Psychiatric Institute and Columbia University Medical Center and drive down the West Side Highway to my private office, to work as a general psychiatrist. For four or five or six hours on those days, long into the evening, I try to apply the latest advances in psychiatry that I have learned in the rarefied world of academia to the people with problems who sit in front of me.

This book is about that process, that practice of psychiatry—the intersection between the latest research advances and the treatment of people who have symptoms and disorders. For want of a better term, I call this approach the "New Neuropsychiatry." One of my predecessors at Columbia, the eminent psychiatrist Jack Gorman, MD, who later became chair of psychiatry at Mount Sinai Medical Center, wrote a book in 1996 called *The New Psychiatry*, which was about the psychiatry of the DSM-IV.

The DSM (*Diagnostic and Statistic Manual of Mental Disorders*) was revolutionary nearly three decades ago, when the third (published in 1980) and then the fourth (published in 1994) editions changed how everyone thought about the treatment of psychiatric disorders. The New Psychiatry was all about making the correct diagnosis, based on specific combinations of symptoms, and then deciding which medicine or therapy approach would give the best outcome. It was a major advance for its time, because before the DSM-III psychiatrists could rarely agree about diagnosis or treatment approaches.

Well, I've been a psychiatrist now for more than twenty-five years, and not long ago it struck me that what my colleagues and I are practicing these days is no longer the New Psychiatry. The best term I could come up with to describe this was the New *Neuro*psychiatry. In this book I'll talk about why that seems to be the best name for this emerging approach and how it works. I'm a little worried that people are going to say, "That can't possibly be true!" or "That's not how it works!"—at least for a lot of it. It *is* the beginning of a new age for psychiatry, though, and a big part of what I am going to do in this book is to explain why that is so.

I have been working at the Columbia University Department of Psychiatry since 2000. I go to conferences and grand rounds and seminars at Columbia every week, and I hear the research presentations by eminent scientists and researchers, brilliant people coming from Johns Hopkins and Massachusetts General Hospital and the like, and a good many of our own researchers from Columbia. They present rat models of psychiatric diseases or genetic research or they show PET scans of the brains of people who have panic disorder or schizophrenia, and it is great stuff. They talk about how the anticonvulsant Lamictal increases "throughput from AMPA receptors" (a class of receptors concerned with synapses in the brain that are involved with the chemical glutamate), possibly accounting for the antidepressant effects of that medication. And how mood stabilizer medicines turn on "neutrotrophic molecules," which help with cell growth and survival.

My colleagues also talk about how depression is related to decreased activity in the prefrontal cortex and to the "hyperactivity of area 25 of the subgenual anterior cingulate," the part of the cerebral cortex that controls blood pressure and heart rate, as well as empathy and decision making, and that may be a gateway between negative thoughts and negative feelings. And how implanting tiny electrodes in area 25 and using tiny doses of electricity to zap this area can relieve intractable depression. I'm fascinated when they talk about mice and prairie voles and about how to measure the formation of memories in aplysia, a form of sea slug that has giant nerve cells. I especially like the brightly colored PET and MRI scans, which show how the brain's activity changes as we think—as we look at sad faces, or as we plan to move a hand, or, even more interesting, how parts of the brain (the mirror neurons) light up when we observe someone else's emotions, when we *literally* "feel for them." I also am intrigued when the speakers talk about other things, such as the epidemiology of mental disorders and phenomenology (which in this context means the main symptoms of various psychiatric disorders).

After a few years of listening to brilliant speakers and to the questions or challenges posed by students and professors in the audience, I began to realize something: all this stuff was starting to connect to what I do when I see patients. After lots of conferences and after innumerable speakers, I was starting to see through people's skulls. Not literally, but figuratively: I was beginning to gain a sense of their brains at work. Herman Hesse once wrote, "The best way to approach the insane is to pretend that you are sane," and in such moments, I would hope that my grip on reality wasn't slipping. Increasingly I began to connect what I see in my office those two or three evenings a week with what is going on in prairie voles and genetically engineered mice and even in that sea slug aplysia.

To put it plainly, I began to sense the connection between brain and mind in my patients. What I mean by this is not only the thinking brain (every word you utter shows that at work), but also the brain as a *physical organ*, as an emotion- and information-processing and perceiving machine. And I am hardly alone in this. For the first time, general psychiatrists are able to look under the hood of the brain, so to speak, and to start to see what is happening in psychiatric disorders. Or, because a certain amount of humility is involved when talking about an organ as complicated as the brain, to start to see what the evidence suggests is happening in the brain, based on our latest technologies.

A word of caution here: this evidence is not always straightforward or simple. Not every study has the same findings, especially when it comes to MRI imaging or genetic studies. And it can be maddeningly difficult to be sure if the brain changes that we see are a cause of the psychiatric disorder, or a result of it. It is also not always clear if people who have similar symptoms actually have the same brain disorder. Nevertheless, we are making rapid progress toward understanding mental and emotional disorders.

My father, Herman K. Hellerstein, MD, was a great cardiologist in the second half of the twentieth century, the heyday of angiography, defibrillation, and coronary bypass operations. As a heart doctor, he was always checking on our pulses when we were kids—he'd suddenly grab our wrists during a concert and palpate our radial pulses, or he'd look at the base of our necks to watch the retrograde pulse of the jugular vein. He would even hook us up to the bicycle ergometer at his cardiology lab, so we could see the 12-lead printout of our hearts' rapid beating as we cycled up imaginary hills.

The brain's activity has traditionally been much harder to measure directly. It's easy to see the *effects* of the brain at work, because nearly everything we do as humans involves our brains. And neurologists, with their reflex hammers and pins and vials of strong-smelling spices, are able to test the functioning of the brain's physical machinery pretty easily. The parts of the brain that I am talking about are those most affected by psychiatric disorders. Only in the past decade or so have we begun to have a clue as to what they are and how they impact daily life. With PET and MRI scans, with gene chips and dozens of other incredible technologies, we now have the tools to study areas of the brain affected by psychiatric disorders. We can now demonstrate how these conditions cause injury to specific parts of the brain that are involved in "stress response systems" and "autobiographical memory," and other functions. And we can see how injury to specific areas of the brain can lead to impairment in the quality of life and in day-to-day functioning. These are remarkable breakthroughs.

Beyond that, as I am going to describe in detail, we have begun to understand how our treatments can slow or stop the process of injury to these parts of the brain and can even, perhaps, begin to repair some of them. This is especially true for people who have had to deal with bouts of overwhelming depression and anxiety.

The New Neuropsychiatry is thus able to begin to describe how specific aspects of brain functioning are affected by disorders, and by our treatments as well. The New Neuropsychiatry is, of course, different from the first wave of neuropsychiatry, which emerged in the late nineteenth century—when psychiatrists and neurologists studied the effects of illnesses such as tuberculosis and syphilis on the brain. That era of neuropsychiatry was able to look at only large injuries to the brain, such as those caused by infection, trauma, or stroke. With our twenty-first-century technologies, the New Neuropsychiatry has returned to the brain but with neuroscience rather than neurology as its basis—and with the ability to look at relatively tiny areas of brain functioning, even microscopic ones.

For instance, today as a general psychiatrist talking to Mrs. Smith who has depression, it is possible for me to realize the effect of her depression on a tiny center of deep within the brain called the hippocampus—or even on a particular type of cell in a specific area, such as those in the dentate gyrus of the hippocampus; that is what is new in the New Neuropsychiatry. Treating Mrs. Smith's depression has a goal of at least partly repairing these hippocampal injuries. And the hippocampus—the brain's learning and memory center—is key to what I'm describing when I talk about the New Neuropsychiatry treatments and how they work.

The biggest realization I've had—in thinking about and trying to practice the New Neuropsychiatry—is how we can begin to use its principles to help many people recover from disorders. I am not claiming any special expertise as a psychiatrist. I'm just talking about being a good general psychiatrist who applies the principles of our twenty-first-century craft to the patients who come through the doors of my office every day. Properly applied, these principles—and these New Neuropsychiatry treatment approaches—can, as I mentioned, lead to positive outcomes. To the control of symptoms that may have tortured people for years, even decades. And to significant—even dramatic—improvement in the ability to have a fulfilling and rich life. These life changes appear to be a result of brain recovery, especially of the vulnerable stress response systems. The tools I am talking about are nothing special in themselves—certain types of clinical assessments and treatment plans, certain types of therapy approaches, the proper use of SSRIs (selective serotonin reuptake inhibitors) and other medicines, and lifestyle changes such as exercise, meditation, and mindfulness. The key—and the subtle art of the New Neuropsychiatry—is in how they are applied and how they are combined. That is what this book is also about.

(I know some people will say, "Well, I heard that a lot of studies recently showed that treatments don't work very well for depression. One that said only X percent of people get better, only Y percent get well, and a lot of those who do get well don't stay well." This is true—but so is my point that, if used properly, present-day psychiatric treatments can work remarkably well and can lead to recovery. I'll discuss this seeming paradox as we go forward.)

This book focuses on two types of common psychological disorders: depression and anxiety, rather than on psychotic diseases such as schizophrenia. This is because the biggest impact of the New Neuropsychiatry so far is on the treatment of these disorders. For many if not most people who have them, it is now possible not only to get better but also to become well. That is why my book has two sections: Getting Better and Getting (and Staying) Well.

One of the effects of going to so many grand rounds at Columbia and of debating, discussing, arguing, and exploring psychiatry with hundreds of colleagues is that I have realized something about brains: they grow. They are always reconnecting and reshaping themselves and pruning and developing new pathways. As neuroscientists put it, the brain is "plastic," always changing and always growing.

One example of this was a study of London cab drivers, who are required to memorize the complex map of the City of London as part of their training. In a landmark 2000 study of London cabbies, Eleanor Maguire and colleagues at the Institute of Neurology in London measured the size of their hippocampi. The hippocampus is part of the brain that, among other things, forms a spatial map of your environment as a result of experience. It is also key for the consolidation of episodic memories, which are memories of personally experienced events and their associated emotions. Memorizing the streets of the City of London, as the cabbies do, is a prodigiously complicated endeavor. Maguire's study found that the posterior part of the hippocampus was larger among cabbies who had been driving for the longest time in London. That is, learning and relearning the map of London as they made their daily rounds caused that part of their brains to grow.

Some of this growth probably resulted from increased connections between brain cells. Other growth was most likely the result of *new cells* growing in the cabbies' brains—what is called neurogenesis. Recent research has shown—contrary to usual belief—that new brain cells *do* appear during adult life in certain parts of the brain, particularly in the hippocampus. The significance of this type of brain cell growth, exciting as it is, remains controversial. Not so another type of brain plasticity—the connections between brain cells, or "synaptic connectivity." This is clearly essential to learning and the development of new skills: how else would we learn a new language if not for synaptic connectivity?

It is not only cab driving that sparks brain growth. Neuroscientists have also shown that the brain is always remodeling itself. Thinking (or learning) causes chemical changes in the brain and changes in brain connections. In a fascinating 2004 study, neuroimager Bogdan Draganski showed that learning juggling measurably changed the brain's gray matter, particularly in the part of the brain related to visual processing. Practicing juggling was required to make these changes, similar to the process of learning a language or other subjects. Psychotherapy of various types also leads to measurable brain changes.

And many of the medicines we use in psychiatric treatment—from SSRIs to lithium to the seizure medication Depakote—actually increase brain connectivity. (In fact, studies suggest that medications *must* make new cells in the hippocampus in order to work as antidepressants!) Exercise also causes neurogenesis in the hippocampus, and so, most likely, do activities such as meditation and yoga. Perhaps this is how psychotherapy and medication are able to halt and even to reverse the types of brain injury caused by psychiatric disorders.

Put simply, depression and anxiety disorders are associated with damage to various systems in the brain, including the ones governing stress response. This damage appears to lead to impaired functioning, which leads to more symptoms and more damage. New Neuropsychiatry treatments—often simple ones—increasingly hope to interrupt these cycles of damage and to help the brain to recover, to remodel itself in a healthy way, even to regrow.

So, in thinking about this beginning of a convergence of science and practice, I wondered whether it would be possible to try to boil down the amazing complexity of the research in the New Neuropsychiatry into some reasonable and simple principles of treatment. This is what I am attempting to do in this book. To show how people can escape from the seemingly interminable suffering of mood and anxiety disorders. And to show how people who have these disorders can use the insights of the New Neuropsychiatry to return to normal life. Or how they can find themselves able to move from disorder to response, from response to remission, and from remission to recovery: from getting better to getting well.

This book is made up of a lot of stories about people who faced—and usually triumphed over—disorders. The characters you will meet are based on people I have treated over the years. Names and other identifying characteristics have, of course, been changed, but I hope to have retained the essence of their experiences with New Neuropsychiatry treatments. I chose this format to some degree because I like stories—telling them, reading them, writing them. Since my Midwestern childhood, hearing my father's tales of growing up in a coal-mining town in southern Ohio and of being a soldier in World War II and then a doctor in the early coronary care units, I have been aware of the power of stories. But to a greater degree it is because stories (or, as my colleagues might put it, "narratives") are essential to the New Neuropsychiatry. Stories—especially the ones about yourself and your life experiences—are a way of organizing your brain. They are the way in which your brain connects and reorganizes itself. In major depression, the access to such "autobiographical memories" is, in fact, impaired—depressed people have trouble connecting to particular memories of their life, especially to ones that can help them recover.

The New Neuropsychiatrist works with you to retell your stories, to break them down into little pieces and help you make new ones. A good part of the getting well in the New Neuropsychiatry results from creating new stories or new scripts about the possibilities and new directions of your life. Storytelling is a brain activity: the repetition of stories and the telling of new ones create connections between brain cells, and recovery from psychiatric disorders involves remapping of your brain in part by telling new stories about yourself. Neuroscientists are increasingly fascinated by subjective experience, because it is a central part of what makes each human an individual and what differentiates the structure and functioning of one brain from the next. And self-narrative is one key part of our individual subjective experiences and of the individuality of our brains.

I'm hoping that my New Neuropsychiatry colleagues will recognize themselves for what they are—pioneers on the edge of exploring new frontiers. It is exciting these days to be practicing as a psychiatrist. No matter what the latest headlines about treatment are—whether SSRIs cause adolescents to become more suicidal, how many negative studies the supposedly nefarious drug companies have hidden, and so on—psychiatrists are now in a position where our treatment approaches can help people who have depression and anxiety, can make a difference in their lives.

For people with depression, the road you face today is much easier than if you had developed an episode of major depression one hundred fifty or two hundred years ago. Best case scenario, you'd have to go to sea and chase whales or head out West and search for gold. Worst case, the sad fact is, you would be housed in a jail along with criminals. Even a century ago, you would not fare much better and would be at risk of either being locked in an asylum for life or of being subjected to crude shock treatment or insulin coma. Forty or fifty years ago, you would have been put into psychoanalysis, which, however fascinating, would not be likely to cure your depression, or you would have been treated with high-side-effect antidepressants such as Elavil and Nardil.

Today, if you have major depression or panic disorder, and you know what to look for, it is possible to get good treatment with medication and therapy.

You are likely to get better. One measure of this is suicide rates, which after a century of increase have dropped significantly since the introduction of SSRIs. Certain (often predictable) problems and complications and side effects may occur with treatment, but we know a lot more today than in past decades. We are more likely to find something to work for you—or, actually, to work *with* you, because your participation is a key part of the New Neuropsychiatry treatment approach.

Back to grand rounds at Columbia: every so often I am foolish enough to raise my hand to ask a question. Once, in a packed auditorium, just as Eric Kandel finished giving a speech summarizing decades of Nobel Prize–winning research, I asked a question. Dr. Kandel had been talking about ongoing research in his laboratory where his colleague Dr. Michael Rogan had discovered something he called "safety centers" in the brains of mice and had conditioned mice to feel safe, to venture into the middle of their cages, free from their fear of predators. Whereas we had traditionally thought only of the brain's "fear center," the amygdala, which becomes active in times of danger, Rogan's work suggests that a different part of the brain becomes activated when things are safe. I began thinking of one of my patients, whom I had seen the night before, a woman with lifelong panic disorder who had had a spectacularly good and sustained response to a combined treatment with SSRI medication and cognitive-behavioral therapy. All her life she had been barely able to leave her home borough of Queens, New York, but after responding to treatment she began to travel throughout the metropolitan area with greater ease. But last evening she surprised me: coming into her session, radiant, telling me about how she had just returned from a trip to Mexico with her fiancé. Her first plane ride. The combination treatment had enabled her to enjoy the plane ride, to sit looking out at the blue waters of the Caribbean far below, feeling a sense of euphoria and wonder.

"I was feeling safe for the first time in my life," she told me, "actually feeling okay, realizing that this is what normal people feel."

So I asked Dr. Kandel if we might see evidence for the activation of the safety center in patients. And that, "with patients who have experienced a prolonged remission of panic disorder, is it possible that their safety centers are being activated again?"

People told me later that they thought it was an interesting question— or, in our academic jargon, "a researchable question." And today's research technology is such that Dr. Rogan is now studying "safety centers" in humans, using state-of-the-art brain imaging techniques. These days, the connection between what is observed in a psychiatrist's office and what can be measured in a research laboratory is closer than ever before. An idea like this, however brash or speculative, can be tested: one can study PET or MRI images of the brains of humans who have been "safety conditioned"—or of people who have panic disorder that successfully responded to treatment. This is the great potential of the New Neuropsychiatry: we can directly study how our treatments affect brain function, and thus can improve them. We can go right from molecule to mouse to man, from laboratory to the doctor's office, and from the doctor's office back to the laboratory. And we can begin to develop personalized treatments that will lead people from disorder back to normal life.

It is a remarkable time, and only the beginning. New Neuropsychiatry is just emerging and being refined, as it comes out of New Psychiatry and neuroscience and psychopharmacology and genetics and other fields. No doubt many of its ideas are oversimplified, perhaps even wrong—but it seems to me to be a compelling and inescapable model, and undoubtedly the future of psychiatry. Clearly, the New Neuropsychiatry will be modified even more over the coming decades, as more is understood about mind-brain-body connections and the effects of existing treatments and as researchers are able to develop and use a wider range of new treatments. This is why, despite the obvious limitations of the New Neuropsychiatry, I am so hopeful. With advances in research and treatment, we are gaining glimpses of an emerging continent—through fog—the first glimpses of something new, the infancy of a new new world, so to speak, and we are likely to be able to better treat, and eventually to cure and even prevent, the mood and anxiety disorders, and other psychiatric illnesses as well.

Part 1

Getting Better

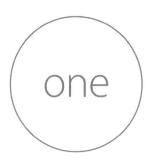

one

Disorder

"Is There Any Hope for Me?"

Misery

IT IS 4 A.M. and you have awakened, startled into deep misery, for the twentieth night in a row. For months, you have delayed, denied, procrastinated, and distracted yourself. Spring vacation, your annual bonus, a weekend away from the kids—day after day, you held out hope that something would do the trick. Now, you realize, it was all an illusion. This state, this misery, is not going away. Four or five years back, you experienced something like this. Then, after months of sleeplessness and agitation, the suffering eventually faded. Not this time. Not only is this episode more severe and more all-pervasive, but every day it seems to be getting worse.

You lie in bed, suffering.

What should you do?

It's complicated, what you're going through. A tangle of old feelings and new, worries about your relationships, your career, problems with your children. Perhaps there is a scandal at work—something being investigated by a federal agency. Or your industry is in a slump and massive layoffs are rumored. Or perhaps your wife has threatened to leave you. Or one of your children is severely ill.

Maybe you have tried exercise to help you cope, or long talks with old friends, or your spouse's sleeping pills. To no end. Now this—whatever it is that is making your suffering even worse than it has to be—is affecting your marriage, your time with the kids. You can't concentrate, you're snapping at everyone. You feel utter despair. Nothing gives pleasure anymore. Except perhaps the increasingly compelling thought of ending it all.

Something must be done.

Finally, just before your alarm is due to go off, you fall back asleep for a last few comforting minutes.

Later that day, in the midst of an endless office meeting or while stuck on the expressway, the feeling of desperation, of unendurable panic, returns. Should you talk to someone? Go on Prozac? End it all?

Is there any hope?

Welcome to the state of disorder—when the mind's natural healing and self-calming processes have failed. For most of us, our psyches ordinarily operate within a broad comfort zone. Time after time, we can screw up. We can push ourselves too far, we can stress out for months—and then we can count on bouncing back. Usually, a quiet weekend, a good talk with a close friend, a funny movie, or just the passage of time returns us to our usual well-being. Not so in the state of disorder. Something, it is clear, is broken. Some mental safety mechanism that worked well for decades has failed.

When people enter this phase, they try desperately to right themselves, to regain the smooth functioning of a vanishing past. They may try to make themselves feel better with exercise, or with marijuana or cocaine or booze. They may pray, or binge on chocolate, or talk incessantly.

Yet past a certain threshold, everything fails. A sort of psychic chaos now threatens their remaining equilibrium, perhaps even their very survival. The idea of suicide can even bring a certain comfort—a solution, a way out. It can seem like the natural choice.

In short, the state of disorder is a desperate place to be. The struggle is not only pragmatic, not only a fight with the world, but it also an internal battle. A philosophical struggle over one's own natural reluctance to admit helplessness, over hopes for spontaneous remission, over the desire to wake up one morning to find that everything is okay.

Eventually, some final line is crossed. It may be a life-threatening event. Ever-blacker moods that make it impossible to go to work. An inability to

> **Depression in the United States**
>
> In a recent large study of more than 9,000 people in the United States, ages 12 to 94, Dr. Ronald Kessler and his co-workers found that 16.2 percent have had major depression at some point in their lives and, of these, 6.6 percent have had major depression in the past year. The greatest risk for depression was among people between 18 and 30 years old, who had three times the risk of people over 60 years of age. The next highest group was women ages 30 to 44, with nearly twice the risk. Not surprisingly, being poor doesn't help things: the risk of depression increased fourfold for people living below the poverty line. It is clear from Kessler's study that depression causes a lot of impairment—those who were depressed over the past year had been unable to work for an average of thirty-five days!
>
> Even though depression is so common, it is still often not well treated. In the early 1990s, only about a third of people who had depression had received adequate treatment within the past year. By 2002, nearly 60 percent of people who had depression had received some treatment. But most people still don't receive *adequate* treatment, which Kessler defined as four or more visits to a physician for medication (and taking an antidepressant or mood stabilizer for thirty days or more) or eight or more visits to a therapist of any discipline. This is better than in the 1980s, when I was training to become a psychiatrist, but obviously is not where we want to be.

stop sobbing. Or strangely enticing dreams of death. Other times it may be more subtle, a realization that some disaster "is happening again"—another damning job evaluation, another bleeding ulcer, another marriage headed down the tubes. The body, the mind, the social system, each has its natural warning system. Each one attempts to transmit an unmistakable message before disaster strikes.

The Toxic Cycle

In recent decades, knowledge we have gained about the human brain has yielded insights both into what types of disorders a person can recover from and into the tools to help them recover. The New Neuropsychiatry has shown that there is a dividing line for human suffering. Most symptoms will pass before becoming disorders; most symptoms will fade away on their own. Get depressed after you break off your engagement or lose your job—that's okay, you'll probably feel better in a few weeks. But if you don't get better, if the symptoms persist for month after month, watch out! Then you may have entered a toxic state, a continual cycle of signals gone awry.

Another facet of disorders that we have learned from New Neuropsychiatry research is that such profound states of disorder are bad for your brain—and for your body. Once they set in, disorders can develop a life of their own, they can create (and reinforce) their own distorted logic, they can take over and even ruin your life. There is an order to disorder—but it is a toxic order, to be sure.

Unequivocally, the New Neuropsychiatry has shown how common, and how devastating, mental disorders can be. Perhaps 15 to 20 percent of the U.S. population at any given time has a psychiatric disorder that significantly affects day-to-day functioning, the most common involving some form of depression or anxiety.

Not only that, but disorder *breeds* disorder. Disordered brain functioning causes impaired social functioning and can set off a chain reaction, causing one disorder (say, clinical depression) to allow another (alcoholism, panic disorder, agoraphobia) to flower. Nearly three-quarters of people who have depression have other disorders as well, especially anxiety and substance abuse. Untreated clinical depression has been shown to lead to suicide as much as 15 percent of the time. And even when there's no impulse toward suicide, depression is devastating—besides poor work functioning, it may lead to financial and health problems and even to more deaths from heart disease. Not to mention the havoc it wreaks on families—marital conflicts, including divorce, problems with kids, and so on. Untreated, depression and other disorders can ruin families.

So, like it or not, once you cross the line of disorder, evaluation and treatment are necessary.

First as a flickering in the back of your mind, then becoming as constant as a pain in your chest, a realization comes over you: *I have a problem. I need to do something.*

Searching for Help

In emergency or extreme situations, the warning signs of a state of disorder may be obvious. A man in his 50s, always healthy, suddenly lusts after death and begins giving away his prized possessions. A woman in her mid-40s hears voices for the first time in her life and sits for days in her living room conversing with people who aren't there. Following her mother's death, a retired teacher becomes entirely unable to sleep, forced into wakefulness for weeks at a time. A stockbroker, always mercurial in temperament, begins to speak with machine-gun rapidity, spending and talking recklessly; setting up meetings with CEOs of large corporations, he proposes impossibly vast business deals.

A woman may have experienced a life-threatening event such as rape. Terrifying flashbacks, startle reactions, an utter inability to calm herself, the hallmarks of posttraumatic stress. At times the seriousness of such situations is more obvious to family or co-workers than to the individual herself, who may be temporarily blinded by the intensity of her suffering. Once identified, though, such extreme situations require prompt action—even a trip to the nearest emergency room or possibly hospitalization.

Many psychological disorders, however, do not announce themselves as acute emergencies but instead creep in as silently as the tide. Almost without notice, feelings grow into symptoms, symptoms become disorders, and disorders impair functioning. Eventually, life seems to be a tangle of dysfunction. Black moods and insomnia and suicidal preoccupations become the stuff of life itself for a person in a major depression. For a person with panic attacks, the tsunami of fear and anxiety overwhelms everything else. And for the person with obsessive-compulsive disorder, the need for symmetry or clean hands or the inextinguishable irrational belief that something bad may happen—may *already* have happened!—swamps the mundane concerns of work and friendships and daily routine. The very idea of doing something about these problems may seem foreign, bizarre, or peculiar, because the symptoms themselves are so compelling, at least at first, and the pain they cause may be almost bracing.

Some disorders are even more subtle. For instance, the young man who has extreme shyness and avoids parties, restaurants, social events, but nonetheless can go to work on most days. Or the young woman with bulimia who manages to hide her vomiting from her family and friends, but spends hours in front of the bathroom sink avoiding glimpses of her pale face in the mirror.

Surely there is a need for help. But life can go on without it. Eventually, one suspects, such problems will catch up with the person who suffers from them, but from one day to the next they can be practically ignored.

In all these instances, the New Neuropsychiatry has much to offer.

What about you?

You are increasingly becoming convinced that you must find a way out of your suffering.

Over the next several days, you plunge into your researches. On the Web, the 144 million Googled pages on depression seem like an endless express-way of drug ads and personal complaints, each contradicting the last. You call your college roommate, who trained to become a clinical psychologist. On the basis of late-night conversations fifteen years ago, he recalls that you had unresolved conflicts. He recommends psychoanalysis. Three times a week, five or six years, that should do it. But, your insurance company, Human Resources informs you, covers only twenty sessions per year. Plus, their new policy is that everyone should go on medication first, to save the shareholders money. And what about medicine? Do medications help or hurt? Don't they cause suicid-ality? Don't they mess up your sex life? The newspapers are full of evidence of the venality of drug companies, how so many doctors are on the take. Who can you trust?

Now you are not only depressed but also totally confused.

Welcome to the bazaar. In your early frantic searches for a cure, you have begun to discover a profound truth about post-Y2K America—as far as the treatment of psychiatric symptoms goes, we are in the midst of the Oklahoma land rush. A vast stampede in which everyone is trying to stake a first claim on your brain—and in which your own needs can easily be ridden over roughshod.

There is no shortage of treatment choices today. Since Prozac was intro-duced in the United States in the late 1980s, innumerable new drugs have entered the marketplace. Some are essentially clones of Prozac (Zoloft, Paxil, Luvox, Celexa, Lexapro), keeping brain cells from reabsorbing serotonin, leav-ing more in the synaptic cleft (the places where neurons connect), to help improve mood and anxiety. Others, such as Serzone and Remeron, work by different means. While also affecting serotonin, Remeron, for instance, is thought to also increase the release of serotonin and norepinephrine farther "upstream" in the brain, and it may be helpful for some people who don't respond to SSRIs. Others work on a combination of transmitter systems—Effexor and Cymbalta, affecting serotonin and norepinephrine, or Wellbutrin, which works on dopamine and norepinephrine. Direct-to-consumer TV ads brag that one compound is better than the next, instilling doubt about them all. Then there are the unregulated food additives and natural supplements that crowd the marketplace. Capsules, powders, teas, soft drinks (even taco chips!) now contain St. John's wort or SAM-e or other putative cures for anxiety and sadness. Plus, countless Web sites offer to ship you the antidepressant of your choice without the inconvenience of ever seeing a doctor.

On the therapy side, over the past few decades, hundreds of thousands of psychotherapists have hung out their shingles across America. Counselors and life coaches and religious therapists (some well trained, others of dubious credentials) practice alongside the more traditional psychiatrists, psychologists, and social workers. Not to mention past-life regression therapists, astrologers, even "psychic chiropractors"!

Caught in this maelstrom, you may begin to perceive—in your alternately desultory and desperate researches—that your brain and mind (and life) have basically become commodified, your suffering bundled with that of a million others to be bought and sold in the open marketplace like shares of YouTube.

What should you do? How can you know when you need help? And where to get it?

The New Neuropsychiatry approach may not be as exciting as what you encounter on the Web or at the health food store, but it has the virtues of being consistent and realistic.

So, as you start, you know that you are *in* a state of disorder. But do you *have* a disorder? For the New Neuropsychiatry, this is a crucial question. And if you do have a disorder, which type is it? These questions must be answered to gain any benefit from treatment. The key is whether you have significant, persistent symptoms. If you persistently have trouble sleeping, if you have suicidal feelings, or panic attacks, or a persistent inability to concentrate or to stop crying, then you are likely to have a disorder. Or if you have symptoms that might vary on a day-by-day basis, but simply won't go away and last for weeks or months—such as continual feelings of agitation or a depressed mood that doesn't lift—then you might have a disorder.

Finding Out What's Wrong

If you think you might have a disorder, you need an evaluation. It's as simple as that. An evaluation by a mental health professional is necessary so that you can understand what the problem or problems may be and can get help in deciding what sort of treatment is appropriate for you.

But how do you get a reliable evaluation? Here's where you are going to have to do some homework. Perhaps, you decide, you'll try going through your insurance company. You call a toll-free number and are given the names of two or three doctors. You pick up the phone, choosing the most confidence-inspiring name. Or, dubious of the methods of managed care, you may opt to step outside the system in search of an impartial assessment.

At this early phase you may discern—accurately enough—that the disorder in your mind is paralleled by an even greater disorder of the American mental health system. However, just as there is an order to psychiatric disorder, there is an order to the mental health system. Competent psychopharmacologists and good therapists can be found, often through networks affiliated with major medical centers and training programs.

Even if you are able to obtain some good referrals, a dilemma comes up. Do you need a psychological evaluation (an evaluation for therapy) or a biological evaluation (an evaluation for medication)? It's usually worth trying to get an evaluation with *both* components—if possible, to find one doctor to evaluate both mind and brain—even though it may be difficult to locate one. One person evaluating both areas is in the best position to make a plan that takes into account both mind and brain. If you don't do this, if you get just a "medication evaluation" or just a "therapy evaluation," then you could end up wedded to one type of treatment without having a chance to consider all the alternatives—or the possible benefits of combined treatments.

As an active partner in your treatment, what can you do? How can you find someone to do an evaluation that will give equal weight to "mind" and "brain"? Perhaps you can try to find a doctor who knows about medications and who *also* "believes in therapy." Maybe your internist or family doctor can make a recommendation. Or you can try word of mouth, via friends who have had good experiences in treatment, or through professional recommendations from your clergyman or from self-help organizations. Alternatively, you may try to guess where your problem lies and get an evaluation of the area of most concern to you.

Sometimes you can get away *without* evaluating the brain. If you are having a relationship problem and neither you nor your spouse has many symptoms of depression or anxiety, perhaps you can do without a biological evaluation. (Though marital therapists tell me that in many couples therapy cases at least one member has depression!) Clearly, many nonmedical therapists—psychologists, social workers, marital counselors—have large caseloads of patients who have never had an evaluation of their psychobiological systems.

To understand both areas, it may even be necessary to consider the possibility of getting two evaluations—one by a therapist, who will presumably focus more on narrative; one by a psychopharmacologist, who will presumably focus more on biology. The New Neuropsychiatrist increasingly handles both types of evaluations. Yet another option: getting a consultation from a clinician who will provide the evaluation but not the treatment and can make a referral to others and thus avoid any conflict of interest.

Most likely, in your suffering, you perceive only a part of the picture described above—like a survivor of some horrible crash who awakens to see a stretch of road, a few signs, a wintry landscape, some broken trees, who groans in pain and wonders where the nearest telephone may be found. *When will help come?* And, *Is there any hope for me?*

In the midst of suffering, of wild disorder, of calamity, it is frequently impossible to see the whole scene at once. Only to realize that your insurance doesn't cover the therapist that your internist referred you to, or that the doctor who participates in your company's plan doesn't have an appointment available until next month.

The Mind-Body Connection

Getting a psychiatric evaluation is not the only essential thing to in dealing with an emotional disorder. You should also see your medical doctor and have a physical exam and lab tests, to rule out the possibility that something is medically wrong with you. It is possible that your psychological symptoms result from some physical ailment. Medical textbooks are full of examples of illnesses that present with psychiatric symptoms, everything from benign and easily treatable conditions such as thyroid disease to serious disorders such as heart disease or cancer. For more about medical issues that can influence the course of mental health treatment, see Chapter 2.

Brain Functioning in Depression

As New Neuropsychiatry research shows again and again, a disorder can result from abnormal functioning of the brain—and recovering from a disorder can repair a significant amount of this damage.

Our knowledge about the effects of disorder on the brain and the workings of the brain itself is constantly being updated. The current understanding of the abnormal brain functioning in depression has come from several different types of research, including the following:

- ► Neuroimaging—such as positron emission tomography (PET) scans and magnetic resonance imaging (MRI)—which provides data about both the anatomy and functioning of the brain
- ► Electroencephalograms (EEGs), which are recordings of electrical activity of the brain
- ► Neurocognitive tests, such as psychological tests of reasoning, perception, and problem solving
- ► Studies of the functioning of neurons themselves, often done in animals such as mice or rats

It is clear that during depression there is reduced activity in some parts of the brain, particularly the dorsolateral prefrontal cortex—the area associated with working memory and executive function, among other things—on the left side of the brain. At the same time, as many studies show, there may be *increased* activity in other parts of the brain, particularly in the right frontal area and the right prefrontal cortex. Neurocognitive tests also have found abnormalities on the right side of the brain—especially in the right temporal-parietal cortex, areas that are associated with processing musical tones and spatial relationships. Besides the decrease in activity in the left prefrontal cortex, there is reduced activity in the dorsal anterior cingulate, which is thought to play a role in emotional self-control, focused problem-solving, and error recognition, as well as in making adaptive responses to changing conditions. Most of these abnormalities are greater the more severe the depression is, and most of them improve when depression goes away.

What about the hippocampus and the amygdala in depression? Most MRI studies of depression have shown shrinkage of the hippocampus, especially in the left side. This shrinkage has been linked with the memory impairments we often see in depression. It is believed that they are related to the elevated levels of glucocorticoids (stress hormones) found during times of life stress or after traumatic experiences. Neuroscientist Robert Sapolsky believes that these elevations cause damage to the hippocampus. The amygdala, the brain's fear center, also appears to be abnormal in depression. The more severe the depression, the more the amygdala is activated. And the more anxiety a depressed person feels, the more the amygdala is turned on.

The secretion of stress hormones appears to be elevated in depression: a depressed person's body puts out more cortisol and a cascade of other hormones. These are particularly increased in people who experienced severe stress during childhood and adolescence. These elevated hormones can damage the brain further, leading to greater impairment in a person's ability to function, causing yet more stress and yet more secretion of stress hormones. This is one of the many vicious cycles of mental disorders—in this case, a toxic interaction among life stress, stress chemicals, abnormal brain activation, and brain injury.

Finally, people who are depressed often develop abnormalities in the rest of their bodies as well—depression leads to elevated cholesterol and glucose levels, which can hurt the heart, blood vessels, and other organs, and even make your blood platelets "stickier." This increased stickiness can lead to more clotting problems, including blockage of the arteries feeding the heart muscle itself. It is no accident that people who have depression have more heart disease—and that depressed people are more likely to die once they have a heart attack! The dysregulation of major depression is profound and involves nearly every organ of the body.

No doubt this sketch does not apply to all people who have depression. Depression is likely to be heterogeneous—to have different causes and to result from different brain abnormalities in different people. The various anxiety disorders also are likely to have somewhat different brain physiology—different from depression and different from each other. Throughout this book, I present a simplified model—similar to the way that Sigmund Freud used the concept of id, ego, and superego to describe the psychodynamic forces of the mind in his model nearly one hundred years ago—of what is happening in the brain during states of disorder and recovery. Nevertheless, it is a useful model, a type that increasingly will underlie our work in the New Neuropsychiatry.

Assuming there's nothing medically wrong, what next? It is hard to argue with the universal desire to call up natural healing mechanisms. New Neuropsychiatry research has proven that depression includes serious dysregulation of body rhythms—everything from the sleep-wake cycle to the body's production of hormones such as cortisol, a stress hormone released by the adrenal glands.

In fact, we are learning that the body and mind are interconnected in depression. Take the endocrine system, our body's hormones. Chemical signals from the limbic part of the brain flow to the hypothalamus, which sends signals to the pituitary gland and then to the adrenal cortex, a gland that sits atop your kidneys. In depression a cascade of stress hormones passes through your bloodstream and bathes all of your organs. These hormones are essential for helping humans respond to stress in the short run but are toxic to your body and your brain in the long run. Not only your hormones are activated but also your immune system, through chemicals called cytokines—which protect you from infection but also can make you feel weak and sick. Over weeks and months, high levels of cortisol can cause actual shrinkage of areas of the brain such as the hippocampus (which is related to personal memory and helps you map your world, locating and orienting you in space). And they trigger the amygdala, the brain's fear center, to stay on high alert.

Overall, in the state of disorder, your body is activated for war. The war mode is a brain-body state that has evolved over millions of years for a reason: it can help with survival. It consists of a constant state of hyperalertness, of battle-readiness in which at any moment you may have to fight or to flee. In the interest of survival, it interrupts your sleep-wake cycles and other circadian rhythms, such as body temperature, melatonin production, and blood pressure. But in psychiatric disorder, the battle never ends; peace never returns. For a brief time, you're ready to fight—but as time passes, this state establishes itself with its own internal logic and order. It can become debilitating and toxic, even fatal.

So, logically, from the beginning of dealing with a disorder, it makes sense to try to normalize your body's functions. It makes sense to cut down on coffee and alcohol, to avoid unhealthy foods, to eliminate so-called recreational drugs. No doubt you've tried regularizing your sleep patterns, aiming for seven or eight hours every night. And getting back into a pattern of regular exercise. You may have even tried buying a CD that has muscle relaxation and deep breathing exercises—hoping to "stimulate alpha-waves." Sometimes old-fashioned clean living can set disordered neuroendocrine and circadian rhythms back to normal. Some people will try the natural route, using melatonin, St. John's wort, or SAM-e in an effort to self-treat.

How often do these efforts work? Probably reasonably often. But if these approaches had been successful, it's unlikely that you'd be considering seeing a psychiatrist.

In any case, for the New Neuropsychiatry it is always essential to set a time limit, to have contingency plans: *if my old stand-bys like exercising, talking to friends, taking a good vacation don't help in the next two weeks, then what? If this herb, potion, or additive doesn't help by next month, what will I do next?*

The Silent Prelude

The difficulty is, by the time a disorder has emerged, by the time prominent symptoms have developed and become a part of your daily experience, they may have a life of their own. There is what could be called "an order to disorder"—all those changes of hormones and behaviors and rhythms can get set in place. Disorder may be painful, or toxic, or destructive, but it has its own rules and logic. It can stubbornly set up house in your brain, refusing to leave. If disorder has moved in and won't leave, despite your best efforts, you have to do something.

How you have attempted to address your symptoms up until now is all a prelude, a beginning phase. Often it is forgotten, unmentioned, brushed aside by the time you arrive at your New Neuropsychiatry evaluation. But it's important. What have you tried already, and what has worked, even partially? What has utterly failed? To know this helps a mental health professional like me to understand your disorder, and it may save time as we proceed. It helps me understand you better as a person as well.

Why couldn't I heal myself? each patient asks as she starts the evaluation, though rarely in so many words. At the same time, each person arrives with a question, an insoluble mystery. *What's wrong with me?* she wonders. *Why is this happening to* me? (*And why not to my boss, my ex-husband, my former mother-in-law, all of whom certainly deserve to suffer more!*) And then, of course, *How can I get better?*

A New Neuropsychiatrist can usually provide some kind of answer to the questions of what is wrong and how to get better—but we often struggle with one question, which is sometimes asked directly, other times only implied: *How can I get my old life back?* Often, the individual seeking treatment wants magical restitution of an ancien regime, the return of lost hopes. Yet, generally, in the New Neuropsychiatry, this can't be done. There is only going forward. Not only is going back often impossible, but in some instances it is positively dangerous. Like it or not, the journey has begun. And because you cannot return to the starting point, you might as well prepare to travel somewhere new.

Mark Is Stuck in Time

The issues of not letting go of the past or living for the present were on my mind a number of years ago when I met a man I will call Mark Maple.

"This has been a long time coming," Liz Weeks had told me when she called to make the referral. Liz is a psychologist who practices on the Upper East Side of Manhattan. Though I have often done medication consults for Liz's patients, we've never actually met—we know each other only from the telephone.

"He's 43 years old, been in therapy for years," she went on. "He has incredible fears surrounding his girlfriend. He needs to know where she is every moment of the day—he becomes frantic if he doesn't know. We've been working on it in therapy, and he's finally come to realize how this relates to his earlier losses."

There had been a horrible disaster fifteen years ago, she informed me, a car accident in which his wife, Corinne, five months pregnant, had been killed. Mark, the driver of the car, had been thrown from the wreckage and had escaped with minor physical injuries. Psychologically, he had been severely traumatized, and he dropped out of law school. After extensive therapy, Mark had been able to finish his education, and then to take a job at a big Manhattan law firm. There he was successful. His personal life was slower to recover, though. Eventually he began dating a woman named Susan, who worked as a marketing consultant. Things gradually got serious, and they moved in together, but he was unable to decide whether to marry her. This had precipitated his return to therapy, and the beginning of a long process of dealing with the psychological consequences of the car accident, which had colored every aspect of his life.

"He's been coming three times a week, and I've been impressed with his progress," Liz said. "I had been, until recently, I mean. Now he's having terrible anxiety, and he's in trouble at work. And recently he's begun to do magic to make sure his girlfriend's okay."

"Magic?" I said.

"Yes. He'll have to arrange things in the apartment a certain way, he'll walk around the block several times before he can go to work. He thinks this will prevent bad things from happening to her." There was a pause. "These things do sound crazy, don't they?"

"Crazy?" I wasn't sure, but I was starting to get the picture of Mark's disorder. These peculiar symptoms had sent roots throughout Mark's life, so every moment of his day was consumed, until it was impossible to know where *he* ended and his disorder began.

"And he's not on medication?"

"He's refused to take anything. He wants only to talk. Finally he's agreed to see you."

So, a week later, my first appointment with Mark Maple.

I must confess to a certain amount of anxiety upon meeting any new patient, a mix of excitement and apprehension. It is not only practical in nature—the pragmatics of appointments and payments and insurance information—but also existential. A stranger will be telling me the intimate details of his life, will be engaging *my* mirror neurons—brain cells that respond empathically when encountering emotions in another person—in the most dreadful or frightening or sad or exhilarating moments he has known. In exchange for these revelations, he will be placing an implicit demand: *be involved with me, help me fix things, help me solve my problems.* It is an obligation, a challenge, a test, and the outcome is never certain. For a New Neuropsychiatrist, practicing a discipline that can and often does achieve profound results, the challenge has only become greater. It is somehow less personal but more intense than what the Old Psychiatrist faced, less predicated on a sharing of difficult moments, of endless silences and wracking tears, than it is an expectation of neurobiological wizardry, a hope for transformation.

About ten minutes after the appointed hour, the clerk at the front desk let me know that Mr. Maple had arrived. I went out to the waiting room. A lanky man with disheveled reddish hair stood near the elevators, cell phone in hand.

"I'm just dialing my girlfriend, Susan," he said, clicking off as I led him into my office. He sat on the edge of his chair. "Look, I don't know why I'm here today," he said. "Basically I'm ready to kill myself. Look, I'm a lawyer but I can't practice law. I used to be a runner, a marathoner, but I can't run. All I can do is think about where my girlfriend, Susan, is, what she's doing." He paused. "Just a moment, let me call her, I'm worried about. . . ." He pushed a single button, speed-dialing Susan.

"Worried about—"

"Safety. Her safety!" he said irritably, waiting for the call to go through.

"Why wouldn't she be safe?"

Angrily he snapped the phone closed. "Because she had to drive to work out in Jersey, because she was supposed to call the moment she arrived and she hasn't. I don't know what may have happened! She might have had a traffic accident!"

He was near tears.

Mark talked about how intensely he had struggled with his demons in therapy, yet how he felt like an utter failure. I listened in silence. In some ways therapy had helped, but now he was stuck in reverberating circuits, obsessing all day about Susan's whereabouts, barely able to focus on his legal cases. The urge to call had started nearly ten years ago, soon after he and Susan met. Now he was up to thirty, forty, fifty calls a day. Recently, the firm's managing partner had formally reprimanded him. The calls were destroying him.

Again he snapped open the cell phone—but stopped himself. "Oh, God! What am I going to do? What if something terrible has happened to me?"

He obviously meant "*to her*"—consciously that is. I considered how to respond. I could see how Liz could spend so much time with Mark searching for "meaning" in his symptoms. Everything he said, every association, every slip, every aside, seemed primed with Freudian significance.

And yet, as a New Neuropsychiatrist, I was already convinced of just the opposite: we weren't talking about an unruly unconscious here—we were talking about the disturbed brain function seen in OCD.

"I don't even know why I came today," he repeated.

"I think that you're here because you *do* care about her," I said.

There is always a moment in the New Neuropsychiatry evaluation (if the psychiatrist is doing the job right!) when what was once a nameless patient becomes a person, when the cascade of symptoms or complaints gives way to an understanding of the suffering human being before you. And it was this moment when I saw through Mark's agitated behavior—I saw anxiety, fear, an indescribable sadness in his eyes. The very essence of his vulnerability.

Though Mark Maple may represent an extreme case, he is hardly unique. Like millions of other Americans since the 1950s heyday of psychoanalysis, Mark tried to seek a way out of disorder through words. He believed in the "talking cure." He loved mulling things over and exploring his feelings. His restless imagination delighted in exploring the meaning of things, symptoms included, in making connections, however tenuous, however painful, and however unlikely to lead to recovery.

Then there is another factor that Mark Maple had in spades: a tendency to view his symptoms—and his inability to control them, to rein them in—as a sign of moral weakness. Talking in therapy meant that you were courageously struggling in a life-and-death battle, with your past, with your demons, with the limits of human capability. Taking medication seemed like a cop-out, an admission of failure. It meant you were "sick." No wonder he had avoided this moment for so many years!

In the old days, when the available drugs were toxic and uncomfortable to use, the stigma of medication was enormous. Indeed, *because* the medications were so toxic and uncomfortable, they tended to be used mostly by those patients whose symptoms were so severe that there was no choice. And, in a circular fashion, needing medications therefore implied that your situation was grave, that there was "something *really* wrong with you," perhaps that you were "crazy."

Therefore disorder often grew in secret for years, until it was vast and pervasive, like some gnawing, cavernous carcinoma hidden beneath a tiny Band-Aid on the skin.

Cindy Rushes In

In recent years, the New Neuropsychiatrist increasingly sees a second type of patient—whose disorder appears in the opposite configuration. Rather than hiding their problem year after year, some people display it as it emerges, almost with pride. Rather than being hesitant or fearful, these folks expect— almost *demand*—a cure. Such was the case for a patient I will call Cindy Prince, who appeared in my office only a few days after I saw Mark Maple.

Cindy Prince was referred by her therapist, whom I will call Will Eastman. A social worker who had gotten extra training in cognitive-behavioral therapy, Will lies at the opposite end of the spectrum from Dr. Liz Weeks. For Liz, medication is often a last resort, after rigorous psychological work, but Will often brings up the idea of a prescription for Prozac or Zoloft early on, giving it little more significance than getting a prescription for Zithromax for an episode of bronchitis.

Cindy Prince rushed into my office, half an hour late for her appointment, a plump, ruddy-faced woman with her clothes all mussed up and her short blond hair in need of a comb.

She perched on the edge of her chair and blurted out: "Sorry I'm way behind schedule. My babysitter got stuck in Hoboken, and I have to get back to pick up Zach, my three-year-old, at preschool and my twin babies from my cousin's house. So, what do I need to tell you? I have a postpartum depression. I need some Zoloft."

"What?" I said. This was fast, even for a Will Eastman referral.

"As I said," she repeated, "Depression, Zoloft, end of story. I brought all my Web searches on postpartum. I diagnosed myself. I have the lab results from my obstetrician, so you can write me the prescription today."

I took a deep breath.

"Well, okay, we'll see," I said. "But why don't you sit back first and tell me something about yourself."

"Do I have to?" she asked.

Clutching her packet of *New York Times* clippings and Web downloads, Cindy Prince had done her own research and had made her own diagnosis; she knew what treatment she wanted. She didn't want to muck around with messy feelings or even to give me a history. It turned out that she had gotten Will's name from a referral service, saw him once, and as soon as she realized that as a social worker he couldn't write a prescription, she asked him to provide a referral to someone who could: me.

"So, what do you want to know?" she asked. "I already told you what my problem is. Isn't that enough?"

Momentarily tongue-tied, I reflected that Will's patients often presented not only with a diagnosis but also holding similar packets of articles clipped from *Science Times* or printed out from Dr. Ivan's Depression Central Web site.

In her first few moments of rushed confession, Cindy Prince managed to reveal that she was 32 years old and lived in New Jersey, that she was a former graduate student in biology who had given up trying to finish her PhD dissertation after the birth of her son, Zach, three years ago. Just two months ago she had given birth to twins, Chloe and Hal. Soon afterward, she had become severely depressed, losing fifteen pounds in a matter of weeks.

Now, she was barely able to care for the babies, toward whom she felt utter revulsion. Night after night, she tossed and turned, her mind racing, unable to sleep. Besides that, her husband Roland was unsympathetic: he "didn't believe in" her depression.

Who could blame her, I thought, for wanting a magic pill?

But by that time I was scarcely listening to the specifics of Cindy's story. I was too struck by the virtual miasma of misery that surrounded her. Whereas Mark Maple had entered my office with a jaunty determination, an agitated willfulness, Cindy Prince soon collapsed in her chair. The disorder of her world—the chaos, the unhappiness, and the confusion—was immense. As soon as she let down her guard, tears began pouring over her cheeks and she sobbed. Poor lady, I thought, you sure do need treatment.

One thing was for sure: she was not going to leave my office without a prescription for Zoloft. Already she was asking me what side effects she might expect from the medication and what was my average recommended starting dose.

Hold on, I wanted to say, what's the big rush?

But I knew she would respond, if I began to ask more about her life, "What difference does it make? I'm just here for the Zoloft. If you can't give me that, I'll go somewhere else."

New Neuropsychiatrists are rightly cautious of such urgent demands. Why? Because we realize that disorder is never so simple as some neurotransmitter being out of whack. Severe disorder affects all areas of life, and medication alone is rarely the answer. The New Neuropsychiatrist rightly resists simple categorization of disorder as biology run amok.

If only I could do a PET scan right that moment and show Cindy a rainbow-bright image of the disturbed rumblings of her brain. I could easily imagine how it might look—the abnormally low activity of her left prefrontal cortex, common to major depression. A furious churning in her brain's anxiety center, the amygdala. Black holes around her hippocampi, her twin centers of working memory. All in all, a brain map of extreme suffering.

Why did I yearn to show Cindy a graphic map of her own brain's disturbances? With the paradoxical hope it would convince her—after all, she was a scientist—that it was *not* all chemical! There were the drops in estrogen and progesterone levels, the rise in prolactin after her baby was born, but also there must be a family history—a mother or grandmother who also had depression after childbirth—and thus a "biological vulnerability" based on as-yet-undetermined genetic factors. But beyond that, some current life stress or conflict must have precipitated her postpartum depression. Perhaps a marriage gone sour, perhaps impossible family expectations. A host of factors might contribute to her broad spectrum of suffering. And treatment might require a lot more than just a pill. As Cindy talked, her reddened fingers shredded one tissue after another. I began to wonder: What were the issues that made her burn so hot? And if we could work together, if medication and therapy lightened the profound blackness around her, where would she end up?

Likewise, I might add, in the first few moments of our evaluation I had a vision of Mark Maple unbound, freed of his profound worries about Susan's well-being, his endless psychic isometrics. He was held back by his severe (yet almost Chaplinesque) symptoms. He seemed to be practically bursting at the seams, desperate to move on. What would happen if *he* responded to New Neuropsychiatry treatment? Would he rise free, like a beached ship lifted by a rising tide? Or would he get stuck again on the next sandbar? I hesitated even to guess.

"Doctor, are you going to help me or not? I need to start Zoloft today!"

What could I say? At that moment, medicine was the only option she would accept. So I broke my usual rule and began to write out a prescription for a week's worth of pills.

"Are you breast-feeding?" That was a complicated issue—even though most pediatricians thought it was okay to breastfeed, even on Zoloft.

"No, I stopped last month."

"Okay, because, you know, the SSRI medicines can be excreted in breast milk."

"I know, I know," she said.

Uneasily, I handed her the prescription. At least she agreed to make an appointment the following week to complete the evaluation. And signed a form okaying me to call Will Eastman.

She began crying as she got up to leave. "I . . . I just don't want to go back home. I don't want my babies, I don't feel anything for them!"

She rushed out before I could respond.

This is the state of disorder—varieties of which every New Neuropsychiatrist sees every day, each time someone new walks through the office door. Mark Maple presented with long-standing patterns of behavior; Cindy Prince came in with a new, urgent, still-evolving crisis. But they were unique, each with particular needs. This is no coincidence. Individuality is key to the New Neuropsychiatry (more about this later). Even with the emerging understanding of underlying common biochemistry of disorder, every person who has a disorder is different and utterly unique.

Perhaps in some similar way you too are lost. Your disorder threatens to swamp you, even destroy your life. But at least now you *know* you are lost. And you are determined to find a way out, a way back that is the same time a way forward. At the very least, you have realized that you can not stay where you are. You know you have a problem, you're starting to get it evaluated, and soon you will have to figure out how to get better.

The Chief Complaint

From time immemorial, young doctors of every specialty have been taught that each new patient presents with a "chief complaint." This is particularly true with the New Neuropsychiatry—which, after all, is a branch of medicine.

Why are you here today? the New Neuropsychiatrist asks. *No, don't tell me what happened twenty years ago or last year, tell me why you came here* today. *What is bothering you? What can I help you with? What's wrong?*

A chief complaint is an essential starting point for the New Neuropsychiatry, a place to begin your travels toward cure. It is the first step in connecting your life to your brain. Some complaints are obscure, others crystal clear. Cindy Prince was awfully clear about her complaint. Perhaps even too clear at this beginning point—when uncertainty, confusion, and a willingness to consider many possible explanations of your suffering are actually helpful for the healing process. Mark Maple, an old-fashioned psychotherapy patient, was overly baffled by his worsening symptoms—his growing and elaborating obsessions, his life-warping anxieties. No amount of talk could cure him, and yet he could not stop talking.

What about you?

What is best for me? you wonder. Medication? therapy? or both? What should I do first? What kind of therapy (or medication) will help most? And fastest, most economically, least painfully? What else can help me? You want an answer specific to your own needs, not the predilections or quirks of your doctor or your insurance plan. So you call around, seeing how best to get a good psychiatric evaluation of your disorder. Perhaps you decide to seek a consultation first, then decide on treatment. You contact the nearest teaching hospital, or your local medical school's department of psychiatry: you want someone who is up to date on new approaches to treatment.

For a brief time, as you begin your search for the best kind of help, such questions—amazingly enough—succeed in distracting you from your suffering. That's good. It means your healing has begun.

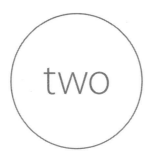

two

The Evaluation

You Are Not Your Diagnosis

Evaluating Mark

"I KNOW I'M PUTTING SUSAN through hell," Mark Maple told me as we started his evaluation. "I wouldn't blame her for leaving me. I mean, I'm not keeping her against her will or anything. But I can't help myself, it's getting to the point that I interrupt her at work, and she won't take my calls, and then of course I get even more worried about her. And then I start trying to control her more, and she gets more furious at me. Sometimes she won't even tell me where she is going, which drives me crazy. But luckily, usually she gives me her complete agenda, so I know exactly where she is going to be."

He reached into his briefcase and pulled out a printout, a week's worth of Outlook schedules. Susan's, of course.

"Let's see, it's 10:15," he said, "So she probably is about to start a meeting with one of her clients. Usually this is when I ring her." He was already reaching for the phone.

"Wait," I said. "What are you feeling?"

"I was fine, but now I—now I need to talk to her!"

"But what are you feeling?"

"Horrible anxiety. It's coming up, just like it always does."

"Just wait for a moment," I said. "Let's see what happens."

But it was too late: Mark could not tolerate his anxiety, and I was the one to wait, as he completed his call, and to overhear her reassurances, that, yes, she had arrived at work, and that, yes, everything was okay.

"Okay, so where were we?" he said, hanging up. He glanced back at Susan's schedule, calmed for the moment. But soon I could see his doubts beginning to rise again. She had arrived safely at work, but what if she went out for lunch? What if she had to drive somewhere for a meeting? And when she said she was okay, hadn't he heard some hesitation in her voice? The instant our session ended, I knew he would be on the phone again.

Susan did work hard to reassure Mark—but maybe that only *worsened* his anxiety. Something to file away for future discussions.

"I want to ask you about your worries, the thoughts that keep coming into your mind," I said. "Then we'll go on to your mood."

"Shoot," he said, "I'm ready."

A guiding principle, something to keep in the back of your mind: the New Neuropsychiatry seeks an understanding of how the biology and psychology, and even the physiology, of your disorder have become part of your life. At times—an acute depression, for instance—a disorder is a thing that has happened to you, a sudden catastrophe (Cindy Prince seemed to be an example of this). At other times—chronic panic disorder, recurrent depression, bulimia—the disorder is more insidious, so that symptoms and abnormal thought patterns and strange behaviors have become interwoven in your daily existence, often to the degree that it is difficult to tell where "you" end and your disorder begins. This seemed to be the case with Mark, in whom trauma led to hypervigilance, which led to frantic behavior.

A second guiding principle of the New Neuropsychiatry: the psychiatric evaluation is something that you participate in and something that changes you. Correct diagnosis is essential, but it is not the end of the story. The psychiatrist and the patient work together to "co-construct" the New Neuropsychiatry evaluation. You, the patient, tell your life story, and your psychiatrist begins to recast it as something in which disorder has played a part of greater or lesser significance. The evaluation is the start of a dialogue.

The New Neuropsychiatry evaluation can be disconcerting—if it reveals to you how much has been lost, how many life choices may have been made under the influence of sadness or agitation or fear. And yet, at best, it is a liberating, even exhilarating process. "I have this disorder—it is not *me*." And: "What if I get it under control? How would it be once the symptoms begin to fade away? How might my life change?" The New Neuropsychiatry evaluation often begins in despair and limitation and often ends in contemplation of new opportunities, of possible changes. Of course, making changes depends on having treatments that work.

During the New Neuropsychiatry evaluation, as I mentioned, your psychiatrist makes an assessment of the biology and physiology and psychology of your mind. By understanding the interplay between these different factors, he or she may be able to improve the quality of your life. The role of biology and physiology in your disorder may have been greater than you realized. As you learn more about this, you may, paradoxically, end up with a *greater* sense of freedom and autonomy. Finally, the New Neuropsychiatry evaluation is a kind of dance. It is agile and focused; it has many purposes that must be accomplished in a short time. The New Neuropsychiatrist must be savvy, able to size up the person before him or her, and figure out how to help. Current history, past history, symptoms, traumas—all must be covered. It is especially crucial to assess your strengths—they will be the key to successful change.

Initially with Mark, I was mainly interested in fear. Not only fear as a psychological symptom but also fear as a symptom of abnormal brain function. Something, I believed, was probably wrong with his amygdala, an almond-shaped set of nuclei at the base of the brain. Like an overly sensitive car alarm that goes off every time a bus goes by, his amygdala was probably setting off false alarms day and night.

So we got down to specifics. What particular types of thing frightened him? What set off his obsessional worries about Susan? How did he *react* to these worries? What were these rituals he did, and how did they relieve his fears, even if temporarily? Mark explained what Liz, his psychologist, had referred to as his "magic" rituals. Soon I was nearly convinced that Mark's symptoms did indeed fall into the category of obsessive-compulsive behaviors. Right after the car crash—and his wife's tragic death—he had symptoms of posttraumatic stress disorder, or PTSD, but these had faded over time. More recently, the obsessive-compulsive symptoms had taken over. At the same time, Mark seemed to have an increasing degree of agoraphobia, an inability to travel on his own and a fear of open spaces. In addition, his compulsive behaviors seemed to be set off by panic attack–like symptoms. When Mark

The DSM

The *Diagnostic and Statistical Manual of Mental Disorders*—the "bible" of the field of psychiatry, which lists mental disorders and diseases—was first published in the early 1950s as a result of a combination of the U.S. government attempts to compile statistics and the U.S. Army's desire to codify psychological disorders among soldiers. The manual was revised in 1968, and soon after the revised edition was published, work began to dramatically overhaul it, resulting in publication of the third edition (DSM-III) in 1980.

In contrast to the 130 pages and 106 disorders of the first edition, the DSM-III, developed under the leadership of my Columbia University colleague Robert Spitzer and published by the American Psychiatric Association, was 494 pages long and listed 265 diagnostic categories. Among other things, the DSM-III included standardized lists of symptoms that were required in order to meet criteria for a diagnosis (for major depression, a person had to have four of nine depressive symptoms, for example). It tried to avoid theory, such as psychoanalytic explanations of mental illness, and instead attempted to focus on observable behaviors. It was also much more scientific than previous editions, using systematic input from scientific studies, and running "field trials" to establish the reliability of new diagnoses. Its effects on the psychiatric profession (and on our wider society) were revolutionary.

Since the introduction of the DSM-III, the U.S. psychiatric diagnostic system has taken a lot of abuse, from both within the psychiatric profession and without. Researchers have had no end of objections to the manual's hodgepodge of categories and conditions. Feminists attack particular diagnoses as gender-biased or homophobic. Conservatives complain that the DSM allows people to evade personal responsibility for the consequences of their

received a message that Susan would be coming home late from work, his heart would start to pound and he would feel breathless, and soon afterward his fingers and toes would get numb and start tingling. The only thing that even temporarily stopped this chain reaction was getting on the phone to Susan and tracking her down.

"I'm even feeling a little of that now," Mark said. A flush spread across his face, and sweat beaded his upper lip. I was tempted to take a few minutes to teach him some relaxation exercises, but we had so much more to cover that I decided to defer that for another visit.

behavior. Psychologists complain of its overly biological bias. And financial watchdogs of all sorts criticize the ever-expanding panoply of classifications, seeing the DSM as the psychiatric profession's proclamation of manifest destiny over the territory of human behavior. This didn't quiet down with later editions, either, with the fourth edition (DSM-IV) in 1994 or the slightly revised DSM IV, text revision (DSM IV-TR) in 2000. (The next edition, which is called the DSM-5 instead of the DSM-V, is currently scheduled for publication in 2013.)

All of these critiques have some validity, I suppose. But as a New Neuropsychiatrist, I must confess that I still find the DSM useful despite all its inadequacies. And usefulness, I think, is the best measure of any diagnostic system.

The American Psychiatric Association's dream is that eventually we will have a true diagnostic manual, based on understanding disease processes, including the effects of genes and specific processes of "pathophysiology" for different conditions. This is still a long way off, even with the progress of the New Neuropsychiatry. So far, we have only a few such gene-based psychiatric diagnoses, such as Huntington disease, Wilson disease, and some rare familial forms of schizophrenia. The DSM-5 will probably be only a small step toward this dream. And yet, our emerging understanding of brain functioning increasingly suggests that the disorders listed in the DSM are often related, that they often share underlying common biological factors. In the 1980s and 1990s, DSM diagnosis was an end in itself, but nowadays a DSM diagnosis is increasingly becoming just a step along the way, one key aspect of trying to figure out what is wrong and how to help someone.

"What about depression?" I asked.

"Oh, *terrible* depression," he answered. "Black moods, dreams of killing myself, of getting it over with! It keeps getting worse, so much that I can't believe it can keep going down!"

I dove into the mood disorders. Of course, if you have a bad case of obsessive-compulsive disorder, or OCD, it might seem natural that you'd be depressed—if only because your life has become so horrible. But that cannot entirely explain why mood disorders so often coexist with anxiety disorders such as panic disorder and OCD. More than half of patients who have OCD *also* have depression. Most likely, a single defect in serotonin or other neurotransmitter systems causes this wide variety of behaviors and psychological functions.

Thus, following the dictates of the New Neuropsychiatry evaluation, I spent some time plumbing the range of Mark's moods: asking the specifics of sleep patterns (especially early morning wakening), energy level, diurnal mood variation (worsening of the mood in the mornings, with improvement later in the day), attention, concentration, physical symptoms, and so on. And, I asked, which symptoms were chronic, and which were related to the current episode of worsening?

The time spent here, cataloging these specifics, is well worth it. As treatment commences, I will often refer back to this list, different for each person, to gain a sense of the degree to which medication or psychotherapy are working. Memory is deceptive, and over time often we (both patient and doctor) will forget the worst symptoms that were present before treatment, so the more specific reminders the better. In a few minutes, I was able to determine that Mark did "meet criteria"—that is, diagnostic criteria in the *Diagnostic and Statistical Manual of Mental Disorders*, or DSM—for major depression, in addition to obsessive-compulsive disorder and possibly panic disorder with agoraphobia.

We next began going through his medical history (no significant problems) and family history (complicated; lots of relatives with anxiety and depression). His family history confirmed the scope of shared suffering, of what probably reflected a "genetic vulnerability"—some gene or combination of genes that made his family more susceptible to anxiety and mood disorders. By his count, at least five members of his immediate family had obsessive-compulsive symptoms or depression of suicidal intensity. One aunt even required numerous operations to repair joints and tendons that were damaged due to her excessive housecleaning: The orthopedist, Mark told me, "said that she had the kind of injuries he usually saw in professional athletes."

Beyond all this, overshadowing everything, was the tragic car accident fifteen years ago. Mark calmly told me the details: How he had had been driving that fateful night, how a drunk teenager at the wheel of a pickup truck had run a red light and smashed into his wife's side of the car, killing her instantly. Indeed, Mark reassured *me* that he knew how to deal with these horrible memories. Only when he began to talk about his current relationship with Susan did his voice began to crack.

The Present Illness: The Teller and the Tale

As you go through your story with your New Neuropsychiatrist, he or she knows that it is crucial to investigate two factors. These factors can have various names, but whatever they are called is woefully incomplete. Every person has psyche and brain, mind and body, the teller and the tale. Every traveler has a tale—a narrative that must be first listened to and then interrupted, so the teller can be examined. The New Neuropsychiatrist is at first sympathetic and then a little bit rude. Both kindliness and impatience are essential to the evaluation. The first thing any doctor says (and this is as true for a surgeon as for a psychiatrist) is, "Tell me, why you are here?" You, as patient, begin with your story. And then the New Neuropsychiatrist tries to figure out what is going on psychiatrically. To take the story of disorder you have told and break it into pieces, and create a different story. So together we can start to create a new, more optimistic, narrative.

By narrative, we mean the story of what is happening in your life. What has happened (in the past or the present) to cause the crisis that you are now in? Where do the current events "fit" in the story of your life? What do they have to do with your development as a person, as an individual, and as a part of a family and community? If you are currently at an impasse, why is that? And—perhaps most important—once you are able to move on, once you are feeling better, what conclusions will you be able to draw from what is happening now to better live your life? (Obviously, at the time of initial evaluation, this may hardly be clear.)

In the New Neuropsychiatric view, narrative is an essential part of treatment even if medication is the "only" therapy prescribed. Your subjective experience is key to who you are—and how you can get better. How you order and explain your world is crucial to recovery. In treatment, changing your story will actually be a part of a process of reintegration of your brain connections. Once you feel better, a key aspect of *staying* better is strengthening these new connections between brain cells.

The New Neuropsychiatrist wants not only to hear your life history but also to understand your biology. By biology, the New Neuropsychiatrist means an assessment of what is going on with your body *and* your brain, and how these physical factors may be contributing to your current life crisis. A good New Neuropsychiatry evaluation will include questions that assess the functioning of your "stress response systems"—their capacities and their limitations, their strengths and their vulnerabilities. It will attempt to determine the possible contribution of your heredity and phase-of-life biological changes (e.g., child-birth, menopause) to the current picture of your life. Medical problems may play a key role in disorders: in fact, they may be the underlying cause of many psychiatric symptoms. However—and this is important—just because the New Neuropsychiatry is "medical" in its orientation *doesn't* necessarily assume that the only treatment is medication. Far from it! After all, as I've emphasized before, thoughts and behavior have an enormous impact on the functioning of your brain and your body. (For more on medical factors and a mental health evaluation, see later in this chapter.)

Evaluating brain and body requires changing gears. At some point in the evaluation (as I did after a while with Mark), I always begin to ask questions, going down lists of symptoms, of depression or panic disorder or obsessive-compulsive disorder. Depending on how you tell your story, they may flow out naturally and spontaneously or they may require repeated interruption and rapid-fire queries. Though these questions may sound routine, in fact they are subtly tailored to what you have already told me, to the outlines of your suffering. My questions help me to clarify among different possibilities, different diagnoses.

Checking Out the Body's Systems

Each psychiatrist focuses his or her evaluation somewhat differently. But we generally agree that it is essential not only to assess the symptoms of various psychiatric disorders but also to explore the function of various systems that link brain and body and mind. These systems are often disturbed by psychiatric disorders, and it is important to take their measure as a part of the evaluation process. In my evaluations, I like to look at

- the emotion regulation system (which controls your mood); this system is regulated by the hypothalamus, the part of your brain that sends chemical messages throughout your body

- the alarm system (which regulates anxiety and relaxation); this results from the functioning of the brain's amygdala (the brain's fear system) and reticular activating system (part of the brainstem that regulates arousal and attention)

- the biorhythms system (which include your body's sleep-wake cycle, circadian rhythms, appetite, and libido); this primarily is regulated through the thalamus

At the same time, the New Neuropsychiatrist is evaluating other mental systems, whose smooth functioning is necessary for our normal lives. These include the reality-constructing system—that is, the parts of the mind that organize our perceptions to create a seamlessly real world—and the cognitive-processing system—the part that resides in the front portion of the brain, which allows us to think in an organized fashion about our world and to plan ahead.

A crucial aspect of this questioning—and a key aspect of the New Neuropsychiatry—is that these "systems" do not exist in isolation from "you." For instance, in asking about his "alarm system," I asked Mark questions not only to gain a sense of how his amygdala was firing but also to discover how he dealt with its signals.

"So after Susan leaves for work," Mark said, "I start worrying about her, whether something bad is going to happen to her. She might get hit by a bus, someone might push her in front of the subway, all these thoughts come into my mind."

"When that happens, what do you do?"

"Naturally, I start getting anxious. So I call Susan right away."

"And how does that make you feel?"

"Much better, right away—until . . ."

I pause. "Yes?"

"Until a few minutes after I hang up. Then I start feeling something's wrong."

"And the cycle starts again?"

"Exactly."

It was remarkable how these exquisitely sensitive fear circuits were driving Mark's behavior.

A key factor would come into play when we started treatment: Just because someone has a hyperreactive stress response system doesn't mean that he or she is doomed to a life of nervousness, fear, and avoidance. People can begin to readjust these systems, initially by making efforts not to act in response to panic when the alarm goes off. Ever since the horrible car accident, Mark was hypervigilant, always on the lookout for bad things to happen to Susan—and to him. Minor worries about Susan's whereabouts set off a huge response in his brain, far out of proportion to the reality. It might take work, but I believed that eventually Mark would be able to recognize—in the very moment that he was about to act—that his fears were false alarms and become able to override his body's signals of fear. Beyond this, the ways in which Mark understood and *thought about* his stress response system could, over time, help to remodel these brain circuits—to block the amygdala's false alarms. Whereas how he currently acted in response to those feelings—picking up the phone and calling Susan—probably ended up strengthening those dysfunctional circuits.

This is another key, indeed revolutionary, aspect of the New Neuropsychiatry: How you *think* and how you behave or react can change your brain itself. *Thoughts themselves* can change brain connections and even brain anatomy! As neuroscientist Joseph LeDoux puts it in his book *The Synaptic Self,* "Psychotherapy is fundamentally a learning process for its patients, and as such is a way to rewire the brain." And changes in behavior, especially in repeated behaviors, can remodel the structure of the brain! Making these brain changes may require a lot of effort, but it is possible. The consequences of these changes can be profound, just as regular exercise at a gym can lead to dramatic changes over time in one's fitness and body shape. Just because New Neuropsychiatry is medical doesn't mean it is reductionistic. There is a "you" independent of your disorder, which can make these changes happen.

Ideas along this line were forming in my mind as Mark continued to give me his history. He was an excellent self-observer, skilled at describing the way in which anxiety and fear had twisted his life. But he was *un*aware of the way in which his own reactions had contributed to his difficulties. As mentioned before, I was willing to bet money that Mark's tendency to call Susan every time he worried about her, and her tendency to drop what she was doing to reassure him, only *worsened* his cycles of amygdala-driven fear. This is where our work would begin. By understanding the interaction between Mark's "mind" and "brain," we could aim for a good outcome. By using biology—that is, medicine—we could alter Mark's life story. And, strikingly, by "retelling" or recasting the story of his life, and getting him to *act* differently, it should be possible even to alter his brain's biology.

Evaluating Cindy

As intense and rushed as things seemed in my first meeting with Mark Maple, my initial meeting with Cindy Prince was so brief that it could fairly be described as a "drive-by" evaluation. For that visit, my main concerns could be summarized by the single word: danger. That day, my main duty (besides keeping Cindy in the office long enough to come up with a tentative assessment) was to determine whether Cindy was dangerous, either to herself or to her children. The most common postpartum reaction is depression, sometimes mild, other times severe. Often depressed women have disturbing thoughts to injure their babies. Sometimes women become psychotic after childbirth; such women may even kill their babies. The depth of Cindy's gloom, the profoundly nihilistic atmosphere that surrounded her, worried me greatly. But she was ahead of me:

"No, I don't hear voices," Cindy told me that first session as I probed her reality-constructing systems. "No, I don't think people are putting thoughts into my mind or that my thoughts are controlled by the CIA. And no, I don't have any intention of killing my baby. Or my three-year-old, usually, unless he's throwing a real tantrum. But my husband, he's a different matter!"

And then the session had ended, and I was left with endless questions.

Our second meeting occurred a week later, after Cindy had begun taking the medication. Whereas the first day she had been brusque and hurried, this next meeting she looked exhausted and drained.

We went through the details of her first week on the SSRIs—selective serotonin reuptake inhibitors—and about how the baby twins were doing. And how her older boy, Zach, was handling things. Her biorhythms were "all screwed up." She'd been almost totally unable to sleep for the past four days because of agitation: was it the depression or a side effect of the medicine? Then there was the extreme, almost leaden fatigue that gripped her throughout the day. But I was struck by one thing: she looked so miserable every time she mentioned the twins.

"You don't seem very happy about being a mother," I said.

A long pause.

"No," she admitted. "Roland wanted them, the twins, I mean, and I thought it might help. Isn't that stupid? Things weren't going well in our marriage. It had been bad ever since Zach was born. We hadn't been getting along, we fought all the time. Roland said he was tired of being married to me. We hardly ever had sex. But then we . . . then I got pregnant."

"And . . . ?"

She went on. I was relieved that she was telling me her story, even though it was not a happy one. At least I could start getting to know her as a whole person.

"And I wanted to end the pregnancy. Roland, he's against abortion, and anyhow he wanted to turn an accident into a blessing. So we went forward. And now it's a curse. My career is over, I'm never going to finish my dissertation, and my marriage . . ." She glared at me, as if to say: *So, haven't I told you enough?*

"Look," I responded quietly, "It's helpful that I get to know you. We need to figure out why you are having such a severe episode now."

"What, now you're going to ask me about my mother?"

I was puzzled. "Well, not specifically—"

"Well, you should. My mother had exactly the same kind of depression."

"She did?"

"Yes!" Since her last visit, Cindy had talked with her mother. Much to her surprise, her mother admitted that had become profoundly depressed following Cindy's birth, and that in fact she had been unable to care for Cindy for the first year of her life. We were leading into one of the most important parts of the New Neuropsychiatry evaluation: the family history.

It Runs in the Family

In recent years the New Neuropsychiatry has definitively shown the great degree to which disorders run in families. Clearly, genes (and family environments) can be a big factor in whether you do or don't develop a disorder. Recent studies show that genes related to the transport of serotonin into the brain are associated with more vulnerability to stress and a greater tendency to develop depression. Other studies have shown that various genes can be related to poorer response to SSRI medications and to the risk of having more side effects. While genetic tests are still not useful for guiding clinical treatment, knowing your parents' history may give important clues to your own treatment. What worked to get your father or sister out of a depression might work for you. A family tendency toward alcoholism might clue me into a risk that you may share.

Cindy's mother was a good example of the influence of genes—and of early life stress. Cindy had been cared for by an aunt for her first year of life, while her mother was hospitalized recovering from depression. Further back, it turned out, Cindy's grandmother also had postpartum depression. Here was a family pattern that had played out again and again over generations.

More immediately, finding out about what had been a family secret had left Cindy shaken and confused. She felt deceived by her mother, who had left her unprotected, unprepared for disaster. And yet this knowledge clarified things as well: it helped to explain what was happening to Cindy now. And it might help us plan for the future.

Your Life, in Ten Minutes or Less

The picture became even clearer when I asked Cindy to tell me the story of her life.

In the Old Psychiatry, exploring your life history was the "meat and potatoes" of treatment. Months might be spent recovering and reviewing your earliest memories about climbing into your mother's lap or falling off the swing set or about the nightmares that woke you in your crib. Often for Old Psychiatry therapists, the present was merely a window into the past.

In contrast, the New Neuropsychiatrist wants to know the story of your life in brief. The goal is to use your past to illuminate your present life. And so, we want to know—in brief—the history of your development as a person: where you come from geographically and culturally and socioeconomically, and who you are now. What previous problems have you faced in life and successfully surmounted? On the surface, the story of your life may be just a recitation of whether you were shy or outgoing as a child, whether you got on well with your parents and siblings, how you met your husband or wife.

But this part of the New Neuropsychiatry evaluation contains the intimations of something more—not just the sources of your disorder but also your temperament, your skills with people, your strengths and interests. We are interested not just in problems or conflicts in your life, which are often all too obvious during a crisis. Knowing your strengths and talents, your positive relationships, provides essential bits of information for the New Neuropsychiatry evaluation. They are often key to your recovery from disorder. Finally, in asking about your current life, we want to get an idea of what the future holds—where things were headed before the current crisis, and what changes might be advisable or necessary, or possible, to help you achieve your goals.

As a child, Cindy had been a bright student, diligent and creative, with a tremendous degree of perseverance. Though she was somewhat shy and introverted, when Cindy set her mind to something, look out—she was certain to accomplish it. In telling me this, about triumphs on the high school basketball team, about writing for the school paper, or winning a science contest, Cindy brightened up, momentarily banishing her despair.

When her parents divorced during her junior year of high school, Cindy had been a great help to her mother. She was 15 then, and had been having a difficult time at home, constantly fighting with her father. She told people that she was glad he had left. During college, she kept living at home, and right after graduating she had married Roland, a fellow student who met with her mother's approval, even though she was not sure she was in love with him. Cindy had gone on to graduate school in biology, and Zach had been born when she was just starting to write up her dissertation.

It was a terrible struggle. Whereas she had previously been sailing through her program, she found herself unable to concentrate on her work. Most frustrating, she couldn't read. Unread papers and journals and books piled up. Then life started getting even harder. Cindy had problems finding good childcare for Zach, her thesis advisor left the university, and Roland was laid off. Try as she might, she couldn't concentrate, and her memory became so bad that she wondered if she was developing early Alzheimer disease. She arranged a leave of absence from the Ph.D. program to take a job as a laboratory assistant. Finances were tight, and she and Roland were fighting all the time. Finally, after nearly a year out of work, Roland got a new job, and, at least financially, things began looking up. So why couldn't Cindy snap out of it? Why did she continually wallow in her misery? Roland was fed up with her anxieties, her low energy, her constant funk. By this time, she was pregnant again.

Should she have an abortion? An ultrasound showed that she was going to have twins—which was even more overwhelming. And now—now that she had three children—her life was falling apart. No, not merely falling apart, it was exploding. I handed her a box of tissues, and she mopped her tear-swollen eyes.

As Cindy saw it, everything had failed her. Her career, her marriage had practically collapsed. Her own mind and body were betraying her! And, to put it mildly, she wasn't sure if I could help her.

The only thing that gave me a slight sense of relief at that moment was that at least Cindy felt comfortable enough to discuss these things with me. Otherwise, I would have been considering putting her in the hospital.

Cindy seemed to feel pressed to go on, to tell me something else, something about her marriage, but for the moment, there was enough detail. Whatever the issues were, Cindy was too depressed now to deal with them in any useful way. So, in an effort to be merciful, I redirected her to the present.

"You have a hard couple of weeks ahead of you," I said quietly. "Is Roland going to be able to help with the twins?"

"I don't know! He does want to help, he is a good father, he loves the kids, but I don't know if I want him near me!"

Another pause: for the first time since meeting her, I was able to understand Cindy's dreadful situation, the feelings of catastrophe that overwhelmed her every waking moment. The New Neuropsychiatrist in me was struggling to find a way to help her. Maybe there was hope.

"Who's with your kids right now?" I asked.

"My cousin Ruth. She lives a few blocks away, she's helping. Oh God! What am I going to do?"

I thought for a while. "Well, that's what we're going to have to figure out."

I was starting to understand Cindy, and I hoped she was beginning to feel understood—which was a relief, because she seemed to feel so alone. With Mark Maple I was also starting to have some ideas. As difficult as things were right now for both Cindy and Mark, my knowledge as a New Neuropsychiatrist gave me an overall sense of optimism. Treatment could help them. I had no doubt of this. For starters, I was pretty sure about their diagnoses. In the New Neuropsychiatry, diagnosis is the beginning of cure. And perhaps you too, as your symptoms have been evaluated, as you have told your life history and reviewed your family's tales and deep dark secrets, perhaps a diagnosis, the beginning of a solution, is emerging for you as well.

Diagnostic Miracles Big and Small

For the New Neuropsychiatrist, an enormous satisfaction comes from sorting through a confusing picture of symptoms and coming up with a right answer, one that will guide treatment. Often we have the experience of reevaluating

Medical Factors

One factor that is woven into the New Neuropsychiatry evaluation is the question of whether your symptoms might come from some kind of medical problem. The New Neuropsychiatry is very aware of medical issues. Let me give some examples.

- Adrienne, who never had enough energy to keep up with her kids, came for a psychiatric evaluation, referred by her longtime therapist. Lab tests showed that she had hypothyroidism, an abnormally low level of thyroid hormone. Her symptoms responded to a small daily dose of Synthroid.
- Robert, a track-and-field coach at a suburban day school, had severe depression but also ongoing joint pain and low-grade fever. He turned out to have rheumatoid arthritis, an autoimmune disease.
- Amelia admitted that she had bulimia, with frequent self-induced vomiting after meals. She was shocked to find that she had scarred the lining of her throat and damaged the enamel on her teeth—and, more dangerously, that her vomiting had led to abnormal heart rhythms because of disturbed electrolyte levels in her blood.
- George, an overweight 57-year-old, complained of poor concentration, severe drowsiness during the daytime, and depression. His internist also noted that his blood pressure was increasingly at dangerously high levels. He was sent to a sleep laboratory, where he was diagnosed as having sleep apnea, with frequent episodes of obstruction of his breathing tubes at night, which led to all of these symptoms. A positive pressure face mask, also called the CPAP, or continuous positive airway pressure, system, as well as a regimen of exercise and a diet to lose weight, relieved his insomnia, depression, anxiety—and his high blood pressure.

people who have been deemed to be hopeless and coming up with an accurate and hopeful diagnosis. Diagnosis can be miraculous and can change lives.

In my residency years, in the waning days of the Old Psychiatry, I met a woman whom I will call Nell. A young woman, an immigrant from Dublin, who had been in and out of state hospitals, Nell had frequently been "noncompliant" with her antipsychotic medications. If she didn't take her meds, she was crazy, but when she did "comply" and swallowed her Thorazine, she entered a state of pharmacological stupefaction.

Other people I have seen for psychiatric evaluation have turned out to have multiple sclerosis, or vitamin D deficiency, or diabetes, or a host of other medical conditions that were the cause of their mental symptoms.

Clearly, the medical history and laboratory testing are crucial to the New Neuropsychiatry. Do medical conditions (known to you or as yet undiagnosed) contribute to your current predicament? When did you last have a physical exam and lab tests? Is further evaluation of medical problems needed? If you *do* have medical problems, are they creating stresses that are making it difficult for you to function? Is it possible some undiagnosed medical problem is causing your current symptoms?

The New Neuropsychiatrist is also acutely aware of the possible effects of substances, both prescribed medicines and recreational drugs, on your mood and on your brain. Frequently, medicines that you take for blood pressure or an infection or a host of other problems may have psychiatric side effects.

- Julius, a graphic designer, had never realized how his daily use of marijuana affected his mood until a month of sobriety during a trip to the Middle East, where pot was not available.
- Ilene's depression (and insomnia) resolved almost entirely when she stopped drinking a bottle of wine every night.

It comes as no surprise that drugs such as alcohol or cocaine can have major effects on psychological functioning and on the above systems, but many are surprised to know that over-the-counter medications, vitamins, food additives, and natural remedies can have an effect as well. So, when you are getting an evaluation for your symptoms, it is always prudent to get a complete medical exam and to give your physician a list of all drugs and supplements that you take.

A senior resident in my hospital was intrigued by Nell's case. He took on the task of thoroughly reconsidering her diagnosis—by obtaining copies of her prior hospital records, by talking with her for hours, and by interviewing family members about the exact presentation of her symptoms, beginning with her first episode in college.

He concluded that Nell did not have chronic undifferentiated schizophrenia, as was originally diagnosed, but instead had an atypical form of manic-depressive illness. Manic-depressive illness, also called bipolar disorder, sometimes presents in unusual ways. Rather than alternating highs with lows, hers was a case of madness alternating with normality. Hence, he inferred, Nell could be effectively treated solely with the mood stabilizer lithium carbonate. What difference would that make? All the difference in the world!

Nell left the hospital taking 1500 milligrams of lithium per day. Initially dubious of the new diagnosis, I had the remarkable experience of watching her reawaken over the following year. Recovering from years of medication-induced haze, Nell returned to a life of relationships and work. For the next decade that I worked with her, Nell remained sane, staying only on lithium. Nell went to graduate school and got a job, and then another, all without a return to madness.

This is what I would call a diagnostic miracle. Like any New Neuro-psychiatrist, I have seen it a hundred times, particularly in a community hospital clinic where I once worked. Take Becca, an elderly woman from Brooklyn. She came into our clinic, having plugged her nostrils with bits of cotton in an effort to block the fantastic odors that overwhelmed her night and day. Or Rob. A house painter in his 20s, Rob would jab his own belly obsessively, leaving deep, dark, and dangerous bruises. All day, while painting kitchens and bedrooms and baths, he cursed and muttered angrily as a madman. Rob had never held a job more than two weeks. And then there was Timothy, a fortyish bachelor who had filled his room, floor to ceiling, with old magazines. He was dragged to the ER by his mother, who wanted him admitted to a state hospital. All three of them had been diagnosed with schizophrenia by the Old Psychiatrists—and doomed to a lifetime of over-powering drugs that would leave them stupefied.

But to me, as a budding New Neuropsychiatrist, none of them was psychotic. I was convinced that Becca had an unusual form of major depression and both Rob and Timothy had obsessive-compulsive disorder.

The test of these diagnoses of Becca and Rob and Timothy was their response to treatment. And all three of them responded beautifully to *antidepressant* (not antipsychotic) medications. The noxious smells that had terrified Becca disappeared on 200 milligrams of desipramine, and she became lively and warm, transformed, a loving grandmother to her many grandchildren. Prozac 80 milligrams a day allowed Rob to stopped muttering and cursing. His co-workers no longer saw him as bizarre or crazy; they even began to like him. And after treatment with Luvox, one of the lesser-known relatives of Prozac, Tim stopped collecting old magazines and began working in a store.

Often the impact of New Neuropsychiatry diagnoses is more subtle than the rescues of Nell, Becca, Rob, and Tim. More commonly, in the New Neuropsychiatry, a diagnosis leads you to a dramatic realization: *I may not be who I thought I was.* The incessant questioning of the New Neuropsychiatric evaluation, the teasing-out of "symptoms" from the fabric of day-to-day life, can lead to strange, at times disconcerting, conclusions. You entered the evaluation feeling badly, wanting relief. You leave with the knowledge that you have "symptoms" and a "disorder." The nervousness that has always prevented you from speaking in public, the restlessness and nightmares that have prevented you from getting a full night of sleep, the continual sadness and despair—all these are not just "who you are." They are symptoms, rather than being immutable givens in your life.

Take diagnoses that are as common as panic disorder or major depression. Even these conditions, properly diagnosed, can be life-changing.

- Betty, a 50-year-old banker, came to see me after having insomnia for a decade. She had used innumerable sleeping pills, Halcion and Restoril and Ambien and Dalmane, with little benefit. She never suspected that awakening every morning at 3 a.m. was a symptom of a biological depression.

- Ricardo, a young computer programmer, became exquisitely sensitive to dust and mold in his office and came close to passing out every time he went to work. He worried endlessly that there was something wrong with his immune system; he never imagined that the problem was panic disorder.

- Stella, a printmaker who lived in the Catskills, had low energy and depression and many aches and pains. Her girlfriend thought Stella was "just neurotic," and both were astonished when testing determined that she had Lyme disease.

It is a strange realization: that you can live life without those continual feelings and symptoms, that these apparent "givens" of daily life can melt away with proper treatment.

Mood and Anxiety Disorders: A Few Cells Have a Dramatic Impact

Because the New Neuropsychiatry is pragmatic and open to new information, insights come unpredictably, often as a result of new medications entering the marketplace. With the introduction of the SSRIs in the late 1980s, we gained a window into the incredible centrality of the serotonin system in all sorts of day-to-day life functions—and became aware how many seemingly unrelated types of problems might arise when that one system was out of whack. Seemingly different disorders might have a common underlying cause. Panic disorder and major depression might be kissing cousins, so to speak. Bulimia, compulsive gambling, and hypersexuality—conditions that are apparently so different—might share a common underlying brain physiology.

Most striking, it became clear how central a role is played by a minuscule number of neurons that make up the essential and yet fragile serotonin (or 5HT, for the chemical name of serotonin, 5-hydroxytryptophan) system, which is present in every mammalian species. It is a tiny system, involving only perhaps 300,000 cells out of billions in the human brain.

Why is it so central? Because it connects nearly all parts of the brain. The giant nerve cells of the 5HT system may be located in the raphe, or bisecting seam, in the brainstem, way down at the base of the brain, but these cells send out a wide net of connections. Their massive axons, like electrical cables, flow both up and down the brain. They trace five routes into the higher brain and three pathways to the spinal cord, which then separate into countless branches. Ranging all the way up to the midbrain and the forebrain and through the spinal cord, these tentacles connect the entire nervous system.

This widespread 5HT system wires the brain for many things, including mood and anxiety regulation, and sexuality and appetite. Let's not forget about hormone secretion, body temperature regulation, breathing, and control over sleep. Even nausea and vomiting are regulated by serotonin.

However, this system is fragile and can easily be set awry by the stresses of modern life. It is easily broken and may be difficult to fix. The stresses of daily twenty-first-century living can easily launch it into abnormal patterns, states of disorder from which it may never recover on its own. Indeed, if you are coming to see a New Neuropsychiatrist for an evaluation of your troubling psychic symptoms of anxiety or depression, the odds are that you have one or another of what one might call the "serotonin disorders."

By this rough categorization of "the 5HT disorders," I do not mean that every person who has mood or anxiety symptoms necessarily has a demonstrable abnormality of the serotonin system and only that system. There is currently no routine psychiatric test to *prove* that there is something specifically amiss with your 5HT cells. Brain scans such as PET scans and MRIs or samples of your spinal fluid, which might well show some abnormalities, would be useful only to researchers. They are not clinical tests to diagnose or treat disorders. Take Cindy and Mark: by this point in their evaluations, I was convinced that each of them had problems in serotonin functioning. And you too—if you are presenting with the kind of depressive symptoms that I have sketched out above, you are likely to have a similar problem. But I couldn't "prove" this to them or to you—there is still no equivalent to the cardiologist's angiogram. Thus, after the introduction of the SSRIs in the late 1980s, it became clear how the many seemingly different mood and anxiety disorders most likely have more in common than not. So many people respond to SSRIs—those with major depression, with dysthymic disorder (described below), with panic disorder, with generalized anxiety disorder, with social phobia, with OCD, and even with bulimia. And now, more than twenty years after the first SSRI was introduced, when all of us—patients and doctors alike—are becoming tired of Prozac, there is still no new breakthrough replacement for this class of medications. They are still the bedrock of treatment of mood and anxiety disorders.

So what are the most common 5HT disorders? There are several forms of depression—one called unipolar major depression, which is an acute condition in which there are fairly severe symptoms of depression (common symptoms include low mood, insomnia, hopelessness and helplessness, and impaired concentration), as opposed to manic-depressive illness or bipolar disorder where a person has both manic and depressive symptoms. If untreated, symptoms of unipolar depression may become chronic. There is also a condition recognized more in the past two decades called "dysthymic disorder," or "dysthymia." Whereas an episode of major depression may have started only a few months ago, dysthymia typically starts in teenage years and may have been present for a decade or more before the person seeks treatment. Our studies and those of other researchers have shown that dysthymic disorder often responds to antidepressant medicines, just about as well as major depression does. Bipolar disorder may also present with depression and does not just affect the serotonin system. It also affects the dopamine and norepinephrine

The Rising Incidence of Depression

Any New Neuropsychiatrist who has even a slightly philosophical disposition can not help but wonder about the veritable tide of people who have come, week after week, seeking medication for panic disorder, for OCD, for depression. And it is not just psychiatrists in the United States who find themselves swamped: worldwide, the sales of antidepressant medications have been rising at a phenomenal rate.

Why do so many people have mood and anxiety disorders these days?

We tend to think of psychiatric (and, for that matter, medical) disorders as having a fixed incidence throughout human history. But a series of studies by my Columbia colleague Myrna Weissman, Ph.D., and her co-workers—and confirmed by other researchers—leads to a startling conclusion: The incidence of depression appears to be soaring around the globe. The World Health Organization predicts that by 2020 depression will be the second most important cause of disability affecting quality of life.

Across the world, the same phenomenon seems to be happening. For decades (until the SSRIs were introduced), the rate of suicide has been rising worldwide. And suicide has been associated with significant changes in serotonin—in particular, decreased serotonin levels. Even bipolar disorder, which seems to be the most "chemical" form of depression we know, is starting earlier in people's lives. It used to first appear in middle age, in the 40s—now it now often first presents in an individual's teens or 20s. Other indicators that have been linked to the rise in depression are increases in alcoholism and drug abuse and in violent behaviors such as murders (which have been shown to be more common among criminals with low serotonin levels in their cerebrospinal systems).

It is not just the serotonin, or 5HT (for its full name, 5-hydroxytryptamine)

systems and probably also the brain's circadian rhythm system, the internal clock that regulates sleep-wake cycles, among other things.

Then there are the anxiety disorders. These include obsessive-compulsive disorder (recurrent obsessions or compulsions that are time-consuming and cause significant distress or impairment) and panic disorder (the presence of repeated and unexpected panic attacks, which are often associated with agoraphobia, the fear of open spaces and crowds), but also social phobia (fear of social or performance situations in which embarrassment may occur) and

system, either. These days, we realized that a whole range of our stress response systems are tied together, into a powerful mind-brain-body response
to stress. Excess stress causes overactivation of the hypothalamic-pituitary-
adrenal axis—the hormonal system that triggers the adrenal gland to release
cortisol, which is essential to coping with stress in the short term but is toxic
to the brain and body in the long term. In situations of high stress, the levels
of the healing protein called brain-derived neurotrophic factor (BDNF) drop.
BDNF is essential to keeping neurons healthy and to maintaining the connections from one brain cell to another. Long-term stress, it is clear, can reshape
the brain—shrinking brain cells, decreasing these cell-to-cell connections.
And of course it can wreak havoc on the body, injuring the heart, the circula-
tory system, raising levels of insulin and cholesterol and triglycerides.

What is happening to the human stress-response systems? What is causing such widespread breakdown of these systems, and at earlier and earlier
ages?

Is there something about postmodern culture, its high pace, its continual
bombardment by electronic stimulation, the instability of employment,
omnipresent fear of terrorism, the shadow of possible nuclear war? Is it
the breakdown of community? a declining belief in God and an increased
secularization of society? the fracturing of the family? the combined effects of
chronic sleep deprivation and a high degree of caffeine consumption? Or is it
something as simple as our twenty-first-century reliance on electric illumina-
tion, our increasing distance from the world's solar and lunar rhythms? Who
can say? Many New Neuropsychiatrists have been drawn to the strange
conclusion that our country—indeed, our world—is in a state of "neurotransmitter crisis."

generalized anxiety disorder (of which the name itself is a good definition).
Then, of course, there is posttraumatic stress disorder (PTSD), a common
response that follows serious trauma (including startle responses, flashbacks,
and emotional numbing).

The 5HT disorders also include many of what are called the "obsessive
spectrum disorders"—conditions such as pathological gambling, compulsive
sexuality, and bulimia (binging and purging with food). Also, certain kinds
of behavior, such as impulsive aggression, have been associated with low

Different Disorders Need Different Medications

Mental disorders may respond to one degree or another to the type of medication called selective serotonin reuptake inhibitors, or SSRIs, but that does *not* mean these medications are identical. Obsessive-compulsive disorder (OCD) will usually respond only to very high doses of SSRIs or to the tricyclic antidepressant Anafranil (clomipramine). And unlike depression, which often responds to placebo, or sugar pills, symptoms of OCD almost never do. Not surprisingly, it has been suggested that OCD has a different physiology from depression. Whereas depression may result from a lack of serotonin, OCD may result from an imbalance between dopamine and serotonin levels.

In contrast to OCD, major depression may respond to a variety of SSRI doses, low *or* high, and to a wide range of medications (like Wellbutrin) that have no effect on OCD. People who have mild, acute depression fairly often respond (at least for a short while) to placebo—but chronic depressions rarely respond to placebo. Panic disorder is different, too: in panic, the serotonin—or 5HT, for 5-hydroxytryptamine—system appears to be exquisitely trip-wired in a way that depressive or OCD brains are not: patients who have panic disorder often have difficulty when they start taking SSRI medications, because they seem to be hypersensitive to side effects of even tiny doses of Prozac or Zoloft. They may need to start treatment with infinitesimal doses and only gradually increase to effective levels. There is an art to treating the varied disorders of the 5HT system.

Finally, as mentioned above, some disorders that include abnormalities in 5HT functioning can be made worse rather than better if treated with SSRIs alone. The most dramatic example is bipolar disorder. People who have bipolar disorder, if treated with only antidepressants, may be pushed from depression into a manic state with elevated mood and agitation. They can even become "rapid cycling," going from high to low mood every few days, or hours, or even minutes. To improve, they usually require treatment with mood stabilizers and cautious use of antidepressants, if that type of medicine is to be used at all.

serotonin levels. Suicidality has also been shown to be linked to low serotonin. Surprisingly, these seemingly unrelated conditions *also* respond to one degree or another to the SSRIs and most other classes of antidepressants.

What You Don't Have

One important (and easily overlooked) part of the New Neuropsychiatry evaluation is deciding which conditions you do *not* have.

For instance, Liz worried that Mark Maple might be psychotic—that he might have schizophrenia or some equally debilitating disorder. I was convinced by this point that Mark did not have an impairment of what are called reality-constructing systems. Neither did Allen Johnson (who you will meet in the next chapter), even though at times of extreme anxiety he tended to become somewhat paranoid. Cindy Prince worried that she was developing "early Alzheimer disease" because her thinking had been so muddled for the past three years. I was almost certain that this was not the case—that Cindy's cognitive-processing systems were intact—and that instead her difficulty concentrating and remembering things resulted from depression and exhaustion.

Other people, though troubled with anxious feelings or low mood, simply don't have a 5HT disorder. Every New Neuropsychiatrist evaluates many people who present with conditions that do not require—and are unlikely to respond to—medication. If you are having problems with your family, or difficulty adjusting to retirement or to life in a new city, you are unlikely to need or respond to medication. You may simply have an "adjustment reaction"—a temporary stress on your coping abilities, but not one that has put you into a closed-loop disordered state.

On the whole, the average person seen for a New Neuropsychiatry evaluation of anxiety or depression will primarily fall into one of the broad categories listed above. For most of these conditions, research over the past twenty years has defined fairly precisely how effective various types of medication will (or will not) be in treatment. For many, psychotherapy studies have been done as well. Thus, treatment can often be started with a reasonable idea of the likelihood of success. This is also new with the New Neuropsychiatry.

In summary, the 5HT system, which regulates mood and alertness and pleasure, all of which are essential to our functioning and our happiness, appears to be a fragile system, easily overloaded by the hustle and bustle of modern life. It evolved in antiquity, eons ago, at the dawn of vertebrate evolution. It was not evolved to deal with the stresses of urban life or with the highly concentrated chemicals (such as cocaine and alcohol) that we bombard it with. And so, it is easily broken and may be difficult to fix. But a crucial note: New Neuropsychiatry treatments often seem to provide at least a partial repair!

What You Might Have

"Wait," said Mark Maple, when I began to bring up the issue of diagnosis with him. "You're telling me that I started out with posttraumatic stress disorder, which then turned into obsessive-compulsive disorder, *and* then depression. *And* I may have a touch of panic disorder too? So, what *else* do I have? That can't be everything, doctor, can it?"

We had shifted gears, from the phase of asking to telling, from getting information to giving recommendations. It was the first step of "What shall we do?"

I drew three partially overlapping circles on the back of a hospital memo, to try to address Mark's rapidly rising discomfiture.

"See, this is what you have. It isn't as complicated as it seems."

Mark warily eyed the circles as I labeled one "PTSD," another "OCD," and the third "Panic."

"Now, some people have symptoms of just one diagnosis," I said. "But a lot of people have symptoms that fit into several different categories. Like you—you're right here in the middle."

"And?"

"Well, all these symptoms may reflect just one type of problem. A problem that manifests itself in several different ways."

"You mean my serotonin being screwed up is why I always want to phone Susan? My incredibly high cell phone bill is a result of my brain chemistry?"

I laughed. "If you put it that way, I guess so!"

He paused, mulling this over. Eventually he said quietly, "So, what next?"

"I *know* my diagnosis," Cindy Prince told me, when she and I began to discuss these issues. "I made it myself! Postpartum depression! I got it two months ago, after the twins were born. Didn't I tell you that within the first minute after I walked in your door?"

She wadded up the tissues she had been mopping her eyes with and dropped them into the wastebasket. Then she sighed deeply and fixed me with a haggard stare.

"Well, yes and no," I said. "You do have postpartum depression, but you've had it for more than three years, ever since Zach was born."

Startled, she was silent for what seemed like an eternity, as I sketched out for her how her symptoms for the past three years were likely to result from untreated depression. Her inability to read was likely to be one of those symptoms. Finally she spoke.

"So—so what does *that* mean? If I've had it for three years, not just a few months? I guess it means that I'll never get better."

"No, you can get better. Much better. It's just . . ." I began to explain how so many of the wide-ranging catastrophes of her life might be explained by that fact. There was her Ph.D., for one thing. Her marriage, for another. But on hearing this—and I did feel she was hearing this—Cindy started getting restless. Clearly, we were not going to be able to discuss the numerous implications of this today. No, not in the midst of her all-enveloping misery. What she needed today was relief.

"Two months, three years, whatever!" she blurted out. "My question is, when am I going to feel better? I've been taking medicine for a week, and I *still* don't feel any better!"

Indeed, what good is a diagnosis? The real question is, what can be done about it? In the New Neuropsychiatry, diagnosis is the wormhole connecting past and present, mind and body, offering a direction for the future. It is a crystallization of suffering, it allows us to make a plan. It explains where you are, so that it is possible to begin drawing a map of where to go. And, most importantly, it enables you to figure out how to get there.

How to get there? More than anything in the New Neuropsychiatry, deciding "how to get there" is a collaborative act. Doctor and patient have to do this part together. Mark was almost ready to move on to that step. Cindy, well, Cindy was going to be a challenge. But I was going to do my best. And I hoped she would help.

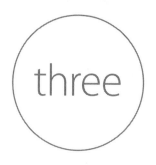

The Treatments

Charting a Course for Recovery

Calming Allen Johnson's Panic

AFTER PEOPLE—LIKE MARK AND CINDY—come to my office looking for relief from their symptoms and I begin to come up with a diagnosis, the next step is what psychiatrists traditionally have called the clinical or case formulation, but I like to call the case synthesis. To put it simply, in a case synthesis we pull together your medical and psychological history, your chief complaint, and my observations and thoughts about your symptoms and strengths and come up with an initial treatment package, or ITP. That way it is clear almost from the beginning how we are going to proceed.

In the old days of psychiatry, an individual might never know what the therapist was thinking of his or her problems or what the best treatment approach might be. In contrast, when I (as a fairly typical New Neuropsychiatrist) make a case synthesis for a person who has a disorder, I want to put practically everything on the table within the first few meetings. Thus, like most New Neuropsychiatrists, I use graphs and drawings and handouts, and I recommend a list of readings and Web sites tailored to each person. I use the language of the DSM, if it is indicated, and I do my best to explain everything. I combine the macro and the micro, the big and the small, trying to connect the goal of achieving day-to-day relief with the overall goal of healing, including brain healing. I ask for feedback; the initial synthesis is very much a collaborative work in progress.

The synthesis can help define treatment. And it can itself be therapeutic. The best example I can think of from the New Neuropsychiatry of "pulling it all together"—of moving from diagnosis toward recovery—is the case synthesis that we make when people have symptoms of panic disorder. It is paradigmatic of the interactions between mind and body that are essential to the New Neuropsychiatry and is key for understanding the power of our new treatments.

Let's look at the story of a man I will call Allen Johnson.

Allen Johnson was a 36-year-old who had haunted the city's emergency rooms for years, in a futile search for help. Heart problems, hepatitis, cancer—the doctors had suspected everything. "He's had the million-dollar work-up," his internist, Dr. Gann, told me. He had undergone MRI scans, stress tests, Lyme disease screens, AIDS tests, and expensive allergy testing, and all had come out negative.

So Allen Johnson came to my office. He looked haggard for his age, as if stressed to the limit by his ever-evolving symptoms. He told me his story. How his terrible anxiety and worries had led to fights (and then a break-up) with his girlfriend and to conflict with his new boss, who reacted sarcastically when he tried to avoid going on business trips. Now he was having severe anxiety attacks every day, sometimes every few hours. At times Allen became paranoid, feeling that people on the subway were out to get him. One ER doctor had even given him the antipsychotic medication Zyprexa. He was terrified to be alone in his Greenwich Village apartment—what if he was unable to call for help?—so most nights he crashed at his brother and sister-in-law's apartment nearby.

"I think I'm losing my mind, doctor," he said. "Literally going crazy."

As Allen Johnson sat before me that first day, trembling in fear, I wondered whether he could be turned around with a synthesis. Not cured, but given a framework for recovery. After perhaps half an hour of discussion, I had become confident that Allen Johnson was not "crazy," that he didn't have an intractable disorder of the dopamine system, such as schizophrenia. There was nothing wrong with his reality-constructing systems. To me, he clearly had panic disorder, a fine-tunable condition affecting his 5HT system—a fear-circuitry disorder.

In working with people who have panic disorder, the New Neuropsychiatrist can discern an amazing, even somehow beautiful, linkage between mind and body, between dysregulated physical systems and extreme psychic unrest. After hearing his symptoms and stresses and delving into his past, I began Allen Johnson's case synthesis.

First I told him the name of his diagnosis. Next I drew some charts and graphs to explain *why* he could never catch his breath, *why* he felt the need to flee from work back to the safety of his apartment. I explained why flight did nothing more than temporarily relieve his anxiety—and yet ensured that the next time he went to work he'd be more panicky than ever.

From childhood, Allen Johnson had been a nervous person. Also (as I could observe from the man sitting before me), he had a tendency to subclinically hyperventilate—to unconsciously breathe too rapidly and shallowly from his upper chest. Exquisitely aware of his body's responses, he tended to react intensely to minor aches and pains (indeed, every time the phone rang in my office, he nearly jumped out of his chair).

That was his physiology, the body he lived in.

And then there was his psychology. Allen had a tendency to catastrophize, to think the worst, to imagine that some disaster was befalling him. His first panic attack seven years ago had transformed him. Whereas someone else might have shrugged it off, Allen had been devastated and had spent the intervening time alternating between dread and panic.

I explained that his "fight-or-flight" response system, governed by his amygdala, was hyperreactive.

"It's the same kind of response that cavemen had to saber-tooth tigers. An adrenaline rush. An incredibly useful response system, but not when it goes off at the wrong times."

I drew upside down on a sheet of paper on my desk between us. "The *A* is the anxiety-provoking situation—say, meeting with your boss; the *C* is your body and mind's responses of fear and terror."

Using my graphs (adapted from the work of renowned researcher Donald Klein, a colleague of mine at the New York State Psychiatric Institute, and of cognitive-behavioral psychiatrist Aaron Beck, of Philadelphia), I did my best to bring order to Allen Johnson's chaotic world. I drew out the rising line of his baseline anxiety level; the upward spikes of his frequent and terrifying panic attacks, which were set off by his boss's irritability or by a smoky conference room or the narrow fuselage of a corporate jet; and the increasing degree of anticipatory anxiety following each attack, a growing fear of each next panic outburst as if it might be the end of his life. And I graphed the gradual increase in his avoidance behaviors and his difficulty traveling over the past several months, making it difficult for Allen to go to work or go out socially.

"Who could blame you for getting depressed? Right now your life stinks!"

I added to the graph a rising line for depression.

As I talked and as I drew, I could see Allen—who had initially seemed reassured—growing more alarmed. It looked pretty terrible, this state he was in. Looking down the timeline I had sketched, Allen was rapidly concluding that he was doomed to a life of agitation and misery. Indeed, when I described how sometimes panic disorder can lead to depression and can increase the chances for other problems, such as alcoholism, he groaned in protest:

"Isn't there anything we can *do?*"

This was the therapeutic moment.

"Exactly the right question," I said. I went back to the drawing of anxiety and reaction, A-B-C. "You see *B*? *B* indicates the automatic thoughts and images that your mind produces. *They* are what cause the intense *C* reactions to occur. You have an incredible ability to make yourself anxious—in fact, to throw yourself into a panic. You're *good* at setting off your anxiety system. You're an expert! All you have to do now is learn to turn the system the other way—to turn *off* the anxiety reaction."

Allen seemed dubious. "You mean you can 'teach' someone not to panic?"

"Sure. Or to set off a panic attack on purpose."

"*Why* would you want to do that?" Allen looked even more terrified, if that was possible.

"To show how it's in your control."

We sat together, going over a possible initial treatment package, and he began to calm down. What we were doing was drawing a map—choosing from the vast array of New Neuropsychiatry treatments to find a package that would work for him. This is the key moment of the New Neuropsychiatry.

Creating a Case Synthesis for You

During the New Neuropsychiatry evaluation, after a great deal of information is gathered—from listening and asking, from silence and from intuition—there

What Is in the Case Synthesis?

In previous chapters, in telling Cindy's, Mark's, and Allen's stories, I have focused primarily on the symptoms of psychiatric disorders. However, the psychiatric evaluation includes many other key elements that are gathered over the first several sessions and that are essential in making a case synthesis, a tool that is used to determine what disorder you might have and the best course of treatment for you.

The evaluation includes the following elements:

- Your chief complaint, or the major reason you are seeking treatment at this time
- Your history of present illness, or the events and psychological experiences leading up to your current difficulties
- Your past history of psychiatric disorders, including previous therapy experiences and medication treatments (and the benefit or side effects of each)
- Your family's history of psychiatric and medical conditions, including what treatments may have been effective for family members
- Your school history, your work history, and your relationship and marital history

A psychiatrist will also want to know your medical history, including hospitalizations, medical treatments, surgeries and accidents, particularly a history of head trauma or seizures. We want a list of the medications you take and any history of medication or other allergies. We do a review of symptoms—asking about physical symptoms in various parts of your body, from your head and neck to your respiratory system to your GI tract, and your cardiac, endocrine, musculoskeletal, and other systems. We ask about your current and previous use of drugs and alcohol, and, probably without asking you directly, we do an assessment of your personality traits, your intelligence, and in particular your coping abilities and strengths, the ways in which you have successfully dealt with problems in the past.

During the evaluation, psychiatrists are also doing what is called a mental status examination, which includes an evaluation of overall presentation, appearance, speech, mood, the organization of your thoughts and your cognitive or thinking ability, as well as the presence of symptoms such as phobias, obsessions, delusions, and hallucinations. We are evaluating whether you appear to be a danger to yourself or others, and therefore whether any emergency measures such as hospitalization might be needed.

One important component of the evaluation (which is too often neglected) is getting information from other important people in your life, including your doctor and your therapist, but also if possible your spouse, friends, or family members. This is particularly important in crisis situations, like Cindy Prince's (and I was sure to meet with her husband, Roland, and to talk to her therapist), but it is also important in less acute situations, not only at the beginning of treatment but also at other phases. Mark Maple's girlfriend, Susan, provided useful information about his behavior at the beginning of his treatment, even though his situation was less dire than Cindy's. Such information can also be useful over the course of treatment: for instance, as Allen began to get close to Donna, we met together with her to get her views on their relationship. Other important people in your life may be able to provide useful information that you might not think of, to provide useful perspectives, or to help your treatment advance more quickly. It can also be helpful to get their input and buy-in to the goals and plan of treatment.

Overall, the psychiatrist uses a case synthesis to work with you to put together a vast array of information and come up with a plan of treatment.

All of the above elements are familiar to clinicians like me who trained in the days of the Old Psychiatry, twenty or thirty or more years ago. In those days, psychiatrists would put their thoughts into a "formulation," which was strongly influenced by the psychoanalytic thinking of the day and therefore focused primarily on your early life experiences, how your parents treated you, and so on. Every time I made such a formulation I would think of a bearded psychoanalyst sitting beside a patient who was lying on an analytic couch! Suffice it to say, the patient was rarely told of our formulation: this was something that we doctors used in discussions among ourselves!

In the New Neuropsychiatry, this certainly has changed. I prefer to use the term "synthesis" for a number of reasons. For one thing, it incorporates not only one's personal history and social environment, but also information about brain functioning, such as your neurotransmitter systems, cognitive functioning, and stress response systems. As the New Neuropsychiatry advances, it can also incorporate relevant information from genetic testing, brain imaging, and so on. Synthesis sounds flexible, being able to use

continued on page 68

different frames of reference where appropriate, rather than being blindly loyal to only one way of seeing things. Second, a synthesis is potentially more collaborative with you as the person who has a psychological disorder, incorporating your input, thoughts, treatment preferences, and your own researches. Over time, you can help to discover what treatment approaches work best for you, and these can be incorporated into the synthesis. Thus, the third reason for using the term synthesis is that it is more amenable to change. This is reflected in the thinking, "Here's our synthesis at this point. It may change as we proceed in treatment." The final reason I prefer to use the term synthesis is that the residents, the young physicians, that I supervise, are practicing the New Neuropsychiatry often without knowing what it is or how it differs from the Old Psychiatry of 30 years ago. What they instinctively do is to develop case syntheses in collaboration with the patient—syntheses that adapt and change over time.

comes an interesting shift. Sometimes it is subtle; at other times it comes as abruptly as the end of a summer rainstorm.

It is a shift from "What is happening?" to "What shall we do?" Or from "What's wrong?" to "Where are we headed?"

In the New Neuropsychiatry, the answer to "What shall we do?" has two parts.

The first thing we will tackle in therapy is making a case synthesis—taking stock of what is going on in the broader picture and examining how to put the current problems into the context of your life. In this, it is essential that your therapist views each person as an individual and sees symptoms and problems as related not only to "disorders" but also to *you*. If we are doing our job right, the New Neuropsychiatrist relates these issues not only to where you currently are (or where you come from) but also to where you are *going*, to your future development as an individual. Your mind (or brain or body) may be telling you that you need to change your life. For the New Neuropsychiatrist, symptoms often *do* have meaning, not so much about deep-seated feelings toward your mother as about your *current* life. You must change either how you live (how you relate to other people, how you work, etc.) or how you relate to yourself (how you deal with your own mind and body), or both. The goal of New Neuropsychiatry treatments is a multimodal reregulation of your life—to reverse the abnormal brain patterns of disorder and to improve the quality of your life to the greatest degree possible—improving relationships, work, satisfaction with your life. So, the aim of New Neuropsychiatry solutions is not only to merely "patch things up," not to return to the status quo, but also to open the possibility of significantly improving your quality of life.

To do this, the New Neuropsychiatrist wants to work together with you to come up with the second part of treatment planning, an initial treatment package. What type or types of psychiatric treatment will be most useful to achieve these goals? medication? psychotherapy? combined treatments? Which sorts of medication? Which kind of psychotherapy? How likely is this treatment approach to succeed? And how will you (and I) know if it works?

Choice Points

In the Old Psychiatry, there was often only one choice point, one major decision to make: "Should I have therapy or medicine?" In the New Neuropsychiatry, the question is, "What treatment package should *we* choose *at this point?*"

Here is the issue: New Neuropsychiatry treatments are definable and finite, yet they proliferate wildly. How can you possibly decide what to do to treat a case of panic disorder or depression when there are dozens of reasonable therapy approaches and potentially effective medications, to mention only the mainstream treatments? And as new treatments emerge, as new research is done, our choices will only grow.

The solution to this problem is what I call "STP"—a series of treatment packages. What this means is that you work with your psychiatrist to choose a treatment package to start with, you test to see whether it works for you. If it doesn't, the two of you move on to another package of treatment. Start treatment, then revise, discard, add, or change approaches, as needed. Simple. Simple but revolutionary, and a marked change from the Old Psychiatry.

The initial aim of New Neuropsychiatry treatment is to relieve suffering quickly and expeditiously—whether through therapy, medication, or other approaches. The New Neuropsychiatry at best is agile and forthright in reevaluating whether a treatment approach has worked—and deciding if changes need to be made, and then in adjusting course as needed.

An ITP for treating your single episode of depression might be an SSRI medicine (Prozac, Zoloft, etc.) as the primary treatment, but also a medical evaluation, regular exercise, and education about the disorder of depression through reading books or magazine articles and researching on the Internet. An ITP for treating panic disorder for an individual who is extremely reluctant to take medicine could be cognitive-behavioral therapy along with mindfulness meditation or yoga classes, and maybe a self-help group for people who have panic disorder as well. An ITP for a person who has a chronic disorder—say, bulimia and repeated episodes of depression—might be both therapy and medicine. Medicine to control potentially dangerous symptoms (self-induced vomiting can damage the esophagus and teeth and lead to life-threatening electrolyte abnormalities) and individual and group therapy to help the person to change behaviors and continue to function.

The ITP can usually be customized in the New Neuropsychiatry—based on your preferences and on what has worked for you in the past. Defining reasonable expectations and setting a time horizon for achieving them is often more important than exactly what treatment is chosen initially. After all, several therapy approaches (including cognitive therapy, interpersonal therapy, and mindfulness training) have been shown to work in treating depression; so have dozens of different medicines. Not only that, the map is not written in stone: it can be revised and redrawn as needed. Decisions made at any point can be rethought, and other types of treatment can be tried.

The key with the New Neuropsychiatry is repeated treatment planning—explicitly drawing a map and coming back to reexamine it regularly once the travels have begun.

This seemingly reasonable and simple process, which is at the heart of the New Neuropsychiatry, is in fact revolutionary in view of the actual *practice* of psychiatry, which is now inventively combining a wide range of treatments with the goal of achieving recovery.

The change in the ability of psychiatrists to use a broad range of techniques to help people in distress is most apparent to me when I supervise young residents in Columbia University's psychiatry residency training program. Typically they present a case history and a case synthesis and then begin assembling an initial treatment package: "a family meeting, acute medication with a benzodiazepine, then start a mood stabilizer, teach some breathing exercises, have a few sessions of behavioral therapy." In contrast, fifteen or twenty years ago, our discussion might have been, "So, should this patient start medicine or go into therapy?"

So it was that Allen and I sat together, going over his treatment plan. At that point, I was seeing Allen Johnson "only" as a psychopharmacologist, because he had been working for more than a year with a gestalt therapist, but medication could end up just as one part of our treatment.

Up front, the important thing was for Allen to radically rethink his behavior. To stop avoiding. To push himself as much as he could tolerate. To stop fleeing from anxiety-provoking situations and places. (Fleeing stressful situations made Allen feel temporarily better—but only increased his fear of the next stress, degrading his staying power. And it increased his urge to escape the next time.) And he could learn a few "tools" to manage his anxiety better. In the long run, we would be working to retrain his brain's fear system, even to shrink his amygdala back toward normal size—basically, to *rewire his brain* so it would not run on fear anymore!

Thus, the way I thought about handling Allen's treatment had several components—including educating him about his disorder, teaching him some cognitive-behavioral techniques, introducing him to various types of exercise, and possibly prescribing some medication. Indeed, this sort of treatment package is paradigmatic of the New Neuropsychiatry—coming up with a sophisticated, personalized strategy that interweaves physical, psychological, behavioral, and emotional approaches. I wasn't just throwing medicine at Allen, and I wasn't just putting him into psychotherapy that would last forever.

We would start here and now. I asked Allen if he wanted to learn "a foolproof way of counteracting the instinctive tendency you have to hyperventilate and set off your alarm system."

"Such as?" he asked.

"Such as deep breathing, such as relaxation exercises." It took only a few minutes for me to satisfy his curiosity—to begin to teach Allen how to do diaphragmatic breathing. ("Breathe in for the count of three, out for the count of three. About ten breaths per minute. Practice this for five minutes, twice a day.") Once Allen had mastered this, we could go on to focusing on other techniques, such as muscle relaxation and cognitive retraining. But he had enough assignments for one day.

One other item remained: were things in such an extreme state that he needed some rapidly acting medication? The only type that works quickly is the antianxiety medications, such as Ativan or Klonopin, which have a risk of addiction. The alternative was to try to live with the "anticipatory anxiety" for the moment. If he was to opt for longer-term medication treatment, the best

Take a Deep Breath and Control Your Anxiety

Many people who have a great deal of anxiety or whose fear circuits are over-reactive can benefit from learning diaphragmatic breathing—taking deep breaths using the diaphragm rather than shallow ones that just barely fill the lungs. This can be particularly helpful for people who (often without knowing it) have had a tendency to hyperventilate all their lives. Many people also benefit from other relaxation techniques that decrease anxiety and stress and can allow them some detachment from overwhelming emotions.

The easiest way to learn to do diaphragmatic breathing is to follow this sequence:

- Take the pillows and blankets off your bed.
- Lie in the bed facedown, with arms up beside your head and your face turned to the side (this may sound strange but lying this way makes it *only* possible to breathe using the diaphragm).
- Breathe deeply and slowly in, to a count of "three Mississippi," then out to a count of "three Mississippi."
- Do this for five minutes, about ten to twelve breaths per minute.
- On a scale of 0 to 10, where 0 is deeply relaxed and 10 is the most anxious you've ever felt, rate yourself in anxiety before having started the breathing, and now, after the five minutes of diaphragmatic breathing.
- Repeat this twice a day.

This lying-in-bed technique (facedown and arms up and to the sides) basically "paralyzes" the intercostal muscles, the muscles between the ribs, which people use for hyperventilating and makes you use your diaphragm for breathing. Almost invariably, people report a sense of breathing-induced relaxation. Over time they can begin to do diaphragmatic breathing while sitting or standing. On a physiological basis, this type of breathing has an impact of normalizing your blood's oxygen and carbon dioxide levels. During hyperventilation, the oxygen level rises and the carbon dioxide level drops, sending a fight-or-flight signal to the amygdala, which then sends

---

choice was the SSRIs—Prozac and the like—which would block the panic attacks. SSRIs would also help with depression, if he continued to be depressed. But SSRIs would take a few weeks to start working.

"I think I can wait," he said. "I feel a little bit better."

out more panic signals. In contrast, during diaphragmatic breathing, you send the "all clear" sign to the brain, which then turns off its alert.

Another useful technique for reversing anxiety cycles is progressive muscle relaxation exercises. It is easy to find a more detailed description in books and CDs found in any bookstore or online. All authors tend to have their own preferred method, not to mention a justification why their method is the best. But basically, all muscle relaxation comes down to a simple physiological fact: muscles become more relaxed after they have been tensed. A muscle that has contracted for a period of time and then relaxes is at a lower level of tension than it was before contracting. If you ever took a college biology course, you probably did an experiment with an isolated frog muscle that was stimulated with electricity and proved this physiological fact for the nth time. In the human body, the easiest way to cause muscle relaxation is to tense a muscle group for several seconds ("as hard as you can"), then relax it completely for several seconds, then tense again as hard as possible. After two or three cycles any muscle will be significantly more relaxed. I demonstrate this to patients; then I ask them to start at the ground and progressively tense and relax each muscle group starting in their feet and working their way up to their head, each muscle group being tensed and relaxed twice before working their way to the next muscle group. For most people, this will cause a deep state of muscle relaxation: many people, doing this exercise at night, will fall asleep before completing it.

Finally, once a person has mastered both the diaphragmatic breathing exercise and progressive muscle relaxation, these two exercises can be combined, which often leads to an even more profound sense of relaxation. Many people who have anxiety and mood disorders who have been convinced that their state of agitation and anxiety was uncontrollable, and resulted from unmanageable external factors, will find that they gain a significant sense of control and mastery over their own state of calm or arousal with these simple exercises.

"But that's only the beginning." I pulled out a second sheet of paper and began drawing a second graph—showing how the panic attacks could decrease in frequency, could be blocked either by medicine or by breathing or relaxation exercises, and how Allen could begin to address the anticipatory anxiety as well as the avoidance behavior. And how, once his baseline anxiety began to drop, the likelihood of having panic attacks would decrease—just like it's less likely for a smoldering cigarette to start a forest fire once the fall rains have begun.

By the end of that session, when I sent Allen out with a slip to get blood tests and a "prescription" to do breathing exercises twice a day for five minutes at a time (plus to go over to the local bookstore to check out some books on panic disorder), he was practically beaming. We would meet again in two weeks—and he was no longer in despair.

Making case syntheses for Mark Maple and Cindy Prince presented different challenges. With Mark, even though his diagnoses were complicated, I was sure that the treatment I was going to recommend was fairly simple. A maximal dose of an SSRI medication (usually required for treatment of OCD), plus some basic education in anxiety and behavior management, might entirely change Mark's life. The complicated thing was not going to be the treatment, but dealing with its consequences. In contrast, at this point with Cindy Prince, the diagnosis (which she had begun making herself, after all) seemed fairly simple. But her life was a mess, and a simple medication regimen would hardly be sufficient to correct her profound, nearly intolerable, suffering. But for both of them, my synthesis was a retelling of the story they had shared with me, as seen through the lens of the New Neuropsychiatry.

A Synthesis for Mark Maple

At our next visit, Mark and I worked on developing a synthesis for him. It was clear by now that Mark had a significant degree of biological vulnerability for depression and anxiety disorders, as seen in his complicated family history. This was affected in a profound way by his life experiences—by the car crash and its traumas. These terrible losses had changed his psychology. And his brain had changed as well. His stress response systems were chronically activated. They turned on various genes in his brain, which produced peptides and other molecules, which further remodeled his brain and kept him in warfare mode.

Mark's initial problem was posttraumatic stress disorder (PTSD), after his wife's tragic death. Studies of PTSD by British researcher Alistair M. Hull show that there is shrinkage of the hippocampus, which, as he puts it, "may limit the proper evaluation and categorization of experience." The increased activation of his amygdala led to increased fear signals. Along with this, in PTSD there is "decreased activity in the prefrontal cortex," which plays a role in "the encoding and retrieval of verbal memories"—making it hard for Mark to put words to his extreme emotions, despite his valiant efforts. Also, as Hull puts it, "the absence of increased anterior cingulate activation . . . may be associated with the inability to extinguish fear"—that is, an inability to return to a state of well-being once the threat is gone. This sure sounded like Mark Maple.

There is no shortage of evidence of brain injury in such conditions. But what can be done about it? Also according to Hull, "the challenge for clinicians is to employ therapies for patients with PTSD that prevent, halt, or reverse these changes."

Mark's story was even more complicated than the usual case of PTSD. Over time, his disorder had morphed, as my kids would say, into OCD and panic disorder, and then into depression. Eventually, not only had Mark's "alarm" system been affected but also his mood regulation system and to some degree the day-night rhythms of his body, his circadian rhythms. It seemed like things couldn't have been worse, but they could have: There no evidence that Mark had any sort of psychosis or manic-depressive illness—also, and equally important, he hadn't started drinking or using illicit drugs to try to control his symptoms. And there didn't seem to be any medical problems, but he agreed to make an appointment with his internist for a physical exam and lab tests.

Even more important than this absence of the worst case scenario, there were a lot of promising signs. Mark was motivated to get better—to the degree that he had spent countless years in psychoanalysis. He had clung to his job despite his life traumas. And he had deep attachments to other people: he had many friends at work (which may have kept him from being fired). Susan loved him deeply, to the point that she tolerated his desperate rituals. In a sense, the possibility of intimacy was stoking the flames of this crisis: Mark was terrified that he would lose Susan, but unable to make a commitment to her.

As strange as Mark's behavior might seem, in our synthesis of his symptoms it all made sense, as his efforts to manage an out-of-control fear system. He had deflected Liz's attention to this by what you might call his "meaningism"—by a pronounced search for meaning in everything. (Believing that *everything* had a deep psychological meaning, Mark had tried heroically to explore his subconscious mind to make his symptoms go away.) In a New Neuropsychiatry view, though, biology—*not* his unconscious mind!—was driving everything. Perhaps even his intimacy problems. My view was a totally different way of explaining his problems—a radical New Neuropsychiatry retelling of his story.

Over about half an hour of that second session, we discussed the synthesis. Mark's eyes welled with tears.

"It makes total sense to me," he said, "but then, I think, how can that be?"

"You mean, how could medicine and behavioral approaches help so many of your symptoms?"

"Well, yes, but also—also how much of my life—" he said. "How—how much effort I've put into trying to deal with this. How much of my life has been totally wasted!"

He looked at once relieved and yet somehow devastated. Diagnosis was one thing; the contemplation of its widespread effects on his life was another. And the idea of trying to undo the damage—that seemed both intriguing and overwhelming to him. This kind of complicated reaction is hardly a surprise: In practice, psychiatrists often see people who have had ten, twenty, even thirty years or more of symptoms of depression, panic disorder, or OCD before seeking treatment. Or who have gone though many years of psychotherapy without *ever* having had an evaluation of biological systems or a consideration of medication or behavioral treatment. Perhaps they are struck less by hope than by the realization that their lives could have been so much different. That many years of suffering may have been in vain.

Mark fell silent as I described the various treatment options—the various SSRI medications, and the possible side effects (sexual problems, weight gain, etc.) he might experience from medication. How he might need to take medication for two years or more to get this under control. I described the importance of the cognitive and behavioral approaches that could help him get better faster, in combination with the medication. Eventually, he gathered himself together and got ready to leave.

"You don't want to start medication today?"

"I—I'd like to talk it over with Susan first. I really—really need to think about all this."

As well he should.

A Framework for Recovery

Mark thought about his treatment options, and on his next visit was ready to make some decisions. In the interim, he had seen his internist for a physical exam and lab tests. Everything came back normal (except for elevated cholesterol and mild high blood pressure, which were nothing new), confirming that his symptoms weren't the sign of some dread disease. Mark had also searched OCD online, especially looking into the use of behavioral therapy and relaxation training, as well as searching out the relative merits of the various SSRI medicines. He had also followed my advice to "try to tolerate your anxiety"—to resist (even for a few minutes) the impulse to call Susan immediately. With only limited success.

"I realized that it's too much to do without medicine," he told me. "I do understand *why* I should hold back, and I try to do it, but even after a few seconds the anxiety is overwhelming!" It could be months, if not years, he felt, before such efforts would pay off. So he had concluded that medication was worth a try.

Any one of the SSRIs would do—Prozac, Zoloft, Paxil. Each had a reasonable chance of working, about fifty-fifty. Side effects were a bit different from one medicine to the next, Paxil being more sedating, Zoloft perhaps causing more stomach upset. Mark was easily sedated by medicines such as antihistamines and had an easily upset digestive system, so we settled on Prozac.

Briefly, we went over what was required: to gain a full response, he needed to reach a full dose of Prozac, 60 to 80 mg/day. He had to take his medicine every day. His symptoms might begin to respond in as little as two weeks, but it could be as much as six months before we saw the full result. We went over possible side effects: stomach upset, slight jitteriness, and possible effects on his sexual functioning, including difficulty achieving orgasm. These were not trivial, but they had to be weighed against the "side effects" of his disorder, which were profound. Even though the behavioral exercises weren't helping much at present, he should continue them, because once his symptoms had lessened, the exercises would be key for helping him to get better. In fact, the combination of medicine and behavioral treatment was likely to bring great relief.

"A few more questions, doc," he said. "How long will I have to take this stuff?"

I told him at least two years, according to the best research on OCD. But there was a chance he might need to take it for a lifetime.

"Oh." A long silence, as I wrote the prescription. Did two years seem a long time to him? or a brief one? He jiggled his phone: I could see that even now he was aching to call Susan, that the question "Where *is* she?" still burned in him.

So, What Kind of Treatment Do You Need?

Now that you have reviewed your diagnosis and your case synthesis with your psychiatrist, what should come next?

You realize that the New Neuropsychiatry goal is not to find the perfect treatment, but to come up with a strategy. What is most likely to help you? What should you do first? What next? And after that? How might you and your doctor best combine treatments to improve the odds—either at the same time or one after another? You have come to understand that we are not seeking a single right answer, so much as putting our heads together to sketch out a reasonable "decision tree."

For major depression, for instance, it is pretty clear that several types of treatment work. Chances are between fifty-fifty and two-out-of-three that any one antidepressant medicine will work for you; literally hundreds of studies with dozens of different medicines show this. Probably the odds are about the same that specific types of psychotherapy can work for you. That is, cognitive therapy or interpersonal therapy, treatments specifically designed to alleviate depression. There are clearly trade-offs. Medicine will work faster, but at the cost of causing some side effects. Most side effects are minor, but others are bothersome, and still others potentially dangerous. On the one hand, therapy is somewhat slower to work and doesn't involve putting chemicals into your body; on the other hand, it requires finding a therapist with the right skills, because not all therapies work to treat major depression. This is not so easy—in some parts of the United States, it's still practically impossible to find a good cognitive therapist! And some kinds of therapy, especially cognitive therapy, require a lot of work—such as doing regular homework assignments.

It is useful to think of this phase in your own treatment as a small case conference—just you and your doctor, considering one case: you.

Simplifying Things

One of the greatest difficulties at this point, as mentioned in Chapter 1, is that there are an enormous number of treatment choices in the world of the New Neuropsychiatry. One can seek single treatments—that is, medicine alone or therapy alone—or one can combine medicine and therapy. Sometimes "serial" treatments are helpful—first one treatment, then another. At other times, one can combine multiple types of treatment, for instance, individual therapy and group therapy or family therapy, as well as medication. Any type of treatment can be short term or long term. Is it possible to simplify this complex picture, and then to apply it to your own situation?

The rule of simplicity would suggest the benefits in many cases of trying a single type of treatment first. For your initial treatment package, you could try therapy alone, *or* medicine. You could make changes if the first approach is unsuccessful, or is only partially helpful. Time limits are a good way to push all of us to make difficult choices. Generally, from the New Neuropsychiatry perspective, "time limits" should mean several months, not several years. The model of STP requires that each treatment package last perhaps two or three or four months before being reevaluated and possibly changed.

Giving Your Treatment a Chance

With medication treatment, it is essential thing to define what is *required* to get an adequate trial of medication, or taking it long enough for it to have an effect. This is determined by the chemistry of the drug and by the way in which the brain responds to medicine, not by what you or I may prefer. Say that you are having your first episode of major depression. You need a full dose of medicine taken daily for six to twelve months of daily treatment—and we don't start counting until *after* the depression has responded to treatment!

Understanding these issues is critically important. Otherwise, there is a high likelihood that you will give up too soon. If you receive an inadequate dosage of medicine, or take it for an insufficient length of time, you will be at a high risk of becoming sick again.

Also, I always try to tell my patients who are starting medication of the "threshold" phenomenon—that they may go through a period, as much as several weeks, when they have side effects from taking medicine, but don't yet

Choosing a Therapist

There is no shortage of reasonable advice available online for finding a good therapist or psychiatrist. If you go online and search for "criteria for choosing a psychiatrist [or psychologist or psychotherapist]," you will be directed to sites from professional organizations such as the American Psychiatric Association, the American Psychological Association, and the National Association of Social Workers, as well as innumerable sites set up by practitioners, such as John Grohol's PsychCentral.com, many of which contain useful advice. It is likely that you can easily get a list of therapists from your insurance company or from doctors, relatives, and friends. However, this is only the beginning of a process of finding someone that you can work with.

There are a number of practical issues, ranging from whether to use in-network therapists (those covered by your insurance company), to sorting out whether one professional can provide both psychopharmacology and therapy, or whether treatment can be successfully split between two practitioners. If treatment is shared or "split" between different clinicians, it is important to find out whether they will communicate regularly with each other. It is also important to find out who will do what parts of the treatment.

To give you an example of the different ways that split treatment can work, here are the ways that I handle it in my practice. Like many New Neuropsychiatrists, I am comfortable working in a variety of ways with patients. Sometimes I do the entire treatment myself, including both medication and psychotherapy. Other times, depending on the situation, I provide only medication treatment, or only psychotherapy treatment. Often there is another clinician, a psychologist or social worker, who provides psychotherapy and I do the medication management. In those situations I will often see the patient once a month for a brief (twenty-minute) visit and they may see a therapist weekly (or more often) for a forty-five- or fifty-minute session. Even when I am "only" doing medication treatment, I often find myself doing some behavioral treatment such as training in diaphragmatic breathing techniques or muscle relaxation. Also when doing medication treatment, I am evaluating the interaction between medical and psychiatric symptoms and illnesses and coordinating care with other physicians on an ongoing basis. These days, however, some New Neuropsychiatrists only do medication treatment, generally because of the way insurance companies pay for care.

Local availability may be more important than finding the best practitioner. However, it essential to find someone with the skills needed to provide the best treatment for you. It is often difficult to find therapists with specific training in evidence-based therapies such as cognitive-behavioral therapy or interpersonal therapy. Research repeatedly has shown the importance of feeling emotionally connected with your therapist in achieving a good outcome. Thus, there is a balance between having a conveniently located therapist who provides a general feeling of good rapport and finding a doctor with the particular skills and expertise you may be seeking.

Important areas to consider in choosing a psychiatrist or therapist include the following:

- What is your comfort level? Do you feel comfortable talking to this person, and feel that he or she understands you?
- What is the therapist's length of practice? Generally longer is better, but being up-to-date in treatment options is increasingly important.
- Has the therapist/psychologist/psychiatrist seen many people who have conditions similar to yours?
- What professional degree does the therapist have? An MD, PhD, MSW, etc.? Generally, the higher level of training, the better, but there are qualified people at all levels.
- What is the therapist's theoretical orientation? Is the therapist's orientation psychoanalytic, behavioral, interpersonal? If you are looking for a focused type of therapy such as cognitive-behavioral therapy, what is the therapist's specific training and experience in that type of treatment?
- Is the therapist or psychiatrist a generalist who can treat a wide variety of problems or does he or she specialize in one area? There may be benefits to each type of approach: a generalist may be best for uncomplicated conditions, for first treatments, and a specialist may be best for complicated conditions and treatment-resistant disorders.
- What are the therapist's practices of communicating with other clinicians, including therapists, primary care MDs, etc.?
- Will your insurance pay for treatment?

continued on page 82

It is important to clarify up front what your insurance coverage is for the proposed treatment: the number of therapy or medication sessions that may be covered, whether there is a need for preauthorization of sessions. Can you get a list of participating psychiatrists or therapists through your health plan? (Unfortunately, these lists are often out of date, and it may be difficult to find practitioners who have openings for patients from a particular insurance plan.) If a psychiatrist or therapist is not part of your insurance plan, can you get partial reimbursement for visits?

Useful Sites for References

www.healthyminds.org/Main-topic/choosing-a-psychiatrist.aspx and www.psych.org (American Psychiatric Association)

www.apa.org/helpcenter/therapy.aspx (American Psychological Association)

www.socialworkers.org and www.helpstartshere.org (National Association of Social Workers)

also see: http://psychcentral.com/therapist.htm (John M. Grohol, PsyD)

have any benefit. Four weeks or more may pass before a medication "kicks in." They may have to "pass through the threshold" of side effects to have a chance for the medicine's benefits to appear.

With medicine, the side effects are often worst early in treatment; only later do they fade and the benefits begin to become apparent.

With psychotherapy, one can ask similar questions about the "dose" and "duration" of treatment. How much therapy is necessary to help you? What type? How often should you meet? Generally, at least a few months of weekly sessions are needed before it is possible to draw any conclusions of whether therapy is helping. Not only that, but in therapy, the ruling order of one's emotions may be upset, and new feelings may emerge unexpectedly. You may feel worse for a time before you begin to feel better. In a way, maybe this isn't so different from the threshold effects of medication!

One cannot list all the possible ways in which treatments can be combined, nor review all the data from all the research studies on combined treatment. There are also many conditions for which combined treatment still hasn't been studied! But it's the general principle that is important—and the New Neuropsychiatry has developed useful paradigms to guide our thinking about these issues.

Psychotherapy Only

As mentioned above, New Neuropsychiatry research suggests that in a number of situations a single treatment may be worth trying initially. Generally, this is when symptoms are not too extreme. Let's first examine the option of instances in which psychotherapy only might be enough to help you recover.

Let's say your depression started after you didn't get a long-hoped-for promotion at work. You're discouraged, angry, feeling helpless and stuck in a dead end. Yet you're sleeping all right, your appetite is fine (if anything, too good!), and your depression goes away when you leave on vacation—only to return when you see your creepy boss and back-stabbing coworkers again. You know you should change jobs, but you keep putting off calling the headhunters and updating your resume. You've talked to your wife and friends and gotten all their well-meaning advice, but nothing has changed. Your disorder, as defined as the DSM-IV, is what would be called an "adjustment reaction" rather than a major depression. In such an instance, medication isn't likely to do much— you probably ought to talk to a therapist and sort things out.

Marsha, a young woman, was having conflicts with her supervisor at work. She had many restless nights and wanted sleeping medicine from the psychiatrist she saw for an evaluation, but when he took Marsha's history it was clear that she did not have anything more than an adjustment disorder. She didn't have major depression, an anxiety disorder, or even a sleep disorder. As she talked to the doctor, she calmed down and felt significant relief. What she had was a problem with her boss, which seemed to be related to her unhappy and conflicted relationship with her parents—her boss was "just like my father." After a few sessions of consultation, the psychiatrist recommended that she try therapy, and that, indeed, taking sleeping pills seemed like a bad idea for her.

Did it work? A review of Marsha's treatment after about three months indicated that her mood was better, she was doing better at work, and that she had largely accomplished her goals. So after a few more sessions, she ended treatment.

Similarly, Allen Johnson eventually decided to try cognitive-behavioral therapy—alone—to treat his panic disorder. He was clearly motivated to do the "homework assignments" required for CBT, to practice relaxation exercises on a regular basis, and to keep track of his thoughts and feelings through a diary. In a way, even though his problems were severe, they were not "complicated"—he had only one disorder.

Medication Only

At times, medication alone may do the trick. Let's say your depression came more or less out of the blue. Your life was going okay, with the usual day-to-day stresses, and suddenly you found yourself wakening at 3 a.m. every night, feeling dreadful. Your appetite dropped, your libido vanished, and you are diagnosed as having a major depression. The most effective plan to help with symptoms would be either medication (no surprise) or cognitive-behavioral therapy. (Cognitive-behavior therapy has been shown in research studies to have significant medicine-like effects on symptoms, unlike most other psychotherapies.)

Or, let's say that you do have a disorder (perhaps, an episode of depression) but you've always done very well at coping with life. In the past, despite difficult life circumstances—your parents' divorce, a serious illness—you've thrown yourself into work and relationships and have emerged stronger than ever. In the current situation, you are depressed, but you have a good support system, helpful friends and family members. You feel that they can be your "therapists." Can't you just try medication, and see how things go?

Or, perhaps resources are limited. Time is short, money is tight.

"I'm traveling a lot. I can't keep regular therapy appointments for the next several months." Or you just plain don't like talking. "If we *have* to choose only one thing," you tell me, "let's choose this. Is it weird to just want to take a pill?"

The data from New Neuropsychiatry depression studies, such as the recent STAR*D long-term study of depression led by A. J. Rush—the Sequenced Treatment Alternatives to Relieve Depression Study, a National Institute of Mental Health study that examined different options for handling depression that appeared to resist treatment—support the decision up-front to provide only one treatment for many cases, for fairly uncomplicated and straightforward situations. These studies have shown pretty clearly that many types of medicine work just as well as the SSRIs—such as serotonin-norepinephrine reuptake inhibitor (SNRI) medicines like Effexor XR, atypical medicines like Wellbutrin and Remeron, and even older medicines such as the tricyclic antidepressants (TCAs) and the monamine oxidase inhibitors (MAOIs). And if the first medicine doesn't work, almost any of the other medicines is equally likely to work. The main difference between these medicines is not how well they work but how well they are tolerated—how many and how severe their side effects are.

Similar to the psychotherapy-alone option, it makes sense to review this decision after two or three months of treatment—and see whether things have worked out as planned.

Making the Switch

Sometimes it makes sense to *switch* treatments entirely. Joan, a 62-year-old office manager, told me that she had been in therapy "for my whole life and then some!" She had spent a small fortune on talk treatments, trying to make her depression go away. For many years, she had gone to her therapist two or three times a week. Two years ago, fed up with her lack of progress, she quit entirely. But that didn't help either. As we talked, it became clear that besides having depressed mood, Joan had suffered also greatly from social phobia—for decades. Joan's extreme shyness in social situations had stopped her from getting a college degree and, later on, from seeking advancement at work. "After all this time, I *know* a whole lot about myself, maybe too much!" she told me. "But I still haven't been able to get over the symptoms."

A friend of hers had responded well to gabapentin (brand name Neurontin), an anticonvulsant that has been shown to be useful for social phobia (but utterly useless for bipolar disorder, a condition that its manufacturer heavily promoted it for in the 1990s).

"I wonder what would happen to me if *I* took Neurontin," Joan she told me. "But I really don't want to go back to therapy. Please don't make me go back!"

So I started her on a course of medication. I told her, "Take a break from therapy for now."

And Joan did well. She began socializing more easily than any time in her adult life.

"It's the first time that I haven't felt agitated all the time," she told me. "I can be calm and enjoy myself at parties. I've started to see how other people experience life."

Practical Issues in Choosing a Medication

Medication choice can be complicated, affected by financial consider-
ations as well as specific characteristics of a particular drug or class of
drugs. Sometimes there are many options within one class of medication:
for instance, there are half a dozen different SSRI medications currently
available. Other times, as with the anticonvulsant lamotrigine (Lamictal) or
the antidepressant bupropion (Wellbutrin), there is only one medication
currently available in that class. Here are some of the issues to discuss with
your psychiatrist. Start with some questions: How effective is this medicine
likely to be? What is the likelihood that I will respond to treatment with
this medicine, and how many weeks will it take to gain full benefit? How
easily will I be able to tolerate this medicine? If a particular antidepressant
causes side effects such as weight gain, sedation, or sexual problems, how
does it compare with other medicines in its class or with other classes of
antidepressants?

Given that you will most likely be taking your medication daily for a number of months, if not years, its side effects will be have to something that
you can live with. So it will be helpful to know which side effects are likely to
be brief in duration and which ones may persist or even worsen over time.

Even within one medication, there may be subtle or not-so-subtle differences in benefits or side effects. The immediate release form of venlafaxine
(Effexor) may be much more difficult to tolerate than the extended, once-
a-day form (Effexor XR). However, you need to find out if it matters which
preparation of bupropion (Wellbutrin) you take—the immediate release,
slow-release (SR), or extended release (XL) forms. And should you take the
brand-name version or the generic?

It is also useful to know if the medication you are prescribed is a controlled substance. Most sleeping medications such as zolpidem (Ambien)
or antianxiety medicines such as lorazepam (Ativan) are in the class of benzodiazepines, which are classified as controlled substances because of their
potential risk of addiction and thus are more strictly monitored. The risk of
addiction is less if these medicines are used for a short time, rather than on
an ongoing basis. On a practical level, controlled substances are given in
limited supplies, often requiring monthly prescriptions, and possibly more
frequent doctor's visits.

Is medication being used off-label? If so, are there medications that do
have an FDA-approved indication for the condition you are being treated

for? However, just because this may be the case for a particular medicine doesn't automatically mean that it will be better for you than a medicine that doesn't have FDA approval for that use. Paroxetine (brand name Paxil) has FDA approval for use in seven conditions (depression, obsessive-compulsive disorder, panic disorder, social anxiety disorder, generalized anxiety disorder, posttraumatic stress disorder, and premenstrual dysphoric disorder), whereas citalopram (brand name Celexa) is officially approved only for treatment of depression. Yet citalopram may be easier for many people to tolerate than paroxetine, because paroxetine is more sedating and causes more weight gain and sexual dysfunction than citalopram or most of the other medicines in its class. And psychiatrists believe that most of the SSRIs have generally similar benefit for a wide range of disorders.

Is the medication covered in your insurance company's pharmacy management formulary? What will your monthly copays be? They may be as little as $5 per month for a generic medication, compared with $40, $50, or even more than $100 per month for a brand-name medicine. If you are taking several medications, these costs can add up! If your doctor is considering prescribing a medication that is not preferred in your insurance company's formulary, is it worth paying a higher copay for that particular medication? For instance, if Lexapro has a higher copay (Lexapro is still under patent as I write this and has no generic form), is it likely to be significantly more effective for you than citalopram, for which generic versions are available?

Be proactive when it comes to your medication. In many cases, choosing the correct medication, or even the correct preparation of a medication, can make the difference between staying in a disordered state and recovering. It is best to learn as much as you can from the beginning.

Why Combined Treatment May Be the Best Choice (or the Only Choice) for You

Despite the benefits of single treatments, there are many situations in which it makes sense to start treatment with a combined approach—with both medicine and therapy.

Take Marianne, for example. Marianne was a fiftyish woman who had had bulimia for more than twenty years. "My whole life has always focused on food," she told her doctor. Most of the time during the day she was thinking about her next meal or about why she couldn't allow herself to eat. Her frequent bingeing and purging had damaged her esophagus and teeth; her social life was in ruins. She desperately needed combined treatment.

People who have several problems coexisting at one time probably need combined treatment. A man who has compulsive gambling *and* alcohol abuse *and* marital problems is unlikely to need only one type of treatment—most likely he will need therapy and AA and possibly medication.

Or, maybe, you've tried therapy alone or medication alone in the past, and that wasn't enough.

Or, you're already in one type of treatment (therapy or medication), and you're stuck, at an impasse, a standstill. You feel the need to get an extra boost by adding a different type of treatment.

It is clear to the New Neuropsychiatrist that certain kinds of conditions cry out for combined treatments. The more complicated things are, the more likely it is that combined treatment will be needed. The major (and most obvious) benefits of combining treatments result from the fact that medication and therapy do different things. Medication can help you to deal with symptoms—to improve your sleep or lift your mood—"to return to the normal *me*." Then, feeling better, therapy can help you to deal with life problems better—to work out relationships with your boss without having angry arguments, to find a way to work together with your husband to discipline your acting-out teenager.

The combination of these different types of effect may be additive, leading to greater benefit than either treatment alone. In a large study of people with chronic depression, lasting more than two years, a psychotherapy called CBASP (a type of cognitive therapy) plus medication led to greater response (about 80%) than either therapy or medication alone (which each helped about 50% of people). This makes sense because severe chronic depression has such widespread effects on a person's life—not only on one's mood, energy, and sleep, but also on one's personal life, one's family, one's capacity for intimate relationships, and even on one's heart, blood vessels, and cholesterol and blood glucose levels!

Sometimes treatments can be combined for the practical—but inelegant—reason that "it can't hurt to do both." The priority may be to get the best response possible as soon as possible. In these situations, combined treatment may be like a broad-spectrum antibiotic: Medication may do something for symptoms; therapy may help you to deal with problems more effectively. And because time is of the essence ("I have to be able to take care of my family, no matter what!"), the possibility that some resources may be spent unnecessarily is of secondary importance.

Conversely, if there is a serious condition but there is a significant chance for a spectacularly good outcome, why not use combined treatment as well? Combined treatments are costly and demand a significant commitment by you as a patient and by your doctor and therapist—but often the benefits will also be great.

Using Your Body and Brain as Well as Your Mind

In a way, the debate in the Old Psychiatry, which pitted therapy against medication, ended up being a false one. I keep emphasizing that the New Neuropsychiatry is a medical specialty. In other fields of medicine, we take it for granted that treatments will be comprehensive, involving medicine *and* behavioral changes *and* lifestyle changes. Heart disease is commonly addressed with a package of treatments including diet and exercise as well as with medication, and possibly surgery. So are high blood pressure, diabetes, asthma, and a host of other medical conditions.

So it is with the New Neuropsychiatry. In reality, *all* New Neuropsychiatry treatments are multimodal. The goals are reregulation of your life—and remodeling of your brain. Renormalization of your mind-body rhythms is one key aspect of this. Regardless of whether therapy or medication is the "only" treatment or are combined, normalizing bodily rhythms and patterns is usually an essential aspect of restoring psychological well-being. In defining each treatment package, it's a question of emphasis.

So let's say you have a "simple" major depression and the only treatment prescribed is a single daily dose, 20 mg of escitalopram (brand name Lexapro). The question of "what to change in my life" is still of crucial importance. Changes in diet, exercise, sleep, and substance use (alcohol, tobacco, caffeine, recreational drugs) and in how you treat your body may have a significant impact on getting you out of this episode of depression, on your risk of becoming depressed again in the future, and even on how your body responds to the medication. They may help to reregulate your brain's 5HT, or serotonin regulation, system, and your body's neuroendocrine stress-response system.

For a person who has a disorder, "get enough sleep!" is no longer just something your mother always told you to do. And getting out and seeing your friends regularly isn't just a matter of fulfilling social obligations: it's part of your recovery. Starting yoga classes or doing a regular regimen of breathing and muscle relaxation exercises may be key to bringing your disorder under control. In almost every case of depression, regular aerobic exercise should be a part of treatment.

Partly this is because, as we all know, exercise makes us feel good and is good for the heart, for cholesterol levels, and so on. Beyond this, fascinating new neuroscience research suggests that there are brain-related reasons to exercise. Recent research suggests that exercise may help your brain regrow, particularly when combined with effective psychiatric treatments such as medication or psychotherapy, and may enhance recovery from psychiatric disorders. Regular physical exercise may specifically help to repair the brain injury that has occurred as a result of the poisonous surges of excessive stress hormones and traumatic experiences, by increasing the levels of the neurotrophic factors—proteins that help maintain brain cells, from the Greek words for brain and nourish—that are crucial to brain cell health, such as brain-derived neurotrophic factor, or BDNF. Chronic stress causes shrinkage of brain cells and atrophy of the interconnections between them. Consequently, exercise and other lifestyle changes have become a significant and essential component of *any* New Neuropsychiatry treatment.

Another key to getting better is decreasing your social isolation, which in the midst of disorder generally means reaching out to friends or supportive family members. Social isolation is often a result of disorder: when you don't feel good, it's often too much trouble for you to see your friends. But social isolation is also a cause of further worsening of disorders, breeding demoralization and despair—increasing the strength of the abnormal brain circuits of disorder. Social connectedness is a key aspect of resilience, of the ability to respond adaptively to stress and trauma. So even when medication is the "only" treatment for a disorder, it is worth asking, "What can I do *today* to feel better?" And, "Who can I talk to? What activity will lift my mood or help me feel calmer or to help me sort things out?" Even without therapy, it can helpful to address these issues in some way—by writing in a journal, discussing them with your friends or spouse.

A Synthesis for Cindy Prince

Often when treatment is starting, the urgencies of the moment can make it difficult to look far ahead. "How do I get through today?" and "What do I do next?" may take precedence over "What are my choices?" and "Where am I headed?" With Cindy, the question became "Why should I live?"

At this stage of her treatment, most of my synthesis of Cindy Prince would remain unsaid.

Indeed, Cindy did have a postpartum depression. She had an increased risk of having this in view of her family history (her mother and grandmother both had postpartum depression) and the many stresses in her current life. After childbirth, there are wide swings of hormones. Estrogen and progesterone fall and prolactin surges. With the pain and emotional turmoil of childbirth and the stresses of returning home to take care of newborn twins—as well as, in Cindy's case, another child—add it up, and you might wonder why *all* new mothers don't become depressed.

What complicated things was that this episode was a second one added to a partially resolved postpartum depression dating from the time of Zach's birth. Over the past three years, during which Cindy had been struggling with an untreated depression, all sorts of problems had developed. Financial, professional, and especially marital. These made it more difficult to get out of this depression. Cindy had fewer reserves; she was more depleted and exhausted. The way I was thinking about it at this point, it seemed that Cindy's treatment might have to be dealt with in stages. First, I'd focus on helping with her most severe symptoms, the insomnia, the agitation, the black moods. And helping her to function as a mother during this time. Then, once things settled down, maybe we could start to deal with other issues, of which there seemed to be no shortage—perhaps marriage next, then career. Perhaps even at some point the issues dating from her childhood might be addressed.

But the most urgent issue was her pain, her overwhelming, moment-to-moment suffering. Everything was at risk of being destroyed today. Her stress response systems had run amok—steroid surges, sleep-wake cycle changes, alarms going off, sprinklers dousing everything. I looked at her, sitting before me; pale, with reddened eyes, clutching soggy tissues, startled by the noise of passing cars.

"First we have to help you get some sleep," I said, "That should help to build your strength back up. Then we have to do something to help your mood."

Silence, a long silence.

"What is it?" I asked.

"I'm terrified. I'm so afraid that I'm just going to end up like my mother's aunt—she's been totally nonfunctional for years, since her youngest child was born. Plus, if what you're saying is true, if I've been depressed ever since Zach was born, and if that's why Roland hates me . . ."

More silence.

"Then?"

"Then I'm going to be depressed for the rest of my life."

"I don't think that's going to happen," I said. "Things can work out fine for you."

"Then what's going to happen with Roland? What about my career? I'm never going to be happy. And the worst thing, the worst thing of all is that I hate my babies."

This just underlined how I needed to focus Cindy's immediate treatment. The question was, did I even have a patient at this point?

"That's a frightening feeling, Cindy. It's part of your disorder."

"It's terrifying," she said, sobbing.

When she stopped crying, I said, "Let's get back to the simplest problem: we have to focus on survival." The worsening physical agitation and sleepless-ness, even the hatred of her new babies, were all part of an evolving disorder that was still not under control, one that was on a worsening trajectory. The symptoms had been moderately bad when she first came in, but her underly-ing disorder was becoming more severe. We had to do what we could to catch up with her disorder. I reassured her that (although it might take some time for the medication to work completely) she was likely to begin to feel bet-ter fairly soon. She had to keep coming to see me, and she had to continue therapy with Will Eastman (I hoped that Will was up for the challenge; this wasn't going to be easy, to say the least. Managing a person with such severe symptoms on an outpatient basis can tax the most experienced clinician).

At that, she quieted down, and we mapped out a plan for the next few days to weeks. I suggested that we increase her antidepressant dose from 100 to 150 mg/day and add Trazodone—a nonaddictive, sedating antidepressant medicine—to help her sleep. The most urgent thing was safety—hers and that of her three children.

"Okay," she said. "So how can we do that?"

Restoring sleep is crucial to recovery from depression—but this would be no easy task for someone with two newborn babies. I hoped she'd need the Trazodone for only a few weeks, until the Zoloft kicked in, and could start reregulating her neurotransmitters, in other words, it could allow her brain to shut down some of its overactive mechanisms.

Beyond medicine, Cindy had to find a way to decrease the stress in her life right now. Could Roland help more with nighttime feedings? Or could she get some help at home—her cousin perhaps, or a baby nurse, someone to lighten her load? Whatever it took for the next few weeks until her symptoms subsided.

Eventually, I said, we could look at the longer-term issues—marriage, career, all that.

As painful as this depression was for her, maybe it could help her to learn something about herself and what her needs were. "But for right now, you just have to focus on survival."

Cindy pulled her things together, tossing her shredded tissues into the wastebasket beneath my desk. Even in her agitation she seemed somehow reassured. She knew that I knew where she was coming from and that I would do what I could to help. For the moment, that was enough.

"Okay," she said. "See you next time."

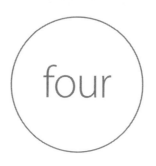

four

On the Road

The Dramatic Beginning of Treatment

The Threshold of Change

"I CAN'T BELIEVE THE CHANGES in Mark Maple," Liz Weeks told me during one of our periodic phone calls. "I saw him just this morning."

"What's different?" I asked.

"Well, his symptoms have begun to melt away. He hardly feels the need to call Susan anymore. I've been working with him for more than five years and I've never seen him like this."

Several weeks had passed. On first starting antidepressant medication, Mark had side effects including an upset stomach, nausea, and agitation—and no discernible benefit. I had dropped the initial dose of Prozac from 20 to 10 mg/day. Once Mark was able to tolerate that, I had instructed him to increase the dose 10 milligrams at a time up to 40 mg/day. Eventually my goal would be to increase the dose to as much as 80 mg/day.

We had last talked two weeks earlier, at which point he felt no better.

Obviously, since then the medication had kicked in.

"For the past six or eight months, he's had to call Susan at least twenty times a day at work. And yesterday he forgot to call her."

"Forgot?"

"Yes! Didn't call her once."

With OCD, Mark's condition, what you usually see is gradual improvement. A man who spends four hours a day washing his hands will note that for the past month or so he has washed for only three; another, who must circle the block two dozen times before entering his apartment building, will find that sixteen or eighteen times suffice. But every so often, someone responds more dramatically.

"The only thing is," she said, "now he wants to quit therapy!"

That I had not anticipated.

"He says he doesn't need it anymore. Because you're seeing him tomorrow, I wanted to ask if you could tell him that he *does* need it." There was a pause. And hesitantly, she asked, "I mean, you *do* think he needs it?"

"Yes, definitely. I'll tell him not to do anything rash."

"That's a relief," she said.

Sometimes New Neuropsychiatry treatment begins without incident. Symptoms begin to melt away: the ragged edge of insomnia fades, there is a return of calm and blessed peacefulness. A good meal gives pleasure once again, and one's spouse's voice seems filled with concern and compassion, not criticism and rage. Yet, often the first several weeks or months of medication or therapy are tumultuous and disorienting. In contrast to the vast landscape of possibilities that may have appeared during the treatment-planning phase, the early days of New Neuropsychiatry treatment revolve around particulars. One waits impatiently for the benefits of medicine to emerge, and yet all that present are side effects, or new symptoms. Is the dry mouth a side effect of Wellbutrin? Or a sign of worsening anxiety? The agitation that you feel on the way to work in the mornings, half an hour after taking your pill—is that from the Cymbalta or does it mean you are more depressed than ever? Or are you imagining things, making a big deal out of nothing? At the same time, remarkable changes may be beginning to emerge.

Similarly, when psychotherapy starts, there may be a sense of relief: "Someone finally understands me!" But there may be a welling up of confusion, an explosion of strong feelings that you didn't even know were there. You may lay into your spouse for an offhand slight at dinner, or angrily berate your boss in a meeting. "Where did that come from?" you wonder. "Why did I do that? What does it mean?"

There is all too much meaning at this point. But the goal is fairly simple.

The goal is response. Whatever else is happening, the goal is to decrease the symptoms of disorder, to help you feel better, to enable you to take care of crucial day-to-day issues, and to get your sleep, appetite, energy, and so on back on track. To help you return to the normal rhythms and patterns of life. In your brain and body, the goal of achieving response is to help get you out of "warfare mode"—to decrease the surges of steroids and adrenaline, to cut back your body's production of cytokines and other stress chemicals, to stop the destruction of brain cells that occurs in the state of disorder.

Often, this requires helping you travel past the basically minor (but sometimes troubling) distractions of medication side effects and the pain of residual symptoms, and helping you persist with treatment until the medicine starts working, which may be several weeks or more. Even these lesser obstacles may derail treatment. For instance, Cecil, a 55-year-old man, came for a consultation after trying nearly a dozen medications for his symptoms. He had concluded that he was "allergic" to the SSRI medicines and that he was unable to tolerate any other class of medication. And yet, in reviewing his history in detail, it became clear that he had *never* had an adequate trial of any medicine. Serzone, Tofranil, Remeron, Effexor, Celexa, he had tried them all—but for only a few days to a week. Not once had he gotten past the threshold of initial side effects, not once had he had the necessary minimum eight-week course of antidepressant medicine at full dosage. So for all intents and purposes, he had never had a medication trial. Once this was clarified, it was a simple matter of choosing a medicine that seemed likely to have lowest side effects for him, and then gradually increasing his dose. This attempt to get him started on yet another medicine required many phone calls and much dosage adjustment to get him past a threshold of severe side effects—but was ultimately successful. Ironically, the New Neuropsychiatry, with its plethora of treatments, makes it all too easy for premature discontinuation or switching to occur.

Other times, the benefits of medication can arrive almost too suddenly, erasing symptoms that seemed fixed and immutable. At such times, therapy can be particularly beneficial, to help you to stay on course. A therapist can guide you through the initial turbulence of starting out, weathering the emergence of powerful feelings or memories, and keeping the focus on getting well (are you beginning to sleep again? are the breathing exercises helping you to block panicky feelings before they turn into full-blown panic attacks?). Again, there is a risk of fleeing treatment before having enough to achieve a stable recovery. Which is what worried me about Mark Maple.

At our next meeting, Mark's cell phone was nowhere in sight.

"I have a confession for you, doc," Mark said.

He filled me in with the events of the past several weeks. The initial jitteriness and upset stomach had faded away, and Mark had grown impatient to see what the Prozac would do. So, overnight, he had increased it from 20 to 60 and then to 100 mg/day per day, to try to gain the maximum effect as quickly as possible.

"I know I should have told you. But I decided that I don't care about the side effects—I just wanted to feel better!"

That began to answer my question—why his symptoms responded so quickly to what seemed an inadequate dose. Abruptly bumping up the dose above the approved 80 mg/day maximum had been tough, even foolish— Mark became agitated and restless. A week later, though, after we lowered his dose to within the therapeutic range, his agitation had faded. And soon afterward, so had his life-pervading fears, his terror about losing Susan.

Mark's other symptoms had begun to fade as well. We had a little discussion about his need to follow the treatment schedule—and not to make dosing changes without consulting me. He promised that he wouldn't do it again. Then, adhering to the ritual of the New Neuropsychiatry medication visit, we began going through symptoms and side effects. His depressed mood had definitely lifted. His sleep was better. And his energy and concentration were somewhat improved. But all those were nothing compared to the changes in his "checking behavior."

"I simply don't *need* to call Susan anymore," Mark said. "I'm not always afraid that something bad has happened. The terrifying thoughts—it's not like they're completely gone, but I can put them aside, I can say, 'Okay, it's just my crazy worries.'"

"You're not so tortured by these thoughts anymore?"

"Much less. It's really a surprise. I didn't expect the medicine to help at all."

There was a long pause. I could tell he was mulling things over, trying to pull it all together.

Often, when medication effects first become apparent, powerful "New Neuropsychiatry insights" can occur. After a month or so of antidepressant treatment, months or years of symptoms may begin to melt away, and you realize, "I haven't felt like this for a long time." Sometimes, there comes a sense of well-being that one may never recall feeling before. What is happening at this point?

Perhaps something novel is happening—a reawakening of brain centers having to do with pleasure, with well-being, with a sense of safety. The amygdala's reverberating alarm circuits have been—at least momentarily—interrupted, and the higher brain's reward circuits, which run on the transmitter dopamine, are starting to send signals that things are okay. For people who have had many years of alarm signals, whose lives have been dominated by fear, these feelings—and associated insights—are indeed "new."

It can be a risky time, though.

"Which gets me to therapy," Mark continued.

The insights attained in the early weeks of treatment may be profound or they may be flawed; the impulses for immediate change may result from cure or from inadvertent side effects. The relief of one form of psychological suffering may lead to the irrational embrace of another.

"I've been thinking about it. I feel like . . . I don't *want* to be in therapy anymore. I'm tired of working on my psyche all the time. I want to enjoy myself."

I reflected on his words. Imagine if you'd been struggling for years, trying to talk your way out of your suffering. And then after taking a few pills and doing a few breathing exercises, they began to fade away. I could understand his perspective, his gut feeling, at least for the short run—though I knew Liz wouldn't be happy, that she would be rightly worried about him.

"So do it," I said. "Quit therapy, take a break—whatever feels right at this point."

"You really don't think I need to be in therapy anymore?"

"Look, you may well have issues to work on. But maybe you should take a break. It's been a long haul for you. I'm sure Liz will understand."

He laughed. "I wanted you to tell me to stay in treatment. Now what am I supposed to do?"

Cindy's Downward Slide

With Mark Maple, the initial psychological response to medication seemed to be a declaration of independence. In contrast, with Cindy Prince, the beginning of treatment was fraught with fear, anxiety, and uncertainty. Her postpartum depression was agonizingly slow to respond to treatment; though her long-term outlook was very good, we had a great deal of difficulty in controlling her initial symptoms. Her sleep would improve for a week or two, then worsen again; her mood would buoy up only to sink like a stone; after an overwhelming night with the twins, the tears would pour again. But finally, there were signs of progress.

At one appointment perhaps six weeks into treatment, Cindy surprised me by coming to the office pushing a double stroller. She maneuvered her way down the hallway. Two tiny pink-faced babies were sleeping side-by-side in the stroller.

"You mind if I come in for a minute?" A man with Elvis Costello black-framed glasses poked his head around the door. "Hi, I'm Roland," he said.

"Sure, come on in."

Cindy and her husband both sat down, and we all admired the sleeping infants, Chloe and Hal, wrapped in their pink and blue blankets.

"Well, this past week, Cindy's starting to sleep again," said Roland. "The Trazodone is helping. I was really worried when she wasn't sleeping at all. Then, after she started the Zoloft, it took her two or three hours to fall asleep and she'd wake up after an hour or so. The past week, though, she's slept five, six hours every night."

Whatever the problems were in their marriage, for the moment Roland and Cindy appeared to be a happy couple, proud of their sleeping twins. I silently praised the pharmacology gods: tragedy averted.

"I've been waking up every night and doing the feedings, to give her a break," Roland said, with a weary smile. "That helps a lot."

"I'm getting my appetite back. And I'm starting to be interested in the babies now." Cindy smiled too. "I feel love for them now, I do."

"That's a relief," I said.

"You have no idea," Cindy replied.

But when Roland left the room, pushing the stroller, it was clear how fragile Cindy still was. "I have some good times, but I feel very tenuous," she said, tears welling up in her large green eyes. "The day will be going great. I'll be on the phone talking to my cousin, and then I'll hang up and burst into tears. I feel like I'm barely holding it together," she said. Indeed, tears poured down her cheeks, as is sometimes seen in profound depression. "I *do* care for the babies, but I'll suddenly burst out crying—for no reason." Plus, despite Roland's appearance here today, despite his support, the marriage was in trouble, big trouble. It wasn't clear if they were going to stay together. He was talking about maybe moving out for a few months. "It's really one day at a time—no, it's one hour at a time."

"Maybe that's the best you can do for now," I said.

"But I'm going to be okay," she said, blotting her cheeks. "I am, aren't I?"

Psychiatric disorder, like other diseases, often has a life of its own. In medical illnesses, this is abundantly clear: Tumors grow inside organs, independent of the body's control, and only reluctantly yield to chemotherapy; so, too, the abnormal rhythms of heart disease maintain their asynchronous beat even when new medicines are added or pacemakers are implanted.

And so, at the beginning of New Neuropsychiatry treatment, disorder retreats, seemingly defeated—and then advances under cover of darkness. Over a period of months, even years, it has imposed its own aberrant order on the brain, its own internal circuits and rewards—focused in the lower brain. The amgydala-hippocampus circuit, the high cortisol and high adrenaline state produced by the stress response are still activated. Even when aggressively treated, these reverberating circuits still dominate the brain's activity. Overcoming their dominance may require a ferocious struggle. That is why at the beginning of treatment the New Neuropsychiatrist spends so much time taking the measure of disorder and asking repeatedly about symptoms and side effects, your strengths and social supports: it is essential to know where we stand, what resources are available when treatment proceeds, especially if our initial efforts fail.

And so it was rough going in those early months for Cindy.

On the next visit, she complained that her appetite had vanished again, and she was again losing weight. Her sleep, better for two weeks, had worsened again. Ten or twenty years ago, she would have been admitted to an inpatient psych unit—but in the managed care era, she was an outpatient case. Why was her response so fragile? This troubled me. She admitted that she hadn't been taking the medicine regularly—some days she "forgot," other days she took only half the prescribed dose. Often she skipped the sleeping pills entirely, even at the cost of staying awake for half the night.

"Taking so many pills makes me feel like I'm really sick," she said. "If I take *less* medicine, then I feel like it's not so bad."

Was that the problem? Perhaps, though I wasn't sure. Starting and stopping antidepressant medicine was similar to starting and stopping antibiotics: surely as a scientist Cindy understood the need for a full course of treatment.

"Call me in a week," I told her. "And take your pills!"

"Okay, okay, I will," she said.

The following Monday she left me a voice mail: things were improving now that she was taking the medicine regularly again, and her mood was much improved. "Finally! I think I'm out of the woods!"

But I was filled with a lingering sense of unease.

At the time for the next appointment, which had been scheduled on a Thursday two weeks later, Cindy didn't appear. I called her home—no response—and left a message on her machine. She called the next morning to apologize ("I'm so sorry, I lay down for a few minutes nap, and overslept! Things are fine."), and we rescheduled for the following Monday. I took her words at face value. It was not until Saturday morning that I learned any differently.

It was a beautiful spring weekend, and I was at the local athletic field with a bunch of other parents, watching our kids play softball, when my beeper suddenly sounded, with the emergency message to call my answering service.

"Doctor," said my service, "You have a call from a Mr. Will Eastman. He says it's urgent, that Mrs. Prince wants to kill herself. Wants to know, what should he do?"

This was, to put it mildly, a surprise. Despite her degree of depression, Cindy had steadfastly denied having any suicidal impulses.

Will picked up right away.

"I think she may need to go to the hospital," he said.

"What's happening?" I asked.

Basically, early that morning, after an argument, Cindy had left her house, saying that she felt like killing herself. Roland, frantic, called Will.

"I've already called the police and given them her description. Is there anything else I should be doing?"

"Let's talk about that. Did she say she was actually going to do anything?"

"Well, no. She said she *might* . . ."

"And where are her kids?"

"At home with her husband. But I can't believe this is happening." He was breathless, and I could hear his anxiety.

"So, take a minute, Will," I said. "Let's think this through."

In Search of a Response

The beginning of treatment thus can be a time of tumult, unpredictable as spring. And yet, with the New Neuropsychiatry there is a crucial fact to be kept in mind: *Almost always, we can get the disorder to respond to treatment.* Response: bringing the main symptoms under control, the first crucial step toward getting better. Improving sleep, decreasing anxiety, improving mood and energy and concentration. Almost always, disorder can be tamed, and symptoms can be controlled. Almost always, you can get better. And then, after that, most of the time you can aim to be *well* again. None of these things was true with the Old Psychiatry: with the Old Psychiatry, remission was the exception, not the rule. Side effects often made medicines barely tolerable. Symptom response was often incomplete. And therapy often took years before any benefit was achieved. With the Old Psychiatry, you might get somewhat better but could not count on getting well.

Now, we know that we can succeed. Success is never guaranteed, but it is achievable.

Take the case of Cindy Prince. That anxious morning, as I stood beside the softball field, listening to Will's account of how he had been working with Cindy Prince over the past several weeks, I wracked my brain to understand why things were going awry.

Now that Cindy was feeling better, Will had encouraged her to talk about the problems in her marriage. And her rage toward her parents for getting divorced. But mostly about the marriage. It turned out that there was a former coworker of Roland's—now living in Texas—with whom Cindy suspected he had an affair back when she was pregnant with Zach. She was obsessing about this woman, and Will encouraged her to vent her feelings, to talk at length— she seemed so eager to talk to sort things out. She seemed strong enough, so he didn't stop her even when she grew increasingly upset.

"Then she called me at 4 a.m.," said Will. "She said she took an overdose of pills."

"What?"

"A small overdose," he added uncertainly. More or less an experiment, three days' worth, just to see what she'd feel. "So, tell me." I could hear his anxiety rising. "What—what are we going to do?"

Lecturing Will wouldn't do much good at this point. Telling him that he was being "Old Psychiatry"—in trying for catharsis, letting out your emotions, and "working through" them at a time when the goal should have been symptom control—what good would that do?

"Will," I answered, trying to search for something remotely useful. "Let's sit tight. You've called the police, the hospitals. Let's hope she'll turn up. Just keep me posted. And if you talk to her husband again, let him know she should call me. Oh, and one more thing, it sounds like it's better to lay off exploring the marriage and the family stuff until things settle down a bit."

There was a pause: I could tell that Will heard the rebuke in my voice. Unwittingly, he had been violating the rules of the New Neuropsychiatry— to treat the current disorder first. To establish reregulation and stabilization. *Response comes first.* The insights of the New Neuropsychiatry, at least during the state of disorder, focus on the present, not the past. There'll *always* be time later on to deal with the past! Uncharacteristically, too, because Will usually focused on behavioral patterns and automatic thoughts.

With Cindy, all sorts of issues—from her husband's possible past affair to her parents divorce years ago—appeared to be churning through her mind, demanding her attention with strange urgency. Major issues, yes, but far too overwhelming to address now, especially given her fragile mental state.

But I'd said enough. Will got the point.

In any case, the cell call broke up, and I lost him. Maybe the gusting wind, maybe the plump white clouds above. I clicked "End" on the dial-pad, and snapped the phone closed, and tried unsuccessfully to reach Cindy. I spoke briefly to Roland, and then, dazzled by the brilliant spring morning, I willed myself to watch my daughter's game.

The Old Psychiatry When Crisis Hits

In the Old Psychiatry, treatment often began with a process of catharsis, or letting loose of emotions. In the New Neuropsychiatry, the psychiatry of disorder, the goal is to find ways to deintensify feelings, to decrease hyperemotional states, to moderate and blunt what has been so overwhelming. Whereas the Old Psychiatry focused on encouraging your "free associations," to allow your mind to travel wherever it wanted, the New Neuropsychiatry often focuses early in treatment on how to stop unproductive lines of thought and to increase self-soothing, evoking any thoughts of "being okay" that you are capable of. In the throes of a major depression, rather than spending hours free-associating, we want to help you to increase your ability to solve immediate problems in a productive way. And to find ways to lower the stress levels in your life and manage your activities to the best degree possible on a day-to-day basis.

Put simply, in early treatment we want to help you achieve control in two ways. One is "top down," from the higher parts of your brain. The other is "bottom up," from the lower brain centers. Top down control is from calming thoughts, asserting feelings of control and mastery. You don't want agitating, stimulating thoughts; you want problem solving, you want reassurance. (Will had the best intentions, but his recent discussions with Cindy may have introduced a level of anxiety that was destabilizing at this point.) Bottom-up control is achieved with meditation, relaxation exercises, breathing exercises, aerobics, normalizing sleep.

Thus, in managing a crisis situation the New Neuropsychiatry focuses on the here and now—on living day-by-day, even hour-by-hour. But it is important to keep the big picture somewhere in mind. For one thing, the ways in which you have successfully coped with adversity in the past can give clues to how to recover this time. Your psychiatrist or therapist may help to put the daily fluctuations of life into the perspective of the overall treatment.

In the Old Psychiatry, there was also a conviction that pain was a great motivator for change and a fear that relieving symptoms too quickly might lead to a loss of motivation for continuing in treatment. In contrast, the goal of the New Neuropsychiatry is to relieve pain. New Neuropsychiatrists are not convinced that suffering is a particularly good motivator to fix things, or to teach valuable lessons about life.

Imagine a doctor saying to a patient in agony from a heart attack or the pain of a splintered tibia: "Go on and feel the pain, it'll be good for you. You'll learn a lot about yourself." The New Neuropsychiatrist knows that psychiatric disorders cause enough suffering in themselves, and that there is no need to prolong suffering or make it worse to increase insight or understanding or to provide you with motivation. Feeling better can be the best motivation for further work.

Changing Course with Cindy

While driving my daughter home from the ball game that Saturday morning, I was paged again. It was my service. I answered the call as soon as I got in the house: Will Eastman again, to tell me that Cindy Prince had surfaced.

"She's all right," he said. She had gone out to the local mall, stayed there for a few hours, and calmed down, and then she called her cousin, who lived a couple of blocks away from her.

"She's still feeling terrible, but she promises that she won't do anything." He sounded greatly relieved. "She's going to stay over at her cousin's house tonight and let Roland take care of the kids, and I'm going to see her to-morrow afternoon. I was wondering something. I know our discussion the other day upset her, but do you think that maybe the medicine is making her suicidal?"

I had to consider that possibility too.

"It could be—there's a whole literature about that topic. Look, have her come by my office. I have some time tomorrow morning."

Cindy arrived first thing the next morning, escorted by Roland and a woman who resembled her, who was introduced as Ruth, her cousin. Cindy alone came into my office. Looking somehow at once abashed and defiant, she slumped down in her chair, and would not meet my gaze.

"Are you okay?" I said.

"Now I am," she said. "But not yesterday."

We began talking: what had happened over the weekend? What led her to make threats, to run out of the house? I tried to keep things calm, low key. But there was no way around it: we had to find some answers.

"Roland's beside himself," she was saying. "He's terrified." She stood by the window—and suddenly burst into tears, trembling and shaking as though she would never stop.

"What's happening to me? Doctor, help me!"

She felt so out of control. It had never been like this before.

What was going on? I wondered, barely able to hold onto my seat in this sudden gale of misery. Was she having a psychotic break? a strange reaction to the SSRI? Just a few weeks ago, she had arrived at my office, in the throes of a moderate depression, presenting similarly to a hundred other postpartum depression cases. Now she was diverging, getting worse—much worse—when she should be improving.

"Why can't I go back to how I was before?" Cindy wailed. "I just want my old life back! I want Roland the way he was when we first got married, I want myself the way I was . . . and I just can't, I can't have it back!"

Cindy had come in that first visit clutching newspaper clippings and Web printouts about better living through Prozac, and she had dutifully begun medication, and even psychotherapy, and here she was, her life blown to pieces. This was not what she had bargained for.

And neither had I. I had not anticipated that her symptoms would become so severe, but sometimes this happens: sometimes you end up playing catch-up to a worsening disorder, trying to bring symptoms under control while the illness itself is becoming more extreme.

"You can't go back," I agreed. "There's no choice, we have to keep going forward."

She calmed down momentarily. "But what's ahead?" she said. "What's next? I can't tolerate this much longer!"

What could we do *today* to help stabilize her situation? I knew the medication *could* work, that *any* antidepressant was likely to work as long as a depressed patient took enough medicine for a long enough period of time. The SSRI medicine should work. And if it didn't work, there was always the decision tree—certainly we could find another one that would. And I knew that psychotherapy—properly focused—should work too. Psychotherapy focused on crisis intervention and symptom relief was an effective way to defuse disaster, to help make things better. Theoretically, everything should be going well right now. And yet, reality was the opposite.

Then Roland knocked on the door. Cindy waved him in.

Roland sat and took Cindy's hand. Cindy let him hold it for a moment; then she pulled her hand away and got up and began pacing around the room. No surprise, I was thinking: a symptom of agitated depression.

Then it hit me: I had been scolding Will for focusing on the wrong things in therapy, but what if I was the one who was wrong? What if Cindy didn't have major depression? What if she really had bipolar II?

Suddenly everything made sense. I could have kicked myself for not having figured it out sooner.

While I explained to them, Roland looked at his wife, his expression conveying equal measures of concern and fear. Whatever the future of their marriage might be, it was clear that he cared deeply about Cindy and wanted to figure a way to help.

For the rest of the session, the three of us worked together to find a plan that would work—to help get her through the next twenty-four hours, the coming week.

Before Cindy came for her visit, I had been planning to make a different adjustment. I had been thinking that Cindy was an "SSRI nonresponder." I had been planning to switch the Zoloft with Effexor, an SNRI, serotonin norepinephrine reuptake inhibitor, medications that act on two neurotransmitters, increasing the likelihood that they will help regulate mood. But what I realized now was that I had to do something entirely different: to back up and rethink her diagnosis.

A significant percentage of people who present for treatment of depression actually have bipolar disorder, or manic-depressive illness. When I first met with Cindy, I had fairly easily concluded that she didn't have classic manic-depressive illness—she had never had a manic episode, she had never been out of touch with reality, or psychotic, or delusional, had never gone days without sleep or engaged in promiscuous sexual activity when in a "high" state. What I hadn't considered and hadn't questioned her about in detail was hypomania, or the symptoms of bipolar II disorder.

Bipolar II is a form of bipolar illness that has been recognized only over the past decade or two. With bipolar II disorder, people have full depressive episodes, but only fairly mild highs. Instead of manic episodes, they have hypomanic episodes. During these times, they have symptoms like increased energy and sociability, are more talkative than usual, have elevated mood, and may be somewhat flirtatious or extravagant with money. But they are not out of touch with reality; they are just a bit too high. Sometimes people who have bipolar II have what are called "mixed states" in which they are both hypomanic and agitated at the same time, or both agitated and depressed, or even both depressed and euphoric at the same time. Some people have rapid switches between high and low moods, which is called "rapid cycling," and may go from depressed to euphoric, from calm to agitated, several times per month, or per day, or even per hour.

Rapid cycling bipolar II disorder. This, I was pretty certain now, described Cindy's state of mind over the past several months. And made it easy to decide what to do.

Basically, it came to this: we would decrease Cindy's antidepressant dose from 200 to 150 mg/day, and start some medicines to help control her mood swings. As I thought over the events of the past two weeks, it was clear that she had been cycling between depression and hypomania—from low mood to a state of agitation and mild euphoria. I would write a prescription for a low dose of Risperdal, an atypical antipsychotic that could help to take the edge off her agitation fairly quickly. And lithium carbonate, the standard treatment for bipolar disorder, both types I and II, starting at 600 mg/day, probably to increase eventually to 900 to 1200 mg/day. This combination would be likely to stabilize her mood within the next week or two. She also had some Valium at home, which she could take only if needed.

Ruth came in for a few moments too. She agreed to take Zach to her house for a few nights. Cindy would also see Will at least twice in the coming week: and I made a note to call him as soon as possible to explain my radical change in thinking—and to apologize a bit. As I saw it now, his explorations of family dynamics weren't crucial to the problems Cindy was currently having, whereas my incorrect diagnosis was. I would also ask his input about how he would be approaching the psychotherapy issues. Obviously, day-by-day coping was the key for now. If she started obsessing about her marital problems, she should try to "turn off" those thoughts, as difficult as it might be. They *weren't* insights; they were intrusive thoughts! Focusing on them at this point was counterproductive. She needed to focus on feeling better. If she felt suicidal again, she was to call me; and if she was getting out of control, Roland could call an ambulance to take her to the nearest emergency room. If all else failed, there was always the hospital.

Cindy and Roland, and Ruth as well, seemed greatly relieved by what I was saying. It was nothing special: I was just following standard New Neuropsychiatry paradigms, which are known to lead to better outcome: in this case, to reevaluate diagnosis if a patient worsens, rather than improves, after a series of reasonable medication trials.

I called Will as soon as they left.

I told him about the changes in diagnosis and the resulting medication changes, and our plans for the next twenty-four hours. He seemed greatly relieved, because this explained a lot of what Cindy had been through for the past several weeks. He agreed that he would put everything into trying to convince her to comply with taking the pills, encourage her to try to block the intrusive thoughts, and reinforce the need for getting regular sleep.

That was the best we could do.

Cindy's Long-Awaited Recovery

In almost every New Neuropsychiatry case, eventually a new stage of stability is achieved. Eventually may mean days or weeks, even months. Given the time that it takes for a medication to achieve adequate blood levels; given the time that it takes for neurotransmitter changes to occur in the brain; given the time that it takes for symptoms and behaviors to change; given the time that it takes for a person to adjust psychologically to these changes; and given the time that it takes for family and friends to adapt to how she has changed— given all that, eventually a new steady state will be achieved. Disorder will be replaced with order.

Eventually, the entire complex system, from chemicals to spouses to therapists, will settle into a new status quo.

So it was with Cindy Prince. Just as I was about to give up and try to have her admitted to the hospital, her disorder melted away. The combination of Risperdal and lithium, plus the lower dose of Zoloft, did the trick. The Risperdal was most helpful early on, enabling her to become less agitated and to get enough sleep. After a few weeks, we got the lithium up to an adequate blood level (0.9 milliquivalents per liter), at a dose of 1800 mg/day, and further tapered the Zoloft to 100 and then 75 mg/day. Cindy kept going to therapy twice a week. Will stuck to his assigned task of helping her cope day-to-day. After a few more weeks, she glided into a normal range of mood: not depressed, not agitated, not excited, just calm. Was it finally a safe landing?

Perhaps a month after starting lithium, Cindy sat by the window in my office, looking at children playing in the park outside. You could see the recovery in her. Her face was no longer puffy with tears and she no longer shredded one tissue after another as she talked. Instead of sitting on the edge of her chair, instead of pacing and sighing, she sat comfortably, occasionally smiling or looking pensive. Even her hair, her nails, her makeup, looked put-together.

"Want to know how I knew I was okay again? Last night, I was able to read a book again. I haven't been able to read books since before Zach was born."

So: she was emerging from the fog of depression—from the obsessive miserable ruminations of despair—and from the agitation of hypomania as well, and the misery of constant cycling from low to high and back again.

She was enjoying being with the kids now, she told me. It was fun being with Zach and the babies.

"Fun." She sounding surprised to hear herself saying that word. She had joined a local group for "new mothers of twins." That was fun too, really fun. "Three pairs of identical, two fraternal. You should see them in action!"

Plus, as she sat in the community room of her local town center, she realized to her surprise that she was much *less* overwhelmed than many of the other mothers of twins. Her relationship with Roland—well, that was on the back burner for now. It was not great, but not terrible either. There had been a few nights he had gone to sleep in the guest room at his brother's house, but then he came back. He wasn't about to move out any day soon; in fact, he was saying how relieved he was to have "the old Cindy back." They were thinking of going into couples therapy.

"When things quiet down with the kids," she said. "If they ever do!"

"Well, you made it," I said.

"*We* made it," she answered.

She was right.

A New Land

Mark Maple responded to treatment in an entirely different way. Prozac—once decreased to the normal maximum dose of 80 mg/day—was a good choice for him. It wasn't perfect, of course: He struggled with increased appetite, a result of the medication, and noted a problem with sexual functioning (a difficulty in achieving orgasm), which lessened when we added a second medication, bethenacol.

But soon the medication began to fade into the background. Instead, over the next several months, Mark started to work on "response prevention"—on training himself not to respond to his fears about Susan's whereabouts, which, though blunted by the SSRI medicine, were still present. He battled against intrusive thoughts and worked on finding other ways to deal with his feelings of anxiety, including beginning to run on a treadmill at lunchtime. At times, he felt positively jaunty. He began to test himself—turning his cell phone off during the day, even leaving it at home. One morning, rushing to court, he even forgot it in a taxi and was almost disappointed when the cabbie returned it to him. Despite having taken a break from therapy with Liz, Mark was starting to see positive effects of his newfound well-being on his relationships with people, including his co-workers, Susan, and his parents—from whom he had been estranged since his accident.

Early on, my concern with Mark's recovery had been akin to that of a doctor treating a cancer patient. The symptoms had been present for so long, and had affected so much of Mark's life, that I had worried that their sudden removal might cause a sort of psychic implosion. After all, in medicine, a patient whose large, slow-growing cancer begins to melt away in response to chemotherapy may actually die from the treatment. The tumor may have ended up providing necessary support to the body, and its sudden disappearance may lead to fractures or infection or bleeding. Psychologically, we are all defined by our quirks and eccentricities: we erase them too quickly at some risk.

So even though Mark seemed to be doing so well over the first several months of treatment, I wondered whether this would last. Every New Neuropsychiatrist has seen smashing successes in which the patient has inexplicably refused to continue treatment—and has chosen to return to the familiar shores of his disorder. And at times I seemed to see a sadness in Mark's eyes, a sense of grief for all that he had lost during the years of his disorder. Perhaps a psychological depression, not a biological one, because with all that SSRI medication on board Mark "couldn't" get depressed. I told Mark what I had been thinking.

"Maybe," he said. "I see what you mean. I do feel twinges of that—of sadness for everything I've lost. But I don't feel overwhelmed by it."

"How do you feel?"

"Mostly good, except for one thing. I'm totally confused about my relationship with Susan."

"How so?"

"Well, in all these years of calling her and checking up on her, and worrying about where she was, I never got to the *real* issue. Which is: do I want to be with her? She wants to get married, she wants to have kids, has wanted this for years. And I've always said I wasn't ready."

"And now?"

He stood at the door, on his way out. He laughed. "Liz would say I'd been using the symptoms to avoid making a commitment."

"And now you have hardly any symptoms," I said.

"Exactly. Which is why I was thinking of making an appointment to see Liz one of these days, just to talk things over."

Afterward, a thought came to me. Maybe Mark had a point. Maybe he *was* avoiding something here. Not something bad, though—something *good*. He had been struggling in psychotherapy for years, unable to achieve his goals, but struggling nonetheless. Mark didn't seem to be some Woody Allenesque character, ever-complaining, never-improving, a therapy addict. Having suffered, Mark had been gamely trying to work his way through his problems. But year after year, he had been stuck. After Corinne's tragic death, he had been frozen in life—sidetracked by a constant need to call Susan, to check up on her. He couldn't be away from her, but neither could he truly be with her.

Now, Mark was freed. No doubt some hyperactive circuits in his brain had been turned down (probably one circuit from the lower brain, including the basal ganglia, containing the caudate nucleus, the putamen, and the amygdala; and another circuit from the higher brain, including the orbital frontal cortex, the cingulate gyrus, and the caudate nucleus), releasing him from the compulsion to check up on Susan. And perhaps some other centers, perhaps, having to do with intimacy, with relationships, with procreation, were now activated. The New Neuropsychiatrist in me wondered this: could Mark use his new energy, his new freedom, to work in therapy with Liz.

I e-mailed Liz: "FYI—you might get a call from MM. As the analysts put it, 'Trust the process.'"

I figured she'd get a laugh out of that.

Parts of the Brain

The brain is such a complicated organ that it is hard to say definitely that one part or another "does" something, particularly since many functions are distributed broadly throughout the brain, and since single areas may play a key role in many (sometimes diametrically opposed, and at other times seemingly unrelated) functions.

Thus any description of the brain is by its nature a vast oversimplification. Nevertheless, studies of brain functioning (such as functional MRI imaging studies and studies of brain lesions or injuries) demonstrate that there is localization of function to particular segments of the brain. Studies also show that the structure and functioning of many of these centers is disturbed in psychiatric disorders—and often is normalized by successful treatment. It is also worth noting that disorders affect not only various parts of the brain but also the circuits or pathways that connect these centers, so that some have greater activity and others have less activity than in states of health. The following is a list of areas of the brain that are thought to relate to psychiatric disorders, in particular to anxiety disorders and depression.

Amygdala: The brain's fear or anxiety center, and a part of the limbic system, the amygdala plays a primary role in the processing and memory of emotional reactions. It consists of several nuclei in the brain with distinct functions. It plays a primary role in the formation and storage of memories associated with emotional events, in particular with fear conditioning. The functioning of the amygdala has been shown to be abnormal in psychiatric disorders including panic disorder, depression, and borderline personality disorder. For instance, people with borderline personality disorder experience increased fear responses from their amygdalas even when they see friendly or neutral faces.

The *anterior cingulate cortex* is the front part of the cingulate cortex, and forms a "collar" around the corpus callosum, the nerve fibers that connect the left and right hemispheres of the brain. The anterior cingulate cortex is involved in regulating blood pressure and heart rate, as well as in rational cognitive functions, such as decision making, empathy, and anticipation of rewards. It plays key roles in detecting and monitoring errors. Its function appears to be abnormal in various psychiatric disorders such as OCD and depression, where its overactivity may account for the overwhelming negative feelings and emotions in these disorders, as well as impaired decision making.

The *cerebral cortex* is the outer layer of the anterior part of the mammalian brain, and plays crucial roles in memory, attention, thought, language, and consciousness.

The *dentate gyrus* is part of the hippocampus, and is thought to play a role in the development of new memories, and in depression. It is one of the few brain areas in which new brain cells grow throughout life. Antidepressant treatment increases brain cell growth in this area.

Dorsal striatum: a subcortical part of the forebrain that includes two main centers, the caudate nucleus and the putamen. It plays roles in the planning and modulation of movement and also in executive functioning, such as self-control and reasoning. This part of the brain is activated by stimuli associated with motivation for rewards, via the neurotransmitter dopamine. Its functioning is thought to be abnormal in drug addiction as well as in disorders like Parkinson disease.

Dorsolateral prefrontal cortex: this area of the prefrontal cortex is responsible for motor planning and organization, and for integrating sensory information and memories. It is also involved in working memory, social judgment, and abstract thinking.

The *hippocampus* is part of the brain's limbic system. It is a paired structure with a seahorse-like shape, and is located in the middle region of the brain's temporal lobes. It plays important roles in long-term memory and in spatial navigation. It is particularly important in the formation of new memories about experiences, or autobiographical memory, as well as for memories of facts, or declarative memory.

The *hypothalamus*, located just above the brainstem, is a part of the brain that links the nervous system to the endocrine system. It secretes neurohormones, or brain hormones, which increase or decrease the activity of the pituitary gland, which in turn regulates glands including the adrenals, thyroid, and sexual organs.

continued on page 82

The *limbic system* is a set of brain structures that includes the hippocampus, the amygdala, the anterior thalamus, the hypothalamus, and the limbic cortex. It plays roles in emotion, behavior, and long-term memory, as well as in olfaction, or the sense of smell. It influences the endocrine system and the autonomic nervous system, and is also tightly connected to the prefrontal cortex.

Mirror neurons are neurons that fire when an animal acts or when it sees the same action performed by another animal. These have been studied in primates and are thought to also exist in humans. They are believed to be located in the premotor cortex and inferior parietal cortex and play important roles in imitation and in language acquisition, as well as in the emotion of empathy.

The *orbitofrontal cortex* is a region in the prefrontal cortex. Its name comes from its location above the skull's orbits, in which the eyes are located. It plays functions in emotional life and in decision making, in particular in relation to rewards and punishments, and its function is often disturbed in depression.

The *pineal gland* is a small endocrine gland in the brain that produces melatonin, a hormone that affects sleep-wake cycles, as well as seasonal rhythms.

The *prefrontal cortex* is located in the anterior part of the frontal lobes of the brain, which lies in front of the motor and premotor areas. It regulates complex cognitive behaviors, decision making, and the orchestration of thoughts and actions. It organizes executive functions of the brain, and is responsible for planning, cognitive flexibility, abstract thinking, and initiating appropriate actions.

The *raphe* or raphe nuclei are a cluster of brain nuclei found in the brain-stem, whose main function is to release serotonin to the rest of the brain. The raphe nuclei have a vast impact on the nervous system, primarily through the transmitter serotonin.

The *reticular activating system* is the parts of the brain associated with arousal and attention, and the transition between sleep and wakefulness. It is composed of circuits that connect the brainstem to the cortex, and includes areas such as the reticular formation, the thalamus, and the hypothalamus. Parts of this system may be damaged in posttraumatic stress disorder, and may account for abnormal waking and startle reactions seen in that disorder.

Subgenual anterior cingulate: Also known as Brodmann's Area 25, this part of the anterior cingulate is highly connected to the serotonin system, and plays a role in sleep and appetite as well as mood and anxiety. It is also closely connected to the hippocampus, which plays a role in memory formation, and to the parts of the frontal cortex that are involved in self-esteem. It appears to be overactive in treatment-resistant depression, and deep brain stimulation near this area appears to be successful in treating such depression.

The *thalamus* is a large structure located on top of the brainstem, which sends nerve fibers widely throughout the cortex. It functions as a relay between subcortical areas and the cerebral cortex, and plays roles in processing information as well as in relaying it between the lower and higher brain. It has major functions for motor and sensory systems. Interestingly, people with a particular genetic variant in the serotonin transporter appear to have enlargement of the thalamus, which may make them more vulnerable to depression, PTSD, and perhaps even suicide.

Invisible Barriers

Medication isn't the only way to bring a disorder under control and to calm the hyperactive stress centers of the brain. Therapy—especially approaches that are targeted toward symptom control—can lead there too. Take the case of Allen Johnson.

After some thought, Allen decided not to use medication to block his panic attacks. He did have a vial with three or four Ativan pills, which he carried with him in case things got bad. "My safety valve," he called it—but he so rarely took the pills that they tended to disintegrate over time, shaken into dust. Allen Johnson had a stubborn streak. Once he discovered that cognitive-behavioral therapy, or CBT, *could* work for panic disorder, that was it. He determined to plunge into treatment without medication. He bought innumerable self-help books and joined Freedom from Fear, a self-help organization for people who have panic disorder. He took a break from his gestalt therapist. He informed me that he wanted me to treat him using cognitive-behavioral techniques.

Not being a "hard-wired" behavior therapist, I wasn't sure if I could give him a rigorous enough course of that approach. Nevertheless, Allen wanted to try. I told him about new research showing that the fear system is controlled by two pathways—the faster amygdala-based system and a slower system controlled by the prefrontal cortex, which can determine whether a situation is truly dangerous or not.

So we began to work together, trying to retrain his fear systems. By committing himself to a program of exercises and behavior therapy—spending fixed periods of time every day practicing diaphragmatic breathing, doing muscle-relaxation exercises, and keeping a log of his panic-inducing thoughts and physical reactions—Allen was able to bring the panic attacks under control.

It was a lot more work than taking a pill or two a day, but Allen had the advantage of discovering how he *himself* could be in control of states of anxiety or calm. Rather than being regulated by some medicine, he could take charge of his own physiology.

A week, two weeks, and then a month passed without full-blown panic attacks. At times, Allen would get twinges of fear, or what are called limited symptom attacks, but there were no more overwhelming explosions of panic, no more terror-ridden visits to the emergency room. Instead, he would continue regular diaphragmatic breathing along with self-calming imagery—and the panic would fade. No longer did Allen have to spend weekends at his brother and sister-in-law's apartment. He moved back to his own apartment downtown and began settling back into his own life. A life marked by milestones that to someone else may have seemed trivial—the first time he was able to take dry cleaning to a store three blocks away, his first bus ride uptown.

And yet, even though the severe panic attacks had stopped, Allen found life constrained. Manhattan was full of invisible barriers that had been erected when he was ill. He was unable to go to previously familiar restaurants, to take the subway, to drop by his favorite video store. Worst of all, his job was in jeopardy because he had so much trouble traveling to see clients. He was unable to travel by plane. By train or car, he could travel to only a few cities. Long transatlantic plane flights seemed entirely beyond him. He was unable to take elevators above the tenth floor. He could travel to and from the office, but if he veered more than two or three blocks off his usual route, the anxiety would begin to flare up.

And, he fretted: would he ever date again?

This in a sense was the true beginning of Allen's recovery. The patient who has panic disorder knows only two states: calm and terror. He or she lives in a binary world. Panic is a monochromatic set, a black-and-white existence, you could say, in a Technicolor world. A psychological state that reflects the biology of the brain. In emergency situations, survival is enhanced by black-and-white thinking: you either flee or fight. You are either safe or at risk of death. A stranger is either an enemy or a friend.

Scientists believe that the brain's structure actually becomes pared down to deal with severe crises—by atrophy of the dentate gyrus and of the CA3 cells in the hippocampus. This brain simplification process occurs in high-stress environments, in wartime, famine, and so on, in which black-and-white thinking enhances survival. In peacetime, however, the world is not binary; continuing to see everything as either black or white, safe or dangerous, creates false dichotomies and often leads to bad choices.

Thus, during the acute phase of his disorder, Allen's world of normality had been transformed to a world of unbearable panic. He had become subject to assaults of dread and fear that seemed irrational, even bizarre, to his friends and family members and the innumerable emergency room doctors, and yet which seem to him to be sure harbingers of death. He had been utterly convinced that "something is seriously wrong with me." He was going to die, to go berserk, his heart was ready to stop beating any instant, his sanity would irretrievably vanish. But as he began to respond to treatment, his view of the world began to change.

Every New Neuropsychiatrist knows the need for referring repeatedly to the map of treatment. But for Allen it was not only the map of treatment we needed to consult, but also the particular map of Manhattan. Allen needed to know how he got lost and then how to turn his course around and get back on track.

The New Neuropsychiatrist, who attempts to integrate our understandings of mind and brain and body, may come to see panic disorder—or depression—as a signal, a wake-up call, an opportunity for growth. An all-or-nothing emotional style, which may have worked for many years, has finally melted down irretrievably. The great opportunity of these disorders is that it indicates that you are ready to grow—to find new ways to deal with emotions, to transcend black-and-white.

Allen and I worked together, week after week, going over the map. It was not a map back to where he was before, but a map of how to get to a better place. Although he might live the rest of his life under the shadow of possible panic attacks (because panic disorder is a regrettably persistent disorder), I tried to help Allen to see anxiety in a new way, at times an enemy, at times an ally or friend. Allen lived in Greenwich Village, around 10th Street. While he was able to take cabs to distant parts of the city (for instance, to my West Side office or to his job in midtown), for years he had been unable to walk around his neighborhood except for a few blocks near his apartment. Over a period of weeks, Allen began to walk up to 14th Street, through Union Square, and actually left the Village and headed toward 23th Street. He also began to make his way downtown, with the eventual goal of Houston Street, and then started facing the challenge of going east and west, on the longer crosstown blocks.

At times it was discouraging.

"What a ridiculous way for a grown man to spend his time!" he would say, full of grief and fury for what had been lost in all his years of captivity.

"Yeah, but right now it's the best thing you can do for yourself," I would say.

We did talk about his losses, his disappointments and struggles and frustrations, but we also ended up talking more speculatively—about how he could be remapping his brain by his travels, making new connections in his hippocampus, helping his newly sprouted pyramidal cells (neurons that help to synchronize brain activity) to grow up and learn their way around, so to speak, so they would develop the right interneuronal connections.

Allen wasn't sure he "could believe all that neurobiology mumbo-jumbo," but he seemed to get a kick out of thinking that there might be something to it.

So he spent a number of months in treatment: retaking Manhattan, one block at a time.

Is Response All There Is?

And so it was that Cindy and Mark and Allen each responded to treatment in a different way. And so perhaps for you—your disorder, whether treated with medicine, therapy, or a combination of approaches, responds to treatment, and most of symptoms eventually melt away.

In the Old Psychiatry, the main goal in treating disorder was to get such a "response."

"His disorder successfully responded to treatment," would be the line at the end of a case presentation. And that was it. The End. Mission accomplished.

To the New Neuropsychiatrist, though, the initial response to treatment is just the beginning. This is a crucial distinction.

In the Old Psychiatry, the stories of Cindy and Mark and Allen would end here. Their—and perhaps your—symptoms were for the most part under control. They no longer "met criteria" for the disorder that had brought them into treatment, and presumably their life was back on track. The only thing to worry about was if they became depressed again at some time in the future, and then the goal would be to get them to "respond" to treatment again.

The New Neuropsychiatry sees things differently.

Response is still the initial goal—in which we want to quiet the brain's and body's overexcited stress-response systems. If we succeed here, we have put out the fire, so to speak. You feel better; your symptoms are "under control." You were in a state of disorder; you have "gotten better." You certainly *feel* better, though some of your symptoms may still be there.

But it has become clear to the New Neuropsychiatry that "better" is not the same as "well." The second stage in the New Neuropsychiatry is remission. Remission, as I will talk about in the second half of this book, is a state in which not only are you better but also your day-to-day symptoms (depression, panic, etc.) are essentially no different from those of a person who does not have a disorder. In remission, your disorder *really* is under control—so for a long period of time you don't have significant symptoms. If response meant putting out the fire, remission means getting rid of the smoldering coals.

Only when remission has occurred for a prolonged period of time does a third stage, recovery, get under way. With the advent of New Neuropsychiatry in the past decade or so, we have had tantalizing glimpses of the processes of both remission and recovery. And with recent advances in neuroscience, we are starting to put the pieces together, to realize that during the phases of remission and recovery, a process of brain remodeling appears to be happening—including changes in brain structure and functional circuits. At the same time as these brain changes settle in, your life is rebuilding and recovering—which I suspect is no coincidence.

That is not to say that the stage of recovery is the same as having never had a disorder. It is clear that a person who has recovered from a disorder, who no longer has significant symptoms of depression or anxiety, may still be more vulnerable to stress in some ways. This makes sense if you think of the recovered brain circuits as more fragile and delicate than never-injured ones. At the same time, a person who has recovered from a disorder may have greater strength, greater resilience, perhaps more empathy or maturity, even wisdom, than a person who has never had a disorder. You may be more of a mensch.

For some people at the "response" phase of treatment, the powerful effects of medications may seem to overwhelm everything else. It may seem that "the medication is doing everything"—an assumption that is worth examining.

If you are taking medication, most likely you have been doing a lot to make the medications work better to help reregulate your systems. Since your disorder was at its worst, you have decreased alcohol use, you worked to increase and regularize your sleep and improve your health through exercise and diet. And now, now that your disorder has responded, you can begin to use your new sense of well-being and optimism to make progress in therapy. The goal at this point, as I will talk about in Chapter 5, is to turn "response" into "remission." To go from "getting better" to "getting well." And eventually, the goal can be to turn the responses to crisis and stress into a higher level of resilience.

The changes that are beginning to appear now thus can open up opportunities for more improvement, for true recovery. You might ask, Are there any changes in how you respond to other people in your life that you could use to improve your relationships? Could your new energy and optimism be put to good use in helping you to deal better with your life issues and problems? Changing how you deal with feelings and emotions, and memories—as Allen and Mark and Cindy were beginning to do—can enhance your recovery.

Insight and the Present Moment

As response to treatment is achieved, one of the most powerful New Neuropsychiatry tools is a form of "insight." Unlike the Old Psychiatry, in which insight was often focused on the past, on excavating old memories and uncovering buried feelings, in the New Neuropsychiatry insight is primarily focused on the present day—observing and reflecting upon your own progress in treatment.

The goal of New Neuropsychiatry is thus not primarily to explore the past more fully in order to understand the present. Rather, it is to see the present more vividly in order to relieve suffering—and, if need be, to loosen the shackles of the past. In early treatment response, the past is often an intrusion, a reminder of old limitations and a distraction from making healthy changes.

The formerly fearful and avoidant woman who is now beginning to take new risks in life tells her doctor, "Whenever I try new things, I hear my mother's voice telling me I'll fail." The Old Psychiatry therapist would say, "Tell me about your mother," and begin to explore the past. The New Neuropsychiatry therapist says, "What is it that you feel *now?* What is it that sets off these intrusive thoughts? Let's focus on how you can find ways to calm yourself to deal better with this new situation." Later in treatment there will be time for the past, but the present comes first.

The primary focus of New Neuropsychiatry insight is thus the present moment itself—and finding ways to use your body's innate abilities to calm itself, and your mind's capacities to relieve its fears. Hence the centrality of mindfulness, self-calming, meditative awareness, of interrupting and stopping ruminative thoughts, of using breathing and relaxation techniques and other body resources for calming. Using these capacities can allow you to deal more capably with your current life. Especially as you change behaviors, as you return to a fuller life.

Allen Johnson was a prime example of this. Often, while he was in the midst of specific "assignments" to improve his ability to travel, his mind would be filled with his stepfather's voice telling him that he was a "loser" and a "weakling" because he was having so much difficulty walking down the street. Initially, Allen agreed with these sentiments. After all, what kind of grown man would be wandering around Manhattan, struggling to make it from 26th to 27th Street while practicing deep diaphragmatic breathing rather than shallow puffing using his rib muscles? Floored by this ignominious situation and convinced that he was a "total wimp," Allen would be overwhelmed by fear. He would stop his uptown trek and turn tail back home.

Over time, with a bit of coaching, Allen was able to block out these "intrusive" thoughts, his stepfather's unhelpful criticisms. When he was a child, his stepfather, a highly aggressive trial attorney, raged up and down the sidelines at football games, yelling if Allen dropped a pass or missed a block, which had hardly helped his game. Seeing the past as an intrusion, Allen worked on calming himself, on "improving mindfulness." He struggled to find an "inner locus of control," whereas in the past he had sought control of his feelings from outside. The muscle-relaxation exercises that he practiced and the deep-breathing exercises both helped, as did "talking back" to his stepfather's voice.

On his treks uptown, as he remapped his city, Allen gradually came to realize to what a great degree he had induced his own anxiety—and hence that he could also make himself calm.

Back to maps for a moment. As I mentioned in the Introduction, Eleanor Maguire's studies at the Institute of Neurology in London, published in the year 2000, have shown that the hippocampus of cab drivers enlarges to allow them to store a detailed mental map of the city. Cab drivers in the city of London—unlike cabbies in the United States—are required to memorize hundreds of city streets, in an intensive process that takes up to two years, before they are allowed to actually carry passengers. Maguire showed that not only do cab drivers have a larger hippocampus than other people but also that their hippocampus *continues* to grow as they spend more time working. Obviously it is not just cabbies we are talking about here. The hippocampus is how all humans orient ourselves in the world and also is the means by which we consolidate personal memories. The functioning of the hippocampus is disturbed in many psychiatric disorders, everything from depression to PTSD to panic disorder. One striking example of this is seen in people who have severe anxiety disorders.

When I was working at an urban clinic in lower Manhattan, we saw many patients who had a history of severe trauma and panic disorder and complained of always getting lost. Invariably, they would get turned around coming off the subway and would wander for many blocks in the wrong direction, eventually ending up in an utter frenzy. My guess now, in view of this recent research, is that they had experienced microscopic brain injury from chronic and severe stress and had lost their ability to access their brain maps of the world. Often they could not find their way even in their own neighborhoods. Recent research on neurogenesis in the hippocampus suggests that this type of injury may be able to be reversed, that with appropriate treatment it may be possible to regrow these crucial areas, both brain cells and brain connections.

Even more amazing, studies show that *all* antidepressant and mood stabilizer medications appear to specifically cause neurogenesis in this part of the brain! Other studies suggest that behavioral therapy, which helps depression and anxiety disorders, does the same thing. Whereas drugs that *don't* help depression—alcohol, sedatives, cocaine, heroin—do not cause neurogenesis!

Neurogenesis and other types of brain regrowth and regeneration seem to be crucial to what makes a medicine an effective antidepressant. These days, I realize how wonderful it would be to have an MRI image of my patients' brains as they began to respond to treatment with medication or therapy, to see whether the hippocampus begins to grow back, and to see if there are measurable increases in connections between other parts of the brain as well. (In fact, my research group has started a study at Columbia that will look at exactly this issue: does medication treatment of chronic depression increase the size of the hippocampus? And does it also help to increase the strength of other healthy brain connections?)

My use of the concept of mapping and remapping in this book is hardly just a metaphor—it is a literal description of what your brain is doing as you make your way through the world! And for Allen Johnson, I am convinced that his explorations, first of Manhattan and later of the five boroughs of New York City and beyond, served the crucial function of remapping and rewiring his brain!

The cases of Mark Maple and Cindy Prince and Allen Johnson, as they began treatment, may be a bit more dramatic than the average. But in essence, they are no different from the situations that every person faces at the beginning of New Neuropsychiatry treatment. The focused, purposeful evaluation and treatment of psychiatric disorders—by a medication, a biological treatment of brain dysfunction, or a focused therapy like CBT, which also affects brain function—inherently introduces new complexities. Disorder causes changes in brain structure and function: it strengthens brain pathways and circuits that maintain a state of suffering, and causes the weakening and withering away of healthy brain circuits. As every psychotherapist knows, and as every neuroscientist also knows (though in a different way), such disorders stubbornly maintain themselves in the human mind and brain and can be difficult to dislodge, frequently reintroducing themselves in different forms, growing back like weeds in a garden. It is almost as if New Neuropsychiatry interventions can set off an effort by your mind (and brain) to return to the status quo of disorder, however painful or maladaptive it may have been. The suffering state may have been a familiar type of homeostasis.

At the same time, events themselves may have made a return to one's past life impossible. Your disorder may have made it impossible to rely on your previously effective coping mechanisms. Take Allen Johnson, for example.

Having experienced unbearable panic, he could never again *not* know: he had an irreversible failure of forgetfulness. He had to learn anew how to become calm, how to gain a sense of well-being and safety in the world. So too Mark Maple, who needed to find a sense of things being okay with Susan. And so too for Cindy, who needed not only to feel better again but also to figure out how to get her life back in order, as a mother, as a wife, as a scientist—to begin to feel normal for the first time in many, many years. And so too perhaps for you, as the symptoms of your disorder begin to fade, as you begin to feel better again for an extended period of time.

So, as your disorder responds to treatment, as "being better" becomes a way of life, something new often becomes clear. Not only is it impossible to go back—it is essential to continue moving toward recovery.

Part 2

Getting (and Staying) Well

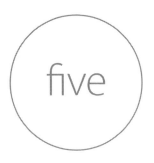

five

A New Vista

Daring to Dream Again

Why Remission?

I HAVE PREVIOUSLY MENTIONED that response is an insufficient goal for therapy of mood and anxiety disorders, and that the goal should be remission. Why is this? Response, you will recall, means that symptoms have dropped about 50 percent and that you are "better." This was the goal of the Old Psychiatry, when I trained in the 1980s. In contrast, remission means that the symptoms of depression or the anxiety disorder are essentially gone.

About 50 to 60 percent of people who have depression will respond to treatment with any one antidepressant medicine and about a third will remit (the numbers are probably roughly the same for depression-focused types of psychotherapy such as cognitive-behavioral therapy or interpersonal psychotherapy). What difference does it make if you respond or remit? The answer: all the difference in the world!

In 2008 Thomas Frodl and colleagues from Munich, Germany, published a fascinating paper on ways that the brain actually changed over three years as a result of depression. Using MRI scans, they compared people with depression and nondepressed people and found differences in the size of numerous areas of the brain both at the time of the initial scan. The "gray matter density" in

Changing Definitions of Response, Remission, and Recovery

When New Neuropsychiatrists talk about a disorder "responding" to treatment, they mean that symptoms have dropped by about half. Treatment "response" thus means you are somewhat better, but may still have significant symptoms like sleeplessness, anxiety, and so on.

In contrast, "remission" means that almost all symptoms are gone for at least three weeks.

And "recovery" is defined as being in remission for four or more months—but it means being well now and for the foreseeable future.

Psychiatrists often use rating scales like the Hamilton Depression Rating Scale (HDRS) to evaluate depression. Individuals rate the most common symptoms related to depression, with scores ranging from 0 (none) to 1 (mild), 2, 3, or 4 based on severity. A person who is significantly depressed may have a score of 25 or 30 or even more. When your disorder has "responded" to treatment, you may still have a score of 12 to 15 points or more. That is still a significant load of depression! For your disorder to go into "remission," though, you would have to have a score of 7 or less on the HDRS, the same as the score of a "normal"—that is, a nondepressed—person.

The Old Psychiatry often had curious attitudes toward symptoms. Back in the 1950s and 1960s, psychotherapists would use your symptoms as a way of getting you motivated to go into therapy, but they might not focus much on relieving them. In any case, the Old Psychiatry psychotherapies—psychoanalysis for example—often didn't focus on early relief of symptoms of major depression or panic disorder. A century after the introduction of psychoanalysis, there is scant evidence that it relieves these symptoms. So you could not count on *ever* getting to a stage where your disorder responded to treatment, much

---

areas such as the hippocampus, anterior cingulate, amygdala, and parts of the prefrontal cortex was lower in people who had depression than in healthy individuals—indicating significant brain damage associated with depression.

Even more interesting, though, Frodl looked at the people whose depression went into remission in comparison to those whose depression did *not* remit. Strikingly, "patients whose depression remitted during the 3-year period had less volume decline than nonremitted patients in most of these areas, including the left hippocampus, left anterior cingulate, and dorsomedial and dorsolateral prefrontal cortex." We have already talked about the hippocampus,

less went into remission. After many years and hundreds of sessions, psycho-analysis might end with your original mood or anxiety symptoms still there!

What about the Old Psychiatry medication treatments? Unfortunately, Old Psychiatry medication treatments focused almost entirely on helping a handful of symptoms. When depressed mood lifted or insomnia subsided, Old Psychiatry medication treatment was done, its goals achieved. Your disorder had "responded." Response of these "vegetative symptoms"—that is, the physical manifestations of psychiatric illness—was the be-all and end-all of Old Psychiatry medication treatment. "Response" alone was a modest goal—it meant that your symptoms were just halfway better. In the Old Psychiatry, you were a responder if your sleep had increased from four hours a night to six rather than your usual eight, or if your mood was "okay" but not "good." The only thing from then on was "maintenance treatment"—keeping up the status quo. Which mostly meant to keep taking your medication. The problem was this: Old Psychiatry medications had many side effects, so the cure was often nearly as bad as the disorder. Lightheadedness, seda-tion, and other symptoms including potentially serious cardiac side effects often interfered significantly with quality of life. Even worse, Old Psychiatry psychopharmacology's emphasis on symptoms as the sine qua non of treat-ment often allowed doctors to ignore continued impairment in functioning, in work, or in social relationships.

In the Old Psychiatry, disorders often did not go into remission. Even if there was a response, a questionable proposition, it was unlikely that remission would be achieved. In the New Neuropsychiatry, we know the majority of people can find relief from their symptoms and a renewed outlook on life.

and its many functions including spatial orientation and working memory. These other parts of the brain are key for making decisions, resolving conflict, and integrating inputs from the senses and other parts of the brain (anterior cingulate), for rapid monitoring for errors (dorsomedial prefrontal cortex), and for a host of functions including motor planning, social judgment, and abstract thinking (dorsolateral prefrontal cortex).

What does this mean? Basically, if your depression doesn't remit, the pro-cess of brain damage continues. This damage occurs in many of the areas I have previously talked about as being related to depression. If depression *is* brought into remission, Frodl's findings suggest that the process of brain damage largely stops! This study, of course, must be "replicated"—its findings must be repeated by other investigators. However, it is consistent with other things that we already know about remission in depression and the risks of nonremission.

People whose depression does not go into remission do worse in a number of areas than do people whose depression does remit. They have worse social functioning, including more absenteeism at work; they have higher medical costs; they have higher risks of illness and death from heart disease; they have worse outcome of diabetes; and they have an overall higher death rate. They also have a greater risk of having a relapse, or a return of depression: in one study, 76 percent of nonremitters got depressed again within 15 months, compared with only 25 percent of those whose depression had gone into remission. Not only is there a greater risk of becoming depressed again, but also there is a risk of having more episodes and a greater likelihood of developing chronic depression. Even having one or two mild symptoms remaining after treatment increases the risk of becoming depressed again! Lewis Judd found that such people stayed well only for an average of thirty-four weeks, compared with more than three years for people who had no remaining symptoms.

Plus, common residual symptoms cause problems themselves. Fatigue, disorganization and low energy, insomnia, poor concentration, social avoidance, and cognitive symptoms such as negative thinking can make it difficult to keep a job or to function as a parent. Clearly, residual symptoms can have a major negative impact on one's quality of life.

How do you know if your depression has gone into remission? The best way is by using rating scales. Some, such as the Hamilton Depression Rating Scale (HDRS) and the Montgomery Asberg Depression Rating Scale (MADRS), are filled out by your doctor and take perhaps ten to fifteen minutes to complete; others such as the Beck Depression Inventory (BDI) or the Quick Inventory of Depressive Symptomatology (QIDS) are filled out by patients, and take from five to ten minutes to complete. Each scale has a different score to indicate whether remission has been achieved: for instance a score of 7 points or less on the HDRS-17 for three weeks or more.

If only about one in three people go into remission with any one medication treatment (and probably the same proportion applies to cognitive-behavioral psychotherapy), what can you do to get into remission? And, if you are in remission, how can you *stay* in remission? These are key questions, the importance of which is being realized within the New Neuropsychiatry. We are just starting to collect data to answer these questions. It is important to recognize that all depression and anxiety disorders do not result from any single cause; rather they are heterogeneous and spring from a variety of causes. Therefore, it is unlikely that any one solution will apply to everyone.

However, some things already appear certain. For one thing, if you have entered remission it is important to stay on your medication or to continue your therapy, and not to stop abruptly. The thought, "Now I'm better so I don't need this medicine anymore," is understandable and natural at this point and also dangerous, because this is the time you need the medicine the most! The mantra of "an adequate dose of medicine for an adequate time" applies even more strongly to the phase of remission as it does to the initial phase of trying to get a treatment response. If there are side effects, it is important to deal with them, because they are a major reason that people go off medications or stop treatment.

What about if your depression or anxiety disorder has responded to treatment but has not yet gone into remission? New Neuropsychiatry research such as Sequenced Treatment Alternatives to Relieve Depression, or STAR*D, has provided some information about this. In STAR*D, as discussed in Chapter 3, about 33 percent of people who had depression went into remission after the first trial of medication. Those who had not done so were then treated with a second medicine, after which about 50 percent had gone into remission, and then a third, and a fourth. With each successive medication trial (either a single medicine or a combination of two or more medicines), more of the people had gone into remission. And this is what is done in clinical practice—a series of treatment trials one after another with the overall goal of first achieving response and then moving toward remission.

This is standard New Neuropsychiatry practice: if the medicine doesn't work one has several choices. One can wait, hoping that it will eventually kick in; one can increase the dose; or "augment," that is, add a second medication; or switch to a different medicine. Not to mention, one can add psychotherapy, switch from medicine to psychotherapy, or add other activities like exercise, relaxation training, light therapy, and so on (see Chapter 7 for more detail about treatment-resistant depression).

The overall point, though, is that remission is key.

Frodl concludes the report of his MRI study by stating, "It is likely that an early start of treatment with antidepressants and psychotherapy may prevent neuroplastic changes that, in turn, worsen the clinical course," in other words, treating depression early can keep your brain from getting worse.

Given that nonremission of depression leads to so much suffering, I believe that it is worth adding, it is essential to try to get depression into *remission* as soon as possible, with the goal of interrupting the toxic effects of stress on the brain.

A New Beginning

In our exploration of the New Neuropsychiatry, we have seen that it doesn't really matter *how* you bring a disorder under control; what matters is that somehow you get there. Medication alone, therapy alone, combined treatment—or unconventional approaches—any which way you can. Most important is that you find a way to get better, to get your brain out of the high-stress disordered state—to turn response into remission. And then to work to keep it there, to maintain and extend your gains. This process, which essentially involves remodeling your brain, requires your active involvement to consolidate and extend these improvements. Then it is possible to move from "getting better" toward "getting well."

Take Alexandra O'Connor. Fifty-four years old, having had an eating disorder for more than thirty years and having seen countless therapists, Alexandra finally got her symptoms under control by an unconventional route. She quit therapy and found a psychiatrist from whom she got a combination of two medications: Zoloft (an SSRI) and topiramate (an anticonvulsant with anti-anxiety and appetite-suppressing properties). She began to read about eating disorders—voraciously, you might say: to the point that she was photocopying medical articles and surfing the Web, downloading abstracts off PubMed, and bringing home stacks of books from the bookstore. Eventually, she became a self-taught expert on eating disorders. She became involved with Weight Watchers—a fine program in itself but not geared to the treatment of bulimia. Initially, Alexandra attended regular meetings in a local shopping center, and then she switched to using their online Web-based weight control program, Weight Watchers Online, which she accessed from work at lunchtime.

The effects of this combined treatment approach, however improvised and unconventional, were dramatic. Alexandra's mood lifted, thanks to the SSRI; her fears and phobias faded away; she lost twenty-eight pounds (the topiramate helped here); and, most important (and this was where Weight Watchers helped), she was no longer obsessed with food. No longer was her mind preoccupied with carbohydrate cravings or overwhelmed by urges to binge and purge or by regret and self-hatred from having succumbed to her hunger. For the first time in adulthood, Alexandra was essentially symptom-free. It was a struggle, but she was able to get her disorder to go into, and to stay in, remission.

From this vantage point, Alexandra O'Connor was able to look over her life—over decades of affliction. Even a year after going into remission, she was still coming to terms with how pervasive and limiting her disorder had been, affecting all areas of her life.

Because of her many-decade, obsessive focus on body weight, her continual worries about "how fat I was," Alexandra had long avoided parties and other social situations. Fearful of failure and of looking foolish, she avoided taking risks. Consequently, she had dropped out of college before getting her BA and worked as an office assistant when most of her friends were pursuing careers in business or the professions.

Entering a prolonged and long-yearned-for remission, Alexandra began to see herself anew. The apparent "givens" of her personality were not as fixed or immutable as she had always believed. Even months and years later, she would arrive at new realizations: how she could travel without crippling anxiety, how she could do "good things for myself" without paying the price afterward of stomach cramps, headaches, and nausea. And how fear and obsessions did not have to dominate her life.

Defining "Better"

One striking thing about the New Neuropsychiatry—in dramatic contrast to the Old Psychiatry—is how recovery can be achieved for many people who have mood and anxiety disorders. That is, people can get better in many areas of their lives, not just having relief from the most obvious symptoms of depression or anxiety. This became clear after SSRIs and other new classes of medications were introduced in the late 1980s and early 1990s and people everywhere began to be able to decrease long-standing symptoms of depression and anxiety.

Psychiatrists soon began observing the results of a massive society-wide natural experiment in the treatment of mood and anxiety disorders. It was similar in some ways to what neurologist Oliver Sacks described in his book *Awakenings,* about the introduction of L-dopa in the treatment of Parkinson disease in the early 1960s. Because the new SSRI medications were relatively easily tolerated, because they were generally nontoxic, and because they helped with a wide variety of disabling symptoms, millions of people took them, and we—professionals and family and friends and the people themselves—saw for the first time the often fascinating process of recovery from these disorders. In a sense, this has given us the opportunity to explore the phases and psychological experiences of recovery, as I will be doing in the second half of this book.

It is important to be clear that here I am moving from the more solid ground of our understanding of disorder (its biology, and the response to treatment) to a more exploratory view of the process of recovery. I am trying to describe something that appears to be increasingly common, but for which we still do not have a clear language or good explanations.

Furthermore, we are just starting to become able to link these changes (in moods, feelings, relationships, and social functioning) with changes that seem to occur in the brain's structure and functioning, even then to speculate about the activation and inactivation of specific genes.

For the New Neuropsychiatry, response is thus essential, but not adequate (for more information, see the sidebar above on the definitions of response, remission, and recovery). Remission is our goal. And it is not the final goal, either. The final goal is recovery. The bar is now set high. Obviously, New Neuropsychiatrists do not always achieve these goals—but at least the goals are clearly in view!

Back to Life?

Alexandra found that remission, however welcome, was somewhat disconcerting. You might also find it disconcerting, especially if you have had a disorder for many years. Perhaps you have been spending much of your energy battling demons, which now—suddenly—begin to fade. Then, who are you? Without your demons, psychic or real, what do you battle against? Achieving and staying in remission can be challenge enough. Then, once attained, the complexity of life comes bursting in. Unfinished business, goals so far unachieved, relationships that need work—all may return full force.

Remission means coming back to life. And life can give you a few slaps in the face. Especially if—like many people—you have had serious symptoms for many years, and have been preoccupied with mere survival. At this point you might well awaken to the realization that you do not *have* much of a life.

Important tasks such as growing independent from your parents or developing close friends, not to mention advancing your career, may have been all but impossible when disorder ruled your life. Now that your symptoms are fading away, the pressure of undone tasks may be intense.

Some people, overwhelmed by remission, stop treatment abruptly, preferring to crawl back into their cave. Toby had that experience. A young man with OCD, Toby, had spent six or more hours per day involved with his rituals. Hand-washing, counting objects, checking cabinets and drawers in his apartment—such activities involved most of his waking hours. Toby had an excellent response to Luvox, an SSRI medication, combined with behavioral therapy. His doctor rated his symptoms on the Y-BOCS (the Yale-Brown Obsessive-Compulsive Scale), the most commonly used rating scaled for OCD. His Y-BOCS score plummeted, and he seemed to be on the verge of a major treatment success. Toby was suddenly free: able to look for (and find) a job, to start dating, and even to fall in love.

After three or four months taking medication, his symptoms firmly in remission, Toby announced that he had had enough. He was going off the pills—he didn't need them.

"Why?" asked his baffled doctor. "You're definitely going to get worse again."

She argued with him, tried every sort of psychotherapeutic technique, but Toby had made up his mind. And he fell back into his rituals, his hermetic and ordered life.

Other people, paradoxically, can have too *few* symptoms, thanks to New Neuropsychiatry treatments. Kevin, a 27-year-old man, had profound relief of severe and disabling anxiety symptoms with Paxil, an antidepressant, so much so that he spent all his time sitting around his apartment building's swimming pool, doing absolutely nothing. Kevin was far too mellow. Although he was rapidly depleting his savings and had made no progress in finding work, he felt virtually no anxiety. His doctor quickly decreased Kevin's medicine dose to bring back some anxiety. Obviously anxiety is not necessarily bad, the human anxiety circuits having evolved over millions of years as an alerting and mobilizing system. Too little anxiety, too little fear, even too little depression may be risky. New Neuropsychiatry medications may at times be all too effective! So the New Neuropsychiatrist strives to find the right balance, trying to help you travel from the initial days and weeks of symptomlessness toward your goal of recovery.

After the Storm

If you sustain a complex leg fracture, you obviously don't just hop out of bed once the bone has been set. You need physical therapy. Likewise, if you survive a serious heart attack, your doctor starts you in cardiac rehabilitation even before you are discharged from the coronary care unit. Rehab is central to the "medical model." Such programs include exercises to strengthen your muscles and increase range of motion, to improve endurance, as well as counseling to change your diet and smoking and other habits.

In the New Neuropsychiatry, a similar rehabilitation process should begin as you start to achieve remission of your psychiatric disorder. It can help to solidify your recovery. In psychiatry the tools we use may be different than those used in orthopedics or cardiology—they include, both mental (and increasingly) physical exercise. The rehabilitation is both of your life and of your brain. (For more on exercise and the brain, see Chapter 6.)

Psychiatric disorder, especially when it has been long-lasting, often leaves a trail of damage in its wake. It is akin to the wreckage left by a twister moving through a Midwestern town. After the storm, amid uprooted trees, roofs blown off, shattered glass, flipped cars, trash-strewn streets, there is often a scene of eerie calm, in which the extent of damage is all too clear. No wonder Toby ran back to his counting and checking! And no wonder Kevin preferred to sit beside his pool in a state of hazy well-being, rather than starting to work on solving life problems.

New Neuropsychiatrists do everything they can at this point to try to help you clear the wreckage from your life. In the words of University of Pittsburgh researcher Michael Thase, MD, at this stage, psychotherapy should focus on here-and-now solutions to remaining problems: "reducing social anxiety, improving assertiveness, forming and/or sustaining satisfying romantic attachments, improving persistence, and enhancing adaptive problem-solving solutions."

Indeed, in the New Neuropsychiatry, the fading away of a disorder is not the end of treatment—it is a beginning. For people who have suffered for decades, it is often a new beginning of a life that may no longer have clearly defined limitations.

Mark Stops Checking and Starts Living

Such was the case with Mark Maple.

Early on, after only about a month of medication, Mark had noted some unexpected changes. These went beyond the most obvious relief of his anxieties about Susan's whereabouts.

"You know, it's interesting," he said. "I actually feel *relaxed* these days. For at least fifteen years, I've never felt calm for any more than a few minutes."

"How does that affect you?" I asked.

"Well, I can look past myself. I feel content, I feel somehow this sense of composure . . ." He paused.

"And what?"

"I realize how my daily life has always been shrouded in anxiety and worry."

"So you weren't just worrying about Susan?"

"That was the worst of it. What I see now is that *every* interaction with people set off anxiety. I was always trying to avoid stirring things up."

Throughout his legal career, Mark had found certain tasks excruciatingly difficult. Giving clients bad news, assigning tough projects to junior lawyers, filing court papers on complex cases—all of these things had caused storms of agitation and fear. As a result, he often procrastinated for weeks or months, even neglecting to submit legal paperwork until too late. Sometimes this had even affected the outcome of cases.

"Now that my anxiety is lessened, these things are much easier. I feel more confident. I can give people bad news without worrying that I'm going to have a panic attack. I can supervise a junior associate without breaking into a sweat." Mark had begun to go back to his most difficult cases, some of which were seriously overdue.

This transformation extended to the home front too. About three months into treatment, Mark realized that he could discuss intimate issues with Susan without panicking. He could even raise things about her that bothered him— her occasional suspiciousness, her tendency to unfairly attack him when she was upset.

"We can actually talk about the future of our relationship," he told me. "Now that I'm not always worrying about her safety every minute, I can think about how I want things to be between us in the long-term."

This was a major change, unprecedented in his recent life.

The Ripple Effect

Remission may mean a change not only in your life but also in the lives of those around you. On more than occasion a few months into treatment a patient will say, as Ahmad, a 46-year-old steamfitter, told me, "My wife thanks you."

"Why?" I will ask.

"Because she says I'm a different person."

Interesting. After all, Ahmad says that as far as *he* is concerned not much has changed. He's sleeping a little better, he's not dragging around as much, but that's it.

"So what does your wife notice?"

"That I'm not impossible to be around. That she actually enjoys being with me."

He explains: she's glad he was not hiding so much down at the shop or in front of the TV, that he is not always irritable and agitated, that he no longer punches walls. He adds: "The kids are saying it, too. They can talk to me, they're not afraid of me."

Since his teenage years, Ahmad had been volatile, irritable, often rageful. In his working-class family, there were no words to quell such feelings, just six-packs of Bud and bar fights on Saturday nights. He punched walls and occasionally people. In recent years, in the clutches of depression, he had been grinding downward, more and more set into these patterns. And now, something strange was happening. He was beginning to feel new emotions—tenderness, sadness, empathy, regret.

"Like I'm finding new rooms in the house that I could never go into before," he said. "It's weird feeling that."

"So what do you want to do about it?" I asked.

Ahmad laughed. "I don't know!" he says. "Nothin', I guess. But now . . . now I gotta be a better person. I guess I can't be such a jerk. That'll be a job and a half."

Understandably, depressed people are often highly self-focused, preoccupied with their own anguish and suffering. As they improve, they commonly can look outwardly again and can connect empathically with others. In recent years, we have learned about the mirror neurons in the inferior frontal and inferior parietal areas of the brain, cells that activate when we observe the emotional responses of other people. Perhaps, now that his depression was in remission, Ahmed's mirror neurons were starting to function again!

The Brain Begins to Heal

These kinds of change arise frequently in the New Neuropsychiatry. As remission sets in, as the initial stage of day-to-day relief is replaced by a new stability, it can be as if a person's very self has changed.

What is happening in the brain at this point?

Research suggests that remission is accompanied by changes in the brain. For one thing, the quieting down of stress response systems. The "fear circuits" have been dampened. The amygdala, the almond-shaped fear and anxiety center tucked away near the base of your brain—one on each hemisphere—is no longer on overdrive. Consequently, the panic sirens no longer are sounding at odd hours; you are not always braced for disaster. From the hypothalamus up in your brain, signals go to the pituitary and then on to your hormonal system through the adrenal glands, renormalizing your body's patterns of sleep and appetite and physical activation. Your body is no longer wired for fight-or-flight responses—no longer do your muscles tremble incessantly and your pulses pound.

As remission settles in, it seems that other areas of your brain begin to awaken. In particular, the hippocampus, the seahorse-shaped center of episodic memory that curls beside the amygdala and the dorsolateral prefrontal cortex, which is central to working memory. In the throes of depression or in the midst of panic attacks, your mind often blanks out—you can't concentrate or keep important thoughts uppermost in your mind. Why? Because disorder impairs the functioning of these parts of the brain! Now, your mind no longer fades into nothingness. No longer are your day-to-day thoughts overwritten with obsessive worries. Again you have enough "working memory" to get the job done—your prefrontal cortex is back online. You can read the *Times* again. You can finish an entire novel. You can prepare all those overdue annual reports at work. Finally, you can use your brain to do more than survive from one day to the next.

On a microscopic level, the brain cells themselves appear to be starting to recover from the damage of acute stress. The shrunken, stressed-out neurons in your medial prefrontal cortex (the thinking and planning part of your brain), have been bathed in high levels of stress hormones for months or years. Now, a surge of brain-derived neurotrophic factor, a protein that helps neurons and other components of the central nervous system, neurons, and synapses start to plump up again, to "re-arborize" and make new connections to neighboring cells. New cells grow in the dentate gyrus of your hippocampus. Other baby

What Do We Mean by Plasticity of the Brain?

There are various definitions of plasticity of the brain, or neuroplasticity. *Mosby's Medical Dictionary* defines it as "the capacity of the nervous system for adaptation or regeneration after trauma," and indeed much research has been done on the ability of the brain to regenerate after injury or stroke. *Merriam-Webster's* dictionary defines plasticity as "the capacity for continuous alteration of the neural pathways and synapses of the living brain and nervous system in response to experience or injury that involves the formation of new pathways and synapses and the elimination or modification of existing ones." And according to Wikipedia, neuroplasticity "is the changing of neurons, the organization of their networks, and their function via new experiences."

The human brain undergoes major phases of development both before and after birth. Before birth, brain cells grow and develop on a massive level, making interconnected branches and forming synapses, or connections between neurons, and they migrate within from one level to another within the brain and develop specialized structure and functions. After birth, the brain continues to grow and mature—as the child reaches milestones such as the development of reasoning and language about age 6, experiences a deepening of emotional experiences in early teenage years, then followed by maturing of the prefrontal cortex in later adolescence, allowing for more abstract thinking, planning, and self-control. (See www.nytimes.com /interactive/2008/09/15/health/20080915-brain-development.html for a graphic demonstrating how different areas of the brain develop between ages 4 and 21.)

The brain also undergoes a process of plasticity after injury or trauma. After a stroke, parts of the brain are destroyed, and over time some functions are able to be reestablished in other locations of the brain, reflecting various types of brain plasticity, including shifting of activation from the damaged area to similar, uninjured areas.

In our discussions of mood and anxiety disorders, we are interested in brain changes that may have occurred in early life, as a result of stress, trauma, and loss, as well as in brain changes that may be a result of head trauma or other brain injury. In terms of psychiatric treatment, though, we are mostly interested in the degree to which the adult brain is capable of plasticity. Until recently, most neuroscientists were convinced that the adult brain had lost all but the most minimal levels of plasticity. And indeed, in comparison to the massive levels of brain cell growth before birth, and the widespread "pruning" of brain cell connections that starts in childhood and continues through teenage years, the plasticity of the adult brain appears to be much more limited. Learning a new language, for instance, is easiest in early childhood and more difficult in adult years.

Nevertheless, adult brain plasticity is essential to human society. Recent research has demonstrated how extensive a level of plasticity can occur in the adult brain as a result of all kinds of behavior, learning, and treatment. Medical students, for instance, have measureable growth in gray matter increased significantly in the posterior and lateral parietal cortex as they learn huge amounts of information about biology, chemistry, and anatomy. Beyond learning, though, it has become clear that plasticity is important both as a cause of psychiatric disorders and as an essential part of their treatment. In a sense, the overactive circuits of depression and anxiety disorders such as obsessive-compulsive disorder represent a type of negative neuroplasticity, in which dysfunctional brain circuits have been strengthened. The treatments of these disorders usually involve trying to stop these destructive processes and even to begin to reverse them by evoking a more healthy form of plasticity. As researcher Paul J. Carlson put it: "We propose that disturbances in neural plasticity and cellular resilience are critical factors in precipitating and perpetuating disruption of the affective circuits. . . . Furthermore, we hypothesize that novel treatment interventions that directly address impairments in plasticity and cellular resilience will both lead to improved clinical outcomes and also show normalization of activity in these circuits." In other words, research bears out the theme of this book: disorder can cause changes to the brain and to the circuits—such as the amygdala—that regulate it. Increasingly, our treatments will attempt to normalize "activity in these circuits," helping the brain to reregulate itself.

neurons, formed in the fluid-filled ventricles of your brain, begin migrating to your prefrontal cortex. Gradually your brain begins a process of healthy reconnection.

And yet, it is worth pointing out, as remission settles in, your brain most likely is different now than it was before your illness. Like it or not, it is—and you are—forever changed by the experience of having gone through the high-stress state of disorder. Research on posttraumatic stress disorder has shown that disorder often irreversibly changes the brain in some ways: trauma leaves some permanent marks. Some genes are irreversibly affected by "meth-ylation"—by the attachment of carbon and hydrogen atoms. One part of the brain, the rostral cingulate, remains hyperactive even when a person is well, perhaps to keep the disorder at bay. And even in people whose depression has remitted, the amygdala may continue to shrink over time.

Nonetheless, as the days of remission turn into weeks and months, even if your symptoms flare up from time to time, this much is clear: once again, all systems are "go."

A New View of Familiar Places

As you enter remission, and you start to come back to your life again, the question is, What do you see? Is your life there waiting for you, untouched, basically unchanged from before disorder hit? Can you just pick up where you left off a few months back at work, and with your family? Or have things irretrievably altered?

Perhaps it is like coming back to your beach house after a hard winter—arriving to find shutters askew, exploded cans in the cupboards, water stains under the eaves, mouse droppings everywhere—a matter of inconveniences that a few weeks of hard work can set right. Or do you awaken to utter wreck-age, to catastrophe? Have you been away from your life for months, even years? Have you been out of touch for so long that the roof has caved in and the stairs have fallen through—or even that the house has burned down and must be rebuilt from the foundation?

Disorder is so variable that any of the above scenarios are possible. The dam-age you've endured may depend on how long disorder has ruled, the number of times it has hit, or perhaps how severe it was. Recovery may be as simple as picking up where you left off—or it may involve years of costly repairs.

In any case, things are likely to be fragile, especially in the first several months. You may fear—rightly or wrongly—that your gains will vanish. You may have to work hard to maintain and enhance them. (This makes sense: that new brain circuits would be fragile, easily disrupted, and require would continual reinforcement and strengthening.) So, you continue your medicine, your individual or couples or family therapy, your exercise regime, whatever has worked to help you out of disorder. Yet, even in the first few weeks, it may be possible for you to look at your life again beyond the tight constraints of day-to-day survival. You can gaze across the landscape of your life once more. The fact that you can dare to dream again may in itself reflect a process of healing.

Cindy Looks over Her Life

It was remarkable to see Cindy Prince as she settled into a sustained state of remission from bipolar II disorder. True, it was long in coming. In the early months, there were weeks when she felt good, virtually back to normal; the next she would feel restlessness and agitation, intimations of despair, and would even worry that she'd never be able to care for her kids. We adjusted the medicines, decreasing the lithium to 1200 mg/day, and the Zoloft to 50 mg/day.

And finally the good feelings took hold. The pudding had set, as it were. About four months into remission, Cindy felt good on a consistent basis. Sleep was again restful for her (though with three young children there was never enough of it), her appetite was back, and all the "vegetative" signs were no more. She didn't have hypomanic or agitated feelings either. More than that, she was enjoying playing with the twins and had an admirable degree of reserves to deal with Zach's antics.

One weekend, I ran into her on the street on the Upper West Side of Manhattan—pushing a double stroller with the twins neatly bundled up. It was a bright and windy early spring day, and Cindy had driven into the city to meet a friend at the Natural History Museum. We chatted for a few moments and then she went on her way, giving me a warm smile.

"You know," she said at our next session, a few weeks later, another blustery afternoon. "Now that I'm better, I see everything in my life so differently."

"How?"

"Well, it all revolves around what you said. How long I've been cycling between being depressed and being hypomanic. When I first saw you I thought I had a postpartum depression since having the twins. But now . . . now I realize that you were right, it did start much earlier, at least three years ago. And my mood cycling probably started a long time before that, maybe when I was a teenager."

"And that changes things?"

"For one thing, it explains why my marriage has gotten so screwed up."

Following Zach's birth three-and-a-half years ago, she was continually tense and agitated. Her moods cycled, she cried over nothing. She and Roland fought constantly. And she had entirely cut off relationships with her friends. "It almost would have been better if it was just a little bit worse, because then I would have had to get treatment. Instead . . ."

We sat in silence as she collected her thoughts.

"So my marriage has almost been ruined. I feel like I've done terrible things to Zach by not being there for him. And I don't know—I hope it's not too late!"

It was painful, this new perspective. But my sense was that she now felt strong enough to start addressing these issues.

Things were difficult right now between Cindy and Roland. They fought, they argued, there were times he stormed out of the house. Perhaps Roland was no longer holding back anymore, now that he sensed she could take it.

"The thing is," Cindy said, "I *know* he's right about a lot of things. But now I feel that maybe I can deal with this. I'm not blown away by what he's saying, like I would have been before."

They had stared seeing Will in couples therapy.

"I'm glad you're doing that," I said.

It seemed likely to me that bipolar II disorder had affected Cindy's PhD program, too. After Zach's birth she had gone on leave from the university. She had abandoned her dissertation and gradually resigned herself to a career as a lab assistant. She called it "going onto the Mommy track," but I had my doubts. While her classmates, PhDs in hand, had landed jobs as researchers and professors (including several female friends with kids), Cindy had been stuck processing lab samples. Not a terrible existence, but a long way down from her previous aspirations.

"Some days," continued Cindy, "I feel like I could even go back to work on my dissertation."

We were on the same wavelength. As Cindy Prince looked over her life from this new vantage-point of remission, her very past had been transformed. What about her future, I wondered, could it be changed as well?

We were going through an odd, and yet common, New Neuropsychiatry moment. Basically, Cindy Prince was no longer cycling between hypomania and depression. And yet, that spring day, along with her optimism and energy there was also an unmistakable feeling of loss. I realized, as Cindy continued to speak, that she was grieving for lost opportunities.

For, now that she felt better, Cindy truly understood what disorder had cost her. Paradoxically, being better, she was almost obliged to grieve these losses. Mark Maple was to experience something similar—though for him, disorder had lasted fifteen years. And Allen Johnson as well: panic disorder, particularly how he found it nearly impossible to travel, had nearly ended his career. For all of them, remission led to a need to come to terms with years of missed opportunities, to grieve their losses—and to figure out what could be done to make up for lost time. Long ago, Sigmund Freud underlined the distinction between depression and grief, between mourning and melancholy. Perhaps in these patients, who "can't" be biologically depressed but who are still grieving, we see this distinction played out.

Another Marriage

Turning response into remission means starting to get your life back. And getting your life back means repairing the damage in your work life and in your family.

Alexandra O'Connor had a lot of work to do. Her combined treatment of medication, self-education, and Weight Watchers led to a solid state of remission. After her eating disorder had been in remission for several months, however, unanticipated issues began to arise. She began to observe how marginalized she was in her family, in particular with the children from her husband's first marriage. At family events—such as christenings and first communions—she was always shunted to the side. During the many years when food obsessions continually occupied her mind, Alexandra had hardly noticed these slights, but now they bothered her.

Alexandra made an appointment with her previous therapist. There, Alexandra worked on being more assertive with her husband so she wouldn't be overlooked. When her stepdaughter began making wedding plans, Alexandra spoke up for the first time, asking to be included in the wedding ceremony. Much to her surprise, her stepdaughter was grateful for her increased involvement—and an always chilly relationship began to become warm, even close.

Challenges during Remission

A New Neuropsychiatry paradox, which Alexandra and Cindy viscerally understood: just because your disorder is better doesn't mean that your relationships will immediately improve. Once your symptoms respond, relationships may get worse before they get better. This is no surprise to New Neuropsychiatrists. Some research studies show that interpersonal problems actually *increase* after symptoms improve! Now that you're not depressed, you may discover that your wife is angry, even enraged—that she has been feeling ignored and mistreated for years. Your kids may act out more now that they have the sense that you can take it, that you won't collapse if they say what's on their mind. If you have a habit of avoidance, you may be tempted to retreat from these problems that emerge early in remission, rather than to persevere and solve them.

But these crises may provide opportunities. The New Neuropsychiatry therapist thus has a crucial role here in helping you face these issues as they appear and to provide hope that there may be solutions out there—that things may indeed improve.

For Allen Johnson, it took a lot of therapy to move from remission toward recovery. It was wonderful to observe. Block by block, he retook Manhattan. After several months of cognitive therapy, Allen was able to travel to Midtown with relatively little anxiety, to venture to the Upper West Side, formerly forbidden territory. Even high buildings, once anathema, weren't daunting. Without SSRI medication, Allen had conquered panic disorder.

And yet, as one panic-free month after another passed, it became clear how much farther Allen had to go to truly recover.

Before panic disorder, Allen had been confident and adventurous, traveling through Asia and Europe to visit clients or to vacation. Now he found himself limited. True enough, he was able to travel more easily throughout Manhattan. But he still found daily activities unexpectedly difficult. While going into a local restaurant or hopping on the subway or even while dropping off DVDs at the local video store, anxiety would surge from nowhere. The panic patterns had spread far beyond traveling—they had infiltrated every area of his life. At his job, he struggled to keep his head above water. He had to brace himself to make presentations in front of large audiences, and he always had a sleepless night or two when leaving the metro area on business. Then there were larger concerns: here he was, 36 years old and unmarried. Panic feelings had surged whenever he got past a certain level of involvement with women. Would he ever get married? Would he ever have children?

Allen even began longingly mentioning the possibility of starting medication as a solution to these fears.

I reminded Allen that he had made so much progress without medication: and that in fact, medicine wouldn't do much for the remaining issues—they were things that were much more likely to be worked out in psychotherapy.

What were Allen's remaining issues at this point?

For one thing, his habitual negative thoughts would emerge, unbidden—telling him that he would fail, that things wouldn't work out. He felt continually "on the edge of an abyss." On a date, critical thoughts would bubble into his head: she was overweight, too old, not amusing enough, not a good match for him. Or, if he *was* interested, informing him that he could never have a successful relationship. These were hardly a surprise—we had talked a lot about these types of thoughts before.

A second issue was what psychiatric researcher Dr. Robert Cloninger, of Washington University in St. Louis, called "harm avoidance," which includes tendencies to worry excessively, and to be pessimistic, easily fatigued, and shy with strangers. Allen was reluctant to push himself, to take risks again, and to face uncertainty. This involved both his personal life, where he had gotten into the habit of avoiding social engagements, parties, and weddings, and his work life, where he found any excuse to avoid going out on work-related outings, trips, and golf getaways.

Third (and most subtle in some ways), was Allen's continuing tendency to see things as black-or-white. This too extended well past his specific problems with traveling. In all areas of his life, either he was a big hit or a total failure. If he approached a potential client and didn't get the business, it was a "strike out" in his eyes. It took an effort to see that a losing pitch for new business might nevertheless be valuable—as a way to practice skills, to make more contacts, or to improve understanding of the marketplace. Regardless of whether he "won" or "lost."

These kinds of thought patterns, more common than not in people who have panic disorder, probably result from the brain changes of chronic stress. With chronic stress, there is shrinkage of areas CA_1 and CA_3 in the hippocampus, which can lead to filtering out of many of the details that normally differentiate experiences and can lead to black-and-white thinking.

All three things were part of the penumbra, or surrounding areas, of Allen's disorder. The disorder had broken out in the most obvious form as panic attacks when he traveled in the city—but in truth the panic was an outcome. An outcome of lifelong habits of how he thought about himself and the world, and how he reacted to his thoughts, and how he acted on his experiences. For Allen turning remission into recovery required great effort at this point. And at the same time, it was exciting for him.

Then there was a fourth issue, the issue of intimacy. By his mid-30s, Allen had become set in his ways. Focusing on a woman's age or physical flaws was a cover for his rusty people skills. It was hard to negotiate intimacy, to tolerate being close to a woman. With prodding, he began dating—and he had many promising first dates, but he was rarely encouraged to call for a second or third date. It took an effort to motivate himself to go back to work on getting into and staying in relationships. For most of Allen's life this had been second nature, something he "just did." Now he had to relearn these seemingly elementary things, the way you have to relearn how to throw a baseball after breaking your arm.

To use New Neuropsychiatry terms, in addressing these issues, we were using what has been called a "top-down" attack on his panic related symptoms—we were working to modify his thought processes, his affective biases (the way his emotions shaped his thinking) and his maladaptive information processing (how the way he interpreted events affected how he felt about them). We were hoping to make changes in the longer fear circuit. We didn't want to change only his amygdala (the brainstem part of the fear circuit) but also the other parts of the brain that regulate responses to fear, which start at the orbital, medial frontal, prefrontal, and cingulate areas of the cortex and then connect to the hippocampus. With this type of approach, we expected that his cognitive symptoms would improve first, before the overactive amygdala-hippocampus cycle could be reversed.

From Remission toward Recovery

As mentioned in Chapter 4, psychotherapy in the Old Psychiatry (at least in the movies) often focused on "letting your feelings out," on cathartic moments of rage or sobbing grief. In contrast, therapies in New Neuropsychiatry often focus on becoming *less* emotionally reactive—on finding alternatives to "emotional reasoning."

While the Old Psychiatry often proceeded with the goal of helping you "get in touch with your feelings," New Neuropsychiatry therapy often works to allow you to have a break from your feelings—to step back, to feel *less* intensely. Mostly, the feelings that are muted are extreme and unpleasant ones coming from the lower brain: anxiety, compulsive urges, despair, rage, and the like. The New Neuropsychiatry therapist also tries to diminish your need to react immediately to these feelings, whether by action or withdrawal. Though the SSRI medications and cognitive therapy work by different means, both have this type of effect. Both have the goal of engaging other parts of your brain—to have you think about and feel other things about situations—before taking action.

In a sense, during disorder, symptoms have largely replaced feelings or emotions. The goal now in New Neuropsychiatry therapies is to decrease symptoms and to allow the emergence of more subtle feelings—to make connections to more varied emotions, in particular, more positive feelings. This can be seen as part of a brain reconnection process. Beyond therapy, useful things include mindfulness, meditation, and talking or writing about one's feelings—and a lot of exposure to other people, to social interactions.

At the same time as it focuses on controlling symptoms, the New Neuropsychiatry tries to help you to increasingly *use* these positive feelings—of well-being and confidence and serenity—so that you can start to repair the damage to your life. In the brain, you could say that the dopamine-based reward systems have been activated, and we want to strengthen and reinforce them as remission settles in. In particular, it is important to start to take reasonable risks again, to try new things. Especially with activities that will be pleasurable, such as sports, socializing, or creative pursuits. So, in contrast to the intense analysis of dreams and early memories of the Old Psychiatry, New Neuropsychiatry treatments often provide a life raft of calm in a storm of feelings.

"Now I can see what I'm doing to myself," said Britta, a 53-year-old real estate agent, a few months after she responded to medication. "Since I've started to feel better, it's like I can step to the side and get a different perspective—I don't have to react right away."

Tony, a Web programmer, told me, "I can see how other people must feel in this situation. I have a kind of perspective on my emotions that I never had before."

And Ivan told me, once he was several months into remission, "I find myself doing the same damn things, just by habit, but I don't *have* to do them anymore."

Changing Thought and Behavior Patterns

Each of these people, in a sense, is describing how a person's disorder affected his or her established patterns of thought and behavior, what could also be called personality.

Fascinating New Neuropsychiatry research suggests how this interaction between disorder and personality may occur. A brief episode of depression, a few months of panic, probably won't do much damage to your habitual thought and behavior patterns, your way of living in the world and relating to other people. Once the symptoms fade, you'll probably bounce back and be pretty much the same person as before you were panicky or depressed. But if depression returns for numerous episodes or anxiety symptoms persist for year after year, your personality is likely to become warped. In the throes of disorder, Mark had become dependent and clinging—and yet, at the same time, emotionally distant and at times even cruel. Cindy had become irritable and insecure, fearful and easily overwhelmed, and utterly uninterested in intimacy, sexual or otherwise. Allen had become incredibly self-absorbed and, as he later put it, "one of the great hypochondriacs of all time."

In brief (as we have seen in Allen's and Alexandra's cases), disorders can have warping effects on thought and behavior patterns, especially if they are recurrent or long-standing. Beyond the excessively negative thinking patterns we have discussed, these include

- Avoidance—including both avoiding relationships, whether platonic or romantic, and general fearfulness of bad outcomes and unwillingness to take normal risks of day-to-day life

- Excessive clinging and dependency in intimate relationships

- Compulsive and impulsive behavior, such as compulsive eating, gambling, sex, or drug use, perhaps resulting from efforts to make yourself feel better

- Irritability and highly reactive (even explosive) behavior

As Cindy and Allen and Mark and Ahmad all discovered in their own ways, when disorder began to recede, there was an opportunity to remake their "selves." Even making small changes in thought and behavior patterns could have a significant impact on the quality of their lives.

"When I was having panic attacks all the time, being afraid made a lot of sense," Allen told me. "That way, I could avoid situations that set off panic attacks. Being afraid all the time was essential to my survival."

"But now that you're in remission, it may be unnecessary."

"Definitely. Fearing the worst definitely stands in my way when I try to change my life. It puts me in a kind of straitjacket."

And thus, when you are in the state of early remission, it may be time to begin working on changing some of these traits.

Conquering Negative Thoughts

Months and years of depression often create a habit of discouragement, a visceral sense that things will always turn out badly. Negative thoughts bubble up from below, perhaps the subgenual prefrontal cortex, as will be discussed in Chapter 6. The best tools we have to fight these thoughts are from cognitive-behavioral therapy—using more positive thoughts to interrupt or replace the compelling negative ones, and replacing avoidance behaviors with reasonable risk-taking.

Herb, a young man whose depression had responded well to medication, nevertheless found himself easily overwhelmed by pessimism. Talking with his girlfriend, he would be convinced that their relationship would never go anywhere. What if they did marry? Then they'd be stuck together for life. Whenever he saw his parents, Herb realized how they had only a few more years to live (despite the fact that they were in their early 60s and in excellent health) and imagined how terrible it would be when they died. Herb wasn't exactly depressed anymore, yet he was still morose and disillusioned.

And then there was Marvin, a former executive whose wife pushed him to get treatment for depression after he spent the first year of retirement sitting at home in front of the television. Recovering from melancholy, he found a new passion for drawing, which he hadn't done since college days. He signed up for an art class and, liking that, soon was taking life drawing classes several days a week. He enjoyed putting chalk to paper, and his teachers praised his work. Marvin downplayed these experiences, though, throwing out most of his drawings because they were imperfect. However good a time he was having, negative thoughts would kick in and make him miserable.

Over the next several months, Allen Johnson worked with me in therapy to address his issues. He had always prided himself for having a lot of "insight"

Cognitive-Behavioral Therapy

Cognitive-behavioral therapy was invented in the 1950s and 1960s by Aaron
Beck and Albert Ellis. Its basic principle is that a person's thoughts about
an event shape their emotions about that event and their subsequent
behavior. By examining faulty thought patterns, people can free themselves
from cycles of unhealthy emotions and counterproductive behavior.

Much can be done to help people manage disorders and other
problems with medication, but medication alone does not erase all the
limitations that individuals face. In using cognitive-behavioral approaches
(sometimes along with medications, and at other times by themselves) the
New Neuropsychiatrist looks closely at cycles of situations and reactions,
often drawing a circle or a triangle like the one below. "From *A* to *B* to *C*," is
our mantra. Perhaps a dozen times a week we go through this simple and
yet powerful exercise.

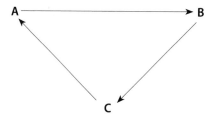

Let *A* be the situation or the activating event and *C* be the endpoint
or behavioral consequence. Between them is *B*, a person's beliefs and
thoughts about the event, including the automatic thoughts, images, and
feelings that come up in the split second before deciding to act.

Making people aware of the existence of *B* is a powerful way to deal with
many of the remaining obstacles to recovery and to help those who are
"better" to get unstuck psychologically and to move forward in life. And it
seems that this process actually helps us to strengthen healthy brain connections and to break the hold of the amygdala's fear system. Interestingly,
MRI studies have shown that cognitive-behavioral therapy has similar (but
not identical) effects on the brain to those seen with antidepressant use.

about his weaknesses. As a New Neuropsychiatrist, I saw that these thoughts were rarely actual insights but were intrusive, negative thoughts. Regardless of whether they contained some grain of truth, focusing on them didn't do him any good. When Allen reported hearing his stepfather's voice telling him how he would never succeed, I discouraged "free association" about his (fairly toxic) relationship with his stepfather. "Rather, you need to think about how to respond to these thoughts, to your stepfather's voice."

"I realize that he was wrong," he said. "I *know* I can do these things. Obviously I can succeed."

"So when these thoughts come into your head . . ."

"I guess I have to keep talking back to them."

Addressing Avoidance

Sometimes after the symptoms of disorder are gone, disordered habits remain. Ryan, a journalist, had recovered nicely from depression, thanks to a course of an SNRI medicine, Effexor XR. Yet, as he frequently complained, "I have no social life!" He was profoundly lonely, but, other than going back and forth to work, he rarely ventured out of his apartment. He avoided work-related socializing and always found a reason to rebuff well-meaning friends who tried to fix him up with women.

If you asked him why, Ryan would come up with a variety of excuses: he was too tired, he didn't feel like it, he forgot to put it in his calendar, and so on. If you probed further, he'd admit that he didn't think it was likely that anything would come out of the effort he put into socializing; if he met anyone, she wouldn't be right for him, the relationship would be doomed.

Like Allen, Ryan had a high level of harm avoidance. Many people who have mood and anxiety disorders have this trait: they tend to fear bad outcomes from taking normal day-to-day risks. Sending resumes around to look for a job, calling a woman you met to ask her out for dinner—these appear to be too risky and too doomed to failure to justify the effort involved. And so, like Herman Melville's character Bartelby the Scrivener, Ryan "would prefer not to" take the chance.

Only after months of therapy did Ryan even begin to contemplate changing his habits. He began looking at online personal ads at Match.com and sending in his responses. He hesitated to post his own profile, but after a fair amount of discussion, he had a photo taken, answered the questionnaires, and uploaded his files. His therapist gave him assignments to approach women for brief chats at the local Starbucks and to make a definitive effort to say "yes" when receiving social invitations. "Even when you feel like 'no.'" And then, regardless of how he felt, his assignment was "to show up"—at the party, dinner, whatever.

This was the beginning of a new phase in Ryan's life.

Improving Relationships

Sometimes avoidance is intertwined with dependency. Take the case of Marietta. A single 37-year-old clothing designer who had depression, Marietta finally agreed to try an SSRI medicine, despite her reluctance about taking pills. On 30 milligrams a day of the SSRI medicine citalopram (brand name Celexa), her mood lifted, she rarely felt weepy or low. She plunged into new assignments at work, and she cleaned up huge piles of bills and tax returns that had accumulated at home during her depressed years. Such cleanup is often a key sign that disorder is fading.

Marietta felt "great—but stuck." What particularly bothered her was her love life. During the course of her depression she had started a relationship with a "sort-of boyfriend" named Rick who sometimes called to ask her out, usually at the last minute, but more often didn't.

"Normally I would be sitting by the phone waiting for Rick's call, totally depressed. Or calling his voice mail and leaving one message after another, asking him to call when he gets back. Now I'm feeling great and I'm *still* sitting by the phone. And I'm wondering, 'What kind of idiot am I to be waiting here?'"

Marietta was a perfect example of being better but not well. Her depression was essentially gone—and yet she still instinctively lived like a depressed person. When sadness and anxiety overwhelmed her, it made sense to cling to Rick and to avoid venturing out to social events. She had been extremely fragile, her life governed by what psychiatrists call "rejection sensitivity," an overactive belief that you are going to be rejected by others, no matter who they are. A hundred times a day, her mood rose or fell depending on others. A friend's dour facial expression proved that "She hates me!" A client's pause on the phone before saying, "That's great!" would mean, "He knows I'm totally incompetent!" During Marietta's depression, such slights, real or imagined, wounded her to the soul. Consequently, she had cut off several friendships and had become deeply reliant on her few remaining contacts. Mostly this had meant Rick, her ever-suffering yet not very nice boyfriend.

This pattern clearly could be charted on the ABC cognitive therapy diagram, with A being the *activating* event, B being the *beliefs* about the event, and C being the *consequences* of those beliefs (for more on this, see the sidebar on cognitive-behavioral therapy above). On Friday nights, Marietta still waited by the phone for Rick to call (this being A, the activating event), and often enough he did not call, evoking her automatic thoughts and feelings (B, her beliefs about the event: "I'm no good, I'm going to be alone the rest of my life," which then set off feelings of panic, hopelessness, rejection, and despair (her emotional responses, C, or consequences).

I asked Marietta, "So he said that '*maybe*' he would call you on 'Thursday *or* Friday' to decide on going out?"

"That doesn't sound so good, does it?" she laughed.

Why did this happen? Because, one discovered, in exploring with her, the B in the equation overwhelmed her logic. Irrational as it might be, she was convinced that "unless I do everything to please Rick, I'll never get married." And marriage, in Marietta's magical equation, equaled Nirvana, a state in which all her problems would be solved and she could find happiness. These automatic thoughts, these irrationalities dating from her childhood years, existed in an otherwise capable, highly independent woman. This was clearly the result of an interaction between her life experiences and her brain's biology.

Now—in an SSRI-induced remission—Marietta was no longer so rejection sensitive. This was a seismic change in her life, in her "self." She was now able to step away from her desperate feelings of abandonment. Perhaps, I wondered, she was in a position to rewrite these circuits, to begin to rewire her brain.

"I'm so pathetic!" Marietta was in epiphany, laughing at herself. "Why do I let him do this to me? I feel like a total idiot waiting for his call! And I realize, I don't deserve this, I don't need to be sitting there anymore."

With my encouragement, Marietta read a book by British psychiatrist Anthony Storr, called *Solitude*. Storr advocates the "return to the self," the virtues of being solitary. He explores how solitude may be essential for creativity among artists and scientists and how it can have a restorative value for ordinary people as well, as it is "linked with self-discovery and self-realization;

with becoming aware of one's deepest needs, feelings, and impulses." At first Marietta found this perspective "bizarre." Then she got it. She practiced reading an entire novel from start to finish without picking up phone to call a friend. She learned how to calm herself using meditative techniques, to feel good without reassurance of having another person around. The key to her success was riding through these cycles without "doing" anything. ("Don't just do something," I would joke with her, "sit there!") Whereas in the past, Marietta had always felt an urgent need to act—including barraging Rick with one phone call after another. Eventually, she learned to *enjoy* being alone—to schedule times of solitude into her weekends. It was a surprise to her that she could become good at calming herself, that she could feel good without reaching out to another person.

In a better baseline mood state, without uncontrollable misery threatening her every moment, Marietta became vastly less clingy and dependent. It didn't take long for her to realize that the relationship with Rick ("that jerk," who, it turned out, had cheated on her with one of her friends) was beyond repair and that she tolerated him only because he would accept her. Feeling better, unafraid to be alone, Marietta was in a stronger position to choose whom she wanted to go out with, and to find a boyfriend who would treat her as she deserved. After four or five years of being single, Marietta met a much nicer and more interesting man named Victor; they started dating and eventually got married.

Thus, when combined with medicine, cognitive-behavioral techniques allowed Marietta to move toward recovery. More important, as for many people, it was only *after* her mood disorder was in remission that Marietta was able to work productively in psychotherapy. For once she could look beyond the immediate feeling states that had preoccupied her for years and could figure out what her life priorities—not just in intimate relationships, but in friendships and at work as well.

Before remission, as Marietta's psychotherapist, I was not much different from her boyfriend: a life raft to cling to in desperation. Now, as Marietta's therapist, I became, well, a *therapist*: someone to help her solve problems.

The cognitive-behavioral approaches I used in Marietta's therapy, although invented in the 1950s and 1960s, have been mainstream since the 1980s. What is new is our understanding of the dynamic nature of brain structure and function and the impact of combined treatment approaches in achieving and enhancing recovery from disorders—the idea that such techniques could be used to enhance your efforts to remodel your brain. New Neuropsychiatry treatment integrates approaches that go beyond medication, and even beyond CBT. Our goal is increasing healthy brain connectivity—integration of the brain and behavior in more adaptive and satisfying patterns, and inducing the brain's capacity for "plasticity"—for remodeling itself in the context of new experiences.

Marietta discovered a variety of things that helped in dealing with her long-standing tendency to have negative thoughts, excessive avoidance, and excessive dependency. She tried meditation, self-calming through mindfulness techniques, and deep-breathing exercises and got back into a program of regular physical exercise as well. Returning to the body, and the body's self-calming reflexes, was a key way for Marietta to exorcise the remnants of disorder.

She also found it useful to keep a journal about her experiences—in her case, a blog on the Web in which the identifying characteristics of her friends and the men she dated were slightly changed, but without removing her essential sense of knowing black humor. Keeping a journal is often particularly useful at this phase, because people who have had disorders often don't register (or recall) positive experiences very well. They often live in a depressive haze of nonspecificity and have difficulty recalling positive experiences. Even though Marietta had many good platonic friendships, she often felt entirely alone and that no one cared about her. She actually had to write them down and then read them later off the Web—along with the various comments and annotations that others added—to "remember" them, to feel that they were real (My guess is that this reflects problems in the vestiges of poor functioning of the subgenual prefrontal cortex, the brain center that integrates inputs from the emotional and thinking parts of the brain, an impairment that that only gradually improves over time).

"I can look back over a week when I feel nobody cares," Marietta told me, "and I see how many people have been in my life, and how many good things have happened."

All these are ways to conquer the remaining limitations of disorder. Obviously, all these things help to decrease stress, but to a New Neuropsychiatrist they may be helping in other ways as well. They may be

• Shutting off overactive brain areas and activating dormant ones

- Helping to decrease the secretion of certain stress-induced hormones in the brain and increase the production of brain healing proteins

- Helping to reregulate your bodily rhythms

- Helping your brain to rewrite its behavioral pathways, to draw new maps

- Even increasing neurogenesis and brain connectivity in key areas of the brain like the hippocampus and prefrontal cortex

Double Vision

It is fair to say that remission is not a given, especially in its early months. Often it is tenuous, even evanescent—probably as fragile as the new brain cell connections that you have developed. For a few weeks, you sleep like a baby, your anxiety is gone, and you burst with energy for new projects. And then you feel a twinge of the old pain—a bad night after a fight with your wife, a presentation at work that goes wrong, or rumors of impending layoffs.

At times, the old disorder beckons. Feelings of panic may surge through your body. You have a sleepless night or two, and before things settle down again, you wonder: is it all starting again?

Or perhaps things have been going so well that you started your remission for granted. You stopped medication for a few days, and then after nothing happened, you "forgot" it for a week. Or, under deadline pressure, you skipped your breathing and muscle relaxation exercises, you abandoned your discipline of exercise and meditation. Or, you decided that things were going so well you could "take a break" from therapy.

The thing is, if you're only a few months into treatment, you may have been lulled into a false sense of security. The disorder's circuits are still there, ready to be reactivated; and the circuits of recovery are fragile and can be easily disrupted. Yes, underneath your recovery, disorder lingers—at stressful times it may reach to assert its pernicious logic into your life.

And so it is early in remission that you are blessed with double vision. You can forget disorder at moments and look ahead to the future, and start to repair your lost life—you can even dream of life beyond mere recovery; you may hope to achieve new heights. And at the same time, you can recall all too vividly your sleepless nights, your days of inertness, your seemingly endless suffering.

The New Neuropsychiatrist is intimately familiar with this phase of treatment, with its perils and opportunities. As is clear from the examples above, a variety of specific approaches can help to move forward at this time, to increase the likelihood of successfully traversing what can seem to be a perilous swamp.

At this time of double vision, a dual approach is needed. First, it is essential to maintain and enhance remission, as Allen and Alexandra and Marietta certainly realized. But second, it is important to start dreaming again. Each of these is both simple and complex.

Daring to Dream Again

Over the first several months of remission, Cindy's therapy with Will evolved from immediate crisis management at the beginning to helping her to get better control of her symptoms. Helping her regulate her mood, to deal with intrusive thoughts, to calm herself, to find ways to empty her mind, to relax and meditate, to stop an endless cycle of critical self-critical ruminations. It seemed at times that there was an incredible synergy of medication with her cognitive therapy. Now that things had settled down within Cindy's mind, the focus had turned to her relationship with Roland.

Couples therapy was an incredible struggle for Cindy and Roland. It was crucial to see if they could rescue their marriage. Over time, the story became clear.

When Zach was a baby, and Cindy was struggling with her depression, Roland had had a relationship with Jill, a co-worker—a platonic relationship, a friendship in which at first "nothing had happened." Jill was "fun," "carefree and spontaneous"—perhaps a touch impulsive. She didn't brood or worry, as Cindy did. Roland had traveled on business with Jill for months before beginning a romance with her. Did he want to leave Cindy—and the kids—for Jill? He and Cindy had been together for so long, ever since college. They had shared so much life experience together. Yet so much bad feeling had emerged during the past three years—most recently, Cindy's pain and rage toward Roland's betrayal and infidelity. This on top of his long-standing resentment of her constant self-doubting, her irritability, her ever-present agitation, and her moods swinging between despair and euphoria. All this had surged out once it was clear that Cindy was stable enough to take it.

And now it seemed that she could take it. She and Roland came every week to their couples sessions with Will Eastman, struggling to see if they could put their marriage back together. It was intense, according to Will. Cindy's parents had divorced when she was a teenager and Roland's parents had separated when he was ten. Neither of them wanted their kids to grow up in a single-parent household. But that didn't seem to be a sufficient reason for them to stay together. The question was this: did they still love each other?

About a year after we'd first met, I was surprised when Cindy came for her medication appointment and brought Roland with her. They were carrying suitcases.

"No kids?" I said.

"We're going to a concert." Roland had bought tickets and booked a room at a Midtown hotel. It helped that they had found a terrific babysitter who could help weekdays and occasional weekends, who took the pressure off. She was watching the kids for their twenty-four-hour getaway.

"Things are really improved between us, we both feel good," Cindy said.

"I feel like the old Cindy is back," Roland added. "This is who I married."

Cindy Prince's focus had changed from "How can I get through the next twenty-four hours?" and "Is life worth living?" to "What could my life be? What could *our* lives be?"

If Cindy and Roland were going to stay together, and it looked like they were, there was no shortage of things to think about and plan for.

Most immediately, now that Cindy and Roland had three children, their apartment had become incredibly cramped. They had to buy a house, which meant figuring out their finances, borrowing money from their parents, and so on. Beyond that, there was the issue of getting Cindy's career back on track. She was now seriously thinking of getting back into academia. The dissertation that she had abandoned in despair after Zach's birth three years ago no longer daunted her. She had started looking back over her notes, sorting out her old data printouts, reading up on the latest techniques in her field. She had noticed that her concentration was better. She could now "start to think linearly again"—and she found that she could "retain the information I need" rather than feeling that her mind was always "skipping all over." She scheduled a meeting with one of her old academic advisors to find out whether she could get back into her PhD program. It looked like she could start again next fall.

Overall, things were looking pretty good for Cindy and Roland Prince.

Buying a Home

After several months of remission, Mark's outlook was also vastly improved. His panic symptoms rarely flared up. And his compulsivity and his checking behavior were becoming a memory—almost like a childhood dream.

His relationship with Susan was also going through major changes. After a several-month hiatus, Mark had returned to psychotherapy with Liz Weeks. As with Marietta, Mark too found therapy was no longer a life raft. It was a means of achieving change.

There was much to work on. The most difficult thing was finding the courage to finish saying goodbye to his late wife, Corinne, to face the reality that life was moving on. Mark had been so emotionally withdrawn for so many years that now it was a struggle to experience intimacy. It wasn't all peaceful; he and Susan had their share of arguments and fights. Through all this, he was finally coming to the conclusion that after so many years of paralysis and mourning, he was ready to embrace the future. One session, as he was on his way out the door, Mark mentioned that he and Susan had begun discussing the possibility of marriage, not to mention the daunting idea of having children.

"Not a trivial issue, given my advanced age of 44."

And then I didn't see Mark for a while. He telephoned shortly before our next appointment to ask if I would renew his medications by phone. Things were going well, he said, really well, plus he was swamped at work and couldn't find the time to come in. Could we meet again two or three months down the line?

Reluctantly, I said okay.

It was just before Thanksgiving when Mark next came in. He tossed his coat on the couch in the corner of my office and sprawled beside it. As usual these days, his cell phone was nowhere in sight. It is hard to describe, but there was something notably less frenetic about him, something *settled*.

"Things are good," he told me. "Good is almost becoming routine." His symptoms rarely bothered him. At the law firm, his work was much improved, his partners even having congratulated him on the timely completion of his cases. "I've noticed that the Klonopin affects my memory."

"That may be a good sign," I said.

He looked puzzled. "What do you mean?"

"This is just a hunch, but it could mean that your anxiety system has started cooling down. The dose you used to need to control anxiety now sedates you.

To me, it says that your amygdala has indeed quieted down, that your fear system is going back to normal."

We started discussing how he could gradually taper the dose, but I could see that he wanted to move on to something else. "What?" I said.

The big news though was that Susan and he were in contract to buy a home. "A kind of raw space, needs a lot of work, but it's reasonably big."

"How big?" I asked.

He smiled. "Big enough for a family."

Driving Lessons

Allen Johnson was also doing well. He was again traveling to see clients, both in the states and overseas.

"I'm going out a lot, too," he told me.

"How much?"

"Every night!"

"*Every night?*"

He laughed. "My friends say that, too. Yeah. To parties, restaurants, shows. It's like I've been in jail for six years. And now that I'm sprung out, I want to get out there as much as I can and make up for lost time."

Allen had gotten back in touch with Donna, a woman he knew from college, who worked at a financial firm in southern Connecticut. He grew flushed in talking about her—how gorgeous she was, was she out of his league?—like an embarrassed teenager. Donna had been divorced recently and was also in therapy. For the past few weekends he had been taking the Metro-North train up to Fairfield County to meet her.

"What a drag that is!" He was always missing trains and having to wait for an hour in Grand Central or on a windy platform up in Connecticut. "So Donna's convinced me to start taking driving lessons!"

Allen had never learned to drive, at first because it wasn't the norm for New York City kids and later on because he had been overwhelmed by anxiety, by consuming fears that he would veer off the road. So far, he had endured four lessons—driving around suburban Connecticut in a Dodge Neon with "N E W D R I V E R" emblazoned on the car.

"And how is that?"

"Not too bad, once you get over the humiliation of driving that stupid Neon!" He laughed. "Actually, I'm not bad behind the wheel. A little overcautious, but I'm working on that. I'm trying to decide what kind of car to buy."

It wasn't just driving either; their relationship was developing rapidly. Allen had introduced Donna to his parents when they came up from Florida for a visit. They'd gone for a weeklong vacation to Vermont (she did the driving) and had a great time. They had even mentioned the word marriage.

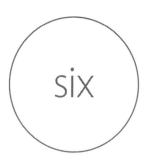

six

Moving Forward
Love, Sex, Relationships, Kids

Mark Postdisorder

WHEN I NEXT SAW Mark, after a several-month delay, he looked good: confident and even, dare I say, happy. He soon made clear that it was a hectic time. He and Susan were facing a host of issues. Everything seemed to be happening at once. They were in the midst of construction on their new home, they were planning their wedding, a mere two months away—and they were thinking of whether to have a child. All huge issues, all of them indications of how well his life was going.

More concretely, though, there were several issues to discuss. For one thing, sex.

"I'm frustrated," Mark said. As he had indicated at a previous visit, he was having sexual side effects from the medicine, in particular, difficulty achieving orgasm. He had tried bethenacol, which helped somewhat but not enough. He tried dropping the medication dose to 60 mg/day, as we had discussed, but had found that he needed 80 mg/day to control his symptoms. He had tried "drug holidays"—skipping the medicine on days that he and Susan were going to have sex, but that didn't help.

"We have to figure this out *now*," he said.

As we talked, it became clear that there were several aspects to this issue. In some ways, it was a positive development. In the midst of disorder, sex had been the last thing on Mark's mind. Depression and OCD had left his libido near zero. Initially as his mood improved and his checking behavior had decreased, sex was not a high priority: there were too many other issues to deal with. Later, he and Susan had had problems in their relationship and *she* had not been very interested. Now, however, they were doing well as a couple, and this was becoming a problem.

"I'm sure we can figure something out," I said. "What else is there?"

He and Susan were thinking of having a baby—and they had realized they should probably start trying to get pregnant soon, if not immediately. But he had a lot of questions, among them whether the SSRI medicine he was taking could affect his unborn child.

Plus, Mark continued before I could even respond, he had been feeling kind of blah lately, not depressed but not feeling very excited about things, and he was wondering if we needed to adjust his medication. There were other things too, including a possible promotion and a job offer from another firm.

"That's it?" I said finally, smiling.

"Sorry, doc, I guess I'm throwing a lot of stuff at you at one time, but it's because I'm feeling good, because things are going so well, and I just want to sort it all out."

"Okay, Mark," I said. "So where do you want to start?"

Some patients, including Cindy and Allen and Mark, achieve good outcomes relatively quickly with New Neuropsychiatry treatments once remission settles in. They begin to move on with their lives. Being postdisorder doesn't mean they are cured, of course. They risk having their disorders reemerge in the future. But they become acutely aware that it is possible to have their lives back. Often they begin making up for lost time, undergoing a process of renewed, even accelerated, psychological development.

Thus, you may find the phase of recovery to be a wild ride. Recovery often raises a flash flood of issues that your friends may have already addressed in their own lives over many years: issues related to dating, sexuality, and developing intimacy; tolerating rejection and uncertainty in relationships; deciding whether to make a commitment to a particular person; planning to get married; and then, in a short time, whether to have children. People who have chronic mood and anxiety disorders have high rates of "single marital status," much to their dismay. So it makes sense that recovery often involves entering relationships.

People who are postdisorder struggle to unlearn habits of thought and behavior that whatever disorder they faced has made second nature and to dare to leave them behind. Being postdisorder, as we will see in the rest of this book, is not a single state or phase—if anything, it is an unfolding, a continual, often surprising, evolution. A series of often-unpredictable developments and unanticipated challenges.

These issues may arise over a matter of months, or even seemingly all at once, and usually are accompanied by a sense of urgency, a feeling they must be addressed ASAP. With pregnancy and childbirth, of course, the biological clock may be a significant reality factor. But it's often more than that.

I have come to think urgency *itself* is part of the recovery phase: a realization that life's possibilities have returned, that opportunities can be seized, yet that time is short and important decisions must be made.

(Re)connections: Bringing It All Together

As is clear from the stories I have told in this book, interesting developments occur during the recovery phase, often after many years of suspended animation. After chronic depression or persistent anxiety fade away, you may return to life, dazzled and astonished by pharmacological treatment, ready to pick up again with things the way you left them years before. I have previously talked about how neurogenesis and other brain recovery processes appear to occur with antidepressant treatment. So, let's take these ideas a bit further. After several months of treatment, let's say your hippocampus has continued growing new cells, that your brain's own healing powers—the proteins called neurotrophic factors that I discussed earlier—encourage your previously shrunken neurons to send out more connections throughout your brain. Then what? Let's say your stress hormones have sunk back toward their normal levels, let's say your amygdala is no longer primed for impending disaster. And your cytokines, which are chemicals spewed out by white blood cells in response to stress and which themselves cause you to feel fatigued and sleepy and downcast (i.e., "sick"), let's say that these too have gone back toward normal.

Why should it be any surprise if, after months of being in remission, other systems began to come back on line? Your sexual functioning, for instance.

The neurobiology of sexual behavior requires that several parts of your cortex—the outermost part of your brain that handles the senses, movement, and association—work in tandem. Remember that in depression or anxiety disorder, your frontal cortex wasn't working very well. It was either underactivated or in a frenzy of hyperactivity, looping over and over through cycles of agitation and fear. Now, all systems are go again: so should it be any surprise that (even despite the sexual-dysfunction-*inducing* effects of the SSRIs) the people coming through my office should be preoccupied with sex?

During the flares of disorder, when the hippocampus was going haywire and the amygdala was locked in flight-or-fight cycles, the process of attachment fails. Most commonly, those who are depressed and anxious withdraw from friends, lovers, and families, though at times they will become unpleasantly clinging and endlessly needy. Now, the newly recovered can make normal attachments again. So our brains' sexual neurotransmitter (whichever chemical it is that governs attachment in humans the way that oxytocin does in sheep and rats and voles) can also play its chemical magic again.

After sustained remission achieved by New Neuropsychiatry treatments, something both prosaic and magical appears to be happening: a process of reengagement in life. I wrote earlier about the elevation in harm avoidance that is found among many people who have psychiatric disorders regardless of diagnosis, the general state of increased fearfulness and conviction of the likeliness of bad outcomes that causes such individuals to shy away from taking risks and often to end up living constricted lives, either devoid of intimacy or caught in repetitive patterns of intimate frustration.

In the phase of recovery, we often seem to see the opposite of harm avoidance—instead, the seeking of new experiences, a willingness to try new things. Then, attachment, bonding, courtship, procreation, parenthood. In all, life goes forward, in all its splendor and complexity! Is it possible that the evolutionarily conserved neurobiological pathways of attachment are coming online again?

The psychiatrist who has articulated this best is Dr. Daniel J. Siegel, a California-based researcher. In his view, the process of recovery has to do with a subtle yet crucial aspect of brain anatomy. He focuses on "integrative fibers," which are long neuronal tendrils that connect distant parts of the brain to each other. These parts include the prefrontal cortex, the hippocampus, the anterior cingulate, and possibly the cerebellum. These integrative fibers are damaged in anxiety disorders like posttraumatic stress disorder and in mood disorders.

For instance, MRI studies using the technique called diffusion tensor imaging have shown that people with depression have a significant reduction of fractional anisotropy (the way that liquids move in the brain) in the frontal lobe, anterior cingulate, temporal lobe, and other regions in treatment-resistant depression patients—which means there is impaired connection between these parts of the brain.

But can integrative fibers regenerate? Siegel's theory (as yet unproven) is that recovery from disorder involves reawakening of, and rewiring of, these integrative fibers. In Siegel's view, during the state of disorder, we are ruled, on one side, by chaos, and on the other, by rigidity. We steer between Scylla (of agitation, despair, terror) and Charybdis (of neurotic rules, peculiar checking behavior, phobic avoidance, intense dependency). During recovery, we find a welcome middle ground—of "complexity." Complexity is good. Whereas disorder is simple, yet harsh, the process of recovery leads to differentiation, to complexity, to growth. The brain has "convergent zones" that are central to self-understanding, and these appear to be able to function properly only when disorder is at bay.

Could this explain what we see in people who are recovering from disorders?

Does recovery reflect the returning functions of the integrative brain?

At present, we certainly do not know the answers to these questions, but they are ones that researchers can begin to explore.

Hannah Begins to Trust

"So, what do you think I should do?" Hannah asked.

We had just had a forty-minute discussion, and at moments it seemed, oddly enough, as if she wanted me to decide for her. But it wasn't going to be so easy. Indeed, it was going to have to be *her* decision, or, more precisely, a consensus between Hannah and her husband—something they both could live with.

Did she want to have a child?

When I first met her in the early 1990s, Hannah Wrenn was a 27-year-old Ivy League–educated woman whose best employment was as a temporary secretary and who had been immobilized for years by panic attacks and profound, agonizing depression. After responding to an SSRI medication, Hannah had emerged from a cocoon of avoidance and withdrawal—so suddenly and frighteningly that, in the resulting psychological turmoil, she had almost quit treatment. Later on, Hannah had successfully addressed many of her fears in therapy and entered a phase of rapid psychological growth. Her work functioning, her personal life blossomed as she settled into the postdisorder state.

For Hannah Wrenn, one major aspect of this process of recovery related to intimacy. Because of her terrible anxiety and depression, Hannah had rarely dated in college, and even less after she graduated. In her secretarial years, there had been the occasional one-night stand and more than one dismal affair with a co-worker, which had only reinforced her belief that relationships were not for her. After she felt well for many months, she began emerging from her cocoon. In the past, psychotherapy had been a crutch for Hannah, something that helped her cope with one setback after another but didn't lead to much progress. Now Hannah was able to use psychotherapy—for the first time—as a way to solve problems.

Within a year, Hannah had saved enough money to go back to art school on a part-time basis. In the studio, she had an impressive burst of creativity, for once being able to work productively on her photography without fearing catastrophe. Her work there was good enough to qualify her for a major scholarship. Later, she joined her neighborhood gym to get back in shape and decided to take a yoga class. This developed into a true passion, a fascination with an ancient art of body and mind (and also helped her toward her goal of being a less-anxious person). Over time, she became friends with some of the other yoga devotees. In particular, a man I will call Jorge, a teacher at a local school who also had gotten into yoga. He wasn't exactly what she had thought of as marriage material—she had always imagined she would end up marrying a handsome stockbroker or lawyer rather than a balding eighth-grade social studies teacher. Her imagination had always tended toward Park Avenue, not Queens. But as weeks passed, she and Jorge grew closer and eventually became lovers.

Hannah had been traumatized early in life, with abusive parents and many losses. When she became anxious and depressed, it was overwhelming for her to become involved in relationships. Now, feeling better, she faced issues of trust, intimacy, compromise, and negotiation, all things that her friends had dealt with many years earlier. Research shows clearly that mood and anxiety disorders often inhibit attachment or cause patterns of insecure or disorganized attachment with others. And insecure or disorganized relationships can worsen mood disorders. Now that she was in remission, Hannah was able to work on attachment and intimacy issues. Feeling okay, her reactions were much less fearful, she had less of a tendency to flee from intimacy, and she conveyed a sense of increasing calm and confidence as she got closer to Jorge.

Jorge Ramos had been a late bloomer as well, living only a few blocks away from his needy and insecure mother for many years, only gradually becoming independent from her influence after she moved to Florida. After half a year, Hannah and Jorge became practically inseparable, spending nights and days and weekends together. With one difficulty: she was afraid to tell him about her years of panic attacks and her reliance on Zoloft.

To make a long story short, Hannah was terrified that Jorge would reject her if she told him she depended on SSRIs, that he would see her as irredeemably flawed. Only after much agonizing did she finally tell Jorge, perhaps a month before their wedding. Fortunately, Jorge reacted positively: he told Hannah that he loved her, so it didn't matter if she needed to take medicine to stay well. His concern was that she have the best outcome, and in particular, he wanted her to be strong enough to be a good mother to their children. They sailed happily through their wedding and honeymoon and their first year of marriage. But then, as the clock ticked and as they grew more serious about trying to conceive, the discussions became more charged. *Did* she need to take medicine to stay well? What would be the risk to the baby if he or she were exposed to Hannah's Zoloft? Plus, was she strong enough to be a mother?

"You know what? Why don't you bring Jorge to the next session? Let's discuss these issues."

So we scheduled a meeting, Hannah and Jorge and me. We had to sort this out. And soon.

Several years ago, a committee of the American College of Neuropsychopharmacology, an organization of psychiatric researchers, defined recovery as something that occurs after a person's disorder is in remission for four or more months. That definition is fine for researchers, but for the purposes of the New Neuropsychiatry we could define recovery based more or less on general understanding: that a person no longer has symptoms of the disorder, and that his or her life is returning to normal. (Note that a recovery is not the same as a cure; in the latter a person has entirely recovered and is no longer at risk of being ill. With psychiatric disorders, one can never be sure that a person is totally cured. In fact, our current treatments rarely provide cures.)

New Neuropsychiatrists don't have good explanations yet for many of the phenomena seen in recovery and haven't developed much of a language for them either. And too little research has yet been done. It seems clear, though, that recovery occurs more often in the New Neuropsychiatry era than in the old days—probably because more effective treatments have enabled a large number of people to enter sustained remission. These changes tend to be most striking in patients like Mark and Hannah who go into remission after a long history of disorder, misery, and dysfunction.

In the New Neuropsychiatry, this phase has two major goals: (1) to do whatever is possible to keep your disorder in remission (because one has not been "cured") and (2) to embrace and expand your life again.

When facing the urgencies of the recovery period, all the exciting developments and urgent decisions that must be made, it is important to keep these two goals in mind.

Phases and Issues

When Hannah's disorder first began to respond to treatment, major issues included the control of her symptoms and then a need to begin managing her life again—solving practical problems (paying bills, house cleaning, etc.) and catching up with deferred maintenance. In these early phases, a lot of her (and my) effort went into dealing with side effects and residual symptoms, and on a psychological level, grieving over lost opportunities.

As people begin to move from remission to recovery, they often describe that they are "feeling like myself again" or "meeting myself again"—often for the first time in many years. Gradually their interests turn outside themselves. They begin to engage again in the world, often with a combination of trepidation as well as excitement and enthusiasm and pleasure. New interests and passions may emerge, and they may begin new relationships. They commonly feel a new sense of security and confidence—as though the world is again safe for them to explore.

Recovery works according to a concentric process. It starts at immediate issues of self-preservation and then moves outward to quality of life and then toward achieving long-term goals and planning for the future. If there is a sequence to the issues that are addressed, it is often something like this:

1. Symptoms, self-care
2. Work performance
3. Home maintenance, paying bills, cleaning house
4. Recreational activities
5. Relationships
6. Children and family

One thing I find fascinating in the recovery phase is the way in which people's attachments develop and change. Often after many years of being stuck in dysfunctional relationships (or without a relationship), things start moving. Hannah met and dared to develop a romantic relationship with Jorge. After many years, Mark was finally moving ahead with plans to marry Susan. Allen met Donna and things quickly became serious. Sometimes a previously stable relationship will go into crisis; other times a new relationship will start or an existing relationship will accelerate toward marriage (or blow up if key issues can't be successfully addressed). Given the sense of urgency and excitement that often accompanies recovery, things often proceed rapidly from dating to marriage to having children. As I was seeing with Hannah and Jorge.

What does the recovery phase look like for people who are not in their childbearing years or for those who cannot or do not want to have children? In some ways it is less obvious, somewhat more difficult to see than what I am describing for Hannah and Mark and Marietta; but it involves more connections to the community, a reengagement with work goals, a greater level of involvement in things that give meaning. Also, a better ability to care for oneself, whether taking care of health issues or planning for retirement. If one is not having children, it can mean developing a greater connection to others—such as nieces and nephews, siblings, or friends and other nonrelatives—or being involved with mentoring or coaching or teaching or volunteer work with religious organizations.

The Unexpected

One aspect that I find particularly fascinating about recovery is how people spontaneously develop new interests and activities. *Indeed, unpredictability is one of the more predictable aspects of recovery.* To me this suggests that recovery is an organic process, not just the result of a doctor's enthusiasm or of a patient's great expectations.

A Fresh Start in Recovery

In the recovery phase, many facets of life that may have been neglected during months or years of disorder can finally be addressed. Exercise, diet, professional advancement, finances—all can now be given due attention. These issues can be broken into a number of areas.

- ▶ *Self-care*: being good to oneself, economic self-care, having one's home in good order (housekeeping, paying bills, etc.), decreasing social isolation, staying healthy (medical care, decreasing self-injurious behaviors, increasing health-enhancing activities such as exercise, healthy diet)
- ▶ *Enjoyment of life*: doing things for fun, social activities, use of leisure, developing new interests and passions
- ▶ *Intimacy*: developing and maintaining positive attachments rather than damaging, self-defeating ones; returning to romance
- ▶ *Sexuality*: focusing on having good sexual functioning and good sexual relationships rather than none (low libido) or unsatisfying (compulsive sexuality); addressing effects of treatment (e.g., SSRI side effects)
- ▶ *Putting your life in order*: getting health insurance; better job/career; more stable income; going back to school
- ▶ *Family matters*: relationships with biological family and/or creating one's own family
- ▶ *Procreation*: pregnancy, childbirth, parenting

Often these new interests will be things your doctor or therapist had *not* predicted, recommended, or prescribed—things that were not discussed in session. You may come in to an appointment and say in an offhand way, "Oh, by the way, did I mention that I . . ." followed by a verb such as *joined, took up, signed up for, started, met, went,* and so on. Indeed, I tend to view the occurrence of these spontaneous new activities as a sign that recovery is under way!

And so we will hear you have taken up softball, tennis, boating, photography, play-writing, painting, vacations, group activities, entrepreneurial activities (such as real estate investment, for better or worse), running, photography, or cooking. Sometimes these are activities that you had considered before, but often they seem to come out of the blue: just something that you now find interesting, that has somehow has become irresistible. Hence, several months into treatment, Allen took up running in the park and Mark became involved with local politics. And Hannah had come to a visit one day to announce that she had started doing yoga, something she had never indicated an interest in before—and perhaps not surprisingly, her relationship with Jorge had developed from this.

Back to Long-Term Goals

Some aspects of recovery, though, are more predictable. Recovery often involves picking up long-term goals where they left off the last time you were feeling well—sometimes years or even decades ago. This may be fairly easy or may present difficulties.

Cindy Prince, for example, found it both easy and difficult. She was picking up life from about four years earlier, before the postpartum depression that followed Zach's birth. After many months in remission, Cindy had begun working on her dissertation again. First she began reanalyzing data from various experiments and meeting with her advisers. Next she started revising the tables and the text. Finally, she was working full-force on the dissertation and even began investigating postdoctoral fellowships that she could apply for. On one occasion she commented to me, almost as an aside, "You know, I feel like I have my self back."

"What do you mean?" I asked.

"I'm feeling a way I haven't felt since I was 15 years old—before all the bad things started happening in my life. I feel confident again, I'm not always afraid. I feel that if I set my mind to doing something, I can do it." Smiling, she said, "I won't fall apart, I won't face disaster, I won't sabotage myself."

It wasn't easy by any means. Now in recovery, there were innumerable issues to address. Since she had last worked in the lab, her field had progressed dramatically: was her work still current? Was she still eligible for competitive tenure-track jobs after being out of the mainstream for several years? And did she have the energy and concentration to do research? Cindy felt able to use psychotherapy with Will Eastman more effectively to deal with these issues.

No doubt the neurotransmitter stabilization that Cindy got from medication contributed to this. *Because* she felt good, she could see how self-focused and overreactive she had often been, and how she had tended to blame other people for her own failings. Experiencing success (especially after years of frustration and failure) led Cindy to feeling greater confidence as she completed her dissertation—and, once she received her degree, that it would lead to still more opportunities.

Interestingly, Cindy's relationship with Roland was now also going well. Their sex life basically had been on hold for months—not a surprise, given all that was going in their lives: life with three young children, their marital problems, her depression. Recently her libido had begun to return.

"We actually have a sex life again," she told me one session.

To me, this seemed like a confirmation that recovery was indeed under way.

When I saw Cindy in those days, I kept thinking about glutamate. Studies have shown that the mood stabilizers, particularly lithium, have a powerful push-pull effect on that neurotransmitter. Glutamate is an "excitatory" neurotransmitter—the higher its levels, the more active and "up" you are. Its level is thought to be too high in mania and too low in depression. In people who have bipolar disorders, mood stabilizers may adjust the level of glutamate into what some researchers describe as a "stable zone"—not too high, not too low, a middle zone in which it can control both the highs of mania and the extremes of depression. Could this be happening in Cindy's brain, now that her bipolar II disorder was under control for the first time? In any case, her *mind* seemed to have entered a stable zone, freed from the constant shrill calls of agitation and despair.

This is what one could call the High Road of the New Neuropsychiatry: your symptoms have gone into sustained remission, and your brain and body are no longer in a high-stress state. On the High Road, your mind is working full-force and your life has again become pleasurable and rewarding. The High Road comes with its own difficulties and problems, of course. It can be overwhelming at times, and disorienting. Yet it is an enviable state. We'll look at the High Road—and the Low Road—more closely in the next chapter.

Maintaining Remission

Staying in remission is an ongoing process and challenge during the phase of recovery. In the STAR*D study, it was clear that many depressed people would go into remission after one or more courses of medication treatment—only to slip back into a partially depressed state, or even back into full disorder. During all the excitement and challenges of life during recovery, it is important not to lose sight of the importance of maintaining remission, which after all is what makes recovery possible.

There are the obvious things, of course, such as continuing treatment that has been helpful, such as staying on medication and in therapy; though

Exercise and the Brain

Everyone knows that exercise is good for you: it helps to decrease stress, improve your physical fitness, strengthen your heart, and so on. What is not widely appreciated yet, though, is that exercise is good for your *brain*. A study by psychologist Arthur F. Kramer showed that normal adults between the ages of 55 and 79 who exercised more had less shrinkage of their brains over time as measured by MRI scans than did those who didn't exercise. People who were more physically fit had more gray and white matter in the frontal, medial, and temporal areas of the cortex, areas that are crucial to higher level intellectual functioning. Conversely, in a study by Antonio Convit, elevated blood sugar (which is associated with poor physical fitness and poor diet) was shown to be associated with impairment of recent memory—and with shrinkage of the hippocampus (the brain center for learning and memory) as well.

Beyond that, it is becoming clear that for people who have psychiatric disorders, exercise can have specific benefits. A. L. Dunn and Madhur Trivedi did a study that determined that exercise may be an effective treatment of major depression by itself. Exercise has also been used as a way of enhancing the effect of antidepressant medications—in a study by A. S. Mather, exercise helped medication work better in a group of elderly depressed patients who had only partially responded to medication. Recently, Trivedi and colleagues also showed that people who have a partial response with antidepressant medicine can have a significant additional benefit if they add a certain amount of exercise—three to five sessions a week of a moderate degree of exercise. They prescribed the degree of exercise that has been recommended by the Surgeon General's Report on Physical Activity and Health. Their findings? Study participants had been depressed an average of nineteen months. Those who completed twelve weeks of this exercise program had a drop in their depression scores from 17.7 to 7.0—from "moderate depression" to "well." This type of exercise "prescription" makes sense not only for people who have depression, but also those who have panic disorder and other anxiety disorders.

Perhaps the most intriguing of these exercise studies comes from research on animals. A. A. Russo-Neustadt and colleagues at the University of California at Irvine studied the effects of adding exercise and antidepressants on depressed rats (not a joke: there are numerous "animal models" of depression—they can involve repeated mild electric shocks or forced swimming in a water tank). Russo-Neustadt's group was able to look at the brain chemicals involved with the improvement of depression in these rats—in particular the protein brain-derived neurotrophic factor (BDNF), one of the brain-growth chemicals whose levels increase during the recovery from depression. What they found was that antidepressants increase the level of BDNF, and that exercise does too. Moreover, they observed that the combination of exercise *and* antidepressants led to a *greater* effect, "in a manner that appears to be both additive and accelerated." They speculate that "physical activity, in conjunction with antidepressant agents, could represent a novel treatment approach for the improvement of behavioral management in depression." So, exercising the body really can help improve the mind—and the brain itself!

medications may need to be adjusted to get the best outcome. And therapy visits may become less frequent too, if only because life becomes otherwise so busy.

There are less obvious things, however. Ideally the New Neuropsychiatrist would be able to use principles from research, practice, and even neurobiology to figure out how to maintain and strengthen remission and even how to improve the functioning of specific brain networks, such as those connecting the prefrontal cortex to the hippocampus, or the hippocampus to the amygdala. Unfortunately, this process is only just beginning. At this point in time, we definitely do not entirely understand how to do such fine-grained rehabilitation.

The model of the New Neuropsychiatry, though, would suggest that this process requires attention to the relation between mind, brain, and body. In the Old Psychiatry, the idea was that if you were in psychotherapy you would "work through" your conflicts through intensive therapy and emerge healthy on the other side. Or if you opted for medication treatment in the Old Psychiatry, once you had "responded" to treatment, there was not much to do other than to keep taking your pills.

Now, with the New Neuropsychiatry, we have a broader view of disorder and recovery. We now see the brain as a dynamic organ that is continually being remodeled in response to its environment, its anatomy and functioning deeply affected by how you act, how you live your life, how you interact with people, and even how you think.

We are also much more aware of how medical conditions are interwoven with the health of your brain and with your psychiatric health. Study after study has shown that the better one controls medical conditions, the better will be the outcome of depression, and the reverse. Better control of blood sugar in diabetes leads to better outcome of depression. The same for control of blood pressure. Better medical health is associated with less likelihood for the development of cognitive impairment in later life—and less depression as well. People who are more depressed are more likely to die of heart disease. The studies go on and on. So obviously, staying physically healthy is one of the best ways to help keep you in remission.

Beyond that, it is becoming clear that other things—that psychiatrists never paid much attention to in the past—may help people keep mood and anxiety disorders in remission: particularly exercise and learning. Neurosciences research has shown that both exercise and learning can have significant effects on brain regrowth.

Exercise clearly has antidepressant effects in both people and in animals. In animal studies it has been shown to have positive effects on neurotrophic factors such as BDNF, which helps neurons and synapses (see Chapter 5), and Bcl-2, which affects cell health. A growing number of studies in humans show that exercise helps treatment of depression and anxiety disorders. So I always recommend that people include exercise in their plan for staying in remission. Allen began running regularly, for instance, which helped significantly with his anxiety; Mark required some pushing but began working out regularly at a local gym; and Hannah was consistently doing yoga four or five times a week.

As discussed in the Introduction, learning clearly is associated with neurogenesis and plasticity in the brain. I previously mentioned the studies of British researcher Eleanor Maguire, who showed that taxi drivers had growth of the hippocampus after studying and memorizing the map of the city of London. An intriguing MRI study of jugglers by Bogdan Draganski and colleagues showed that learning to juggle and then practicing regularly caused growth of an area of the brain related to the processing of visual movement. It makes sense that learning can play a significant role in brain recovery, although at present it is not clear how we should apply this to the recovery from mood and anxiety disorders. Logical ways to try to harness these processes would include learning more adaptive new behaviors, changing your thought patterns, and learning about disorders. Thus New Neuropsychiatrists encourage everyone to learn more about their disorders, whether major depression, bipolar disorder, or PTSD. Creating more satisfying social connections would seem likely to help too. In particular, having positive intimate relationships: learning to be closer to others seems likely to help stimulate the functioning of "integrative fibers." But does doing *New York Times* crossword puzzles or learning a new language help to prevent depression or stave off Alzheimer disease? Who knows?

Adjusting Medication to Stay in Remission

During your recovery phase, your doctor may need to make various sorts of medication adjustments. You may have side effects like weight gain and drowsiness. Or if symptoms of your disorder start to return, your doctor may have to do things like increasing the dose of your medicine, or switching medications, or augmenting with a second medicine. As always, the goal is to get the best response to medicine with the fewest side effects and to keep your disorder in remission.

Thus, I would be adjusting Mark's meds to decrease sexual side effects and to try to get more antidepressant effect. I tweaked Hannah's meds to help manage her anxiety and took her off the benzodiazepine Ativan once she decided to get pregnant. And I stopped Cindy's Risperdal as soon as it became apparent she no longer needed it to help her sleep.

Sexual Side Effects of Medication—and of Disorder

The recovery phase of the New Neuropsychiatry almost inevitably leads to discussions about sexuality. Sexual functioning is often poor during periods of depressive illness. It gradually improves once disorder fades. The very success of treatment leads to difficult decisions and uncomfortable dilemmas. How can people who have mood and anxiety disorders improve their sex lives? Clearly, just recovering from depression or anxiety disorders could help, because sexual interest is often decreased by disorder, either directly or indirectly. Cindy was a good example of this: her recovery from bipolar II disorder allowed her to improve her relationship with Roland and then to focus on their sexual relationship. Then there are all the pregnancy issues that Hannah had raised. Should a soon-to-be-pregnant woman stop taking the medicine and risk having her disorder return? Or, should she stay on the medicine and

Sexuality, Disorder, and Recovery

Psychological disorders often have a negative effect on sexual functioning. Sometimes this manifests itself in decreases in the levels of desire, arousal, and, to a lesser degree, the ability to reach orgasm. People who have depression and anxiety disorders are often socially withdrawn, which can affect their ability to find sexual partners. Libido is often particularly decreased in depression or anxiety disorders. For instance, a woman I was treating named Luanne had chronic depression and described *never* feeling sexual desire during her entire lifetime before starting therapy. After her depression went into remission with an SNRI medication, she experienced sexual desire for the first time and had the first orgasms of her life.

In some people, disorders have the opposite effect and lead to compulsive sexual behavior. Antidepressant medicine has been shown to decrease their levels of compulsivity. The brain's wiring for sexuality clearly overlaps with the wiring for mood and anxiety regulation.

When the SSRI medications first were introduced, sexual side effects were barely listed in the *Physicians' Desk Reference*, or PDR. Only after the SSRIs were in widespread use did it become clear that they often cause sexual side effects, sometimes decreased arousal but more commonly delayed orgasm—or even the inability to reach orgasm. Why is this? Probably because the SSRIs have an impact on nerve cells in the spinal cord, and on spinal reflexes that are related to sexual functioning. The sexual side effects of SSRIs may result from effects on the spine, not in the brain. The SSRI medicines cause problems most commonly with orgasm, and less often with arousal or desire.

When sexual side effects do occur with medication treatment, there are a number of options. Commonly, medication dose or timing may be changed. For a person I was seeing named Bob, who was treated with Paxil but had sexual side effects, changing the time he took the medicine (later in the day, after sexual encounters) made it somewhat easier to achieve orgasm, but skipping a day of medicine (a "drug holiday") was more effective. This worked because the blood level of Paxil dropped enough during these times that sexual functioning returned temporarily to normal. Another option is to change antidepressants: some of the SSRIs seem to have higher sexual side effects (Paxil, for instance) than others (such as Lexapro). Some antidepressants (Wellbutrin, Remeron) rarely have sexual side effects. Sometimes doctors add a second medication to an SSRI: it may be another antidepressant (like a small dose of Wellbutrin) or another psychiatrically active medicine (the antianxiety agent Buspar, the stimulant dextroamphetamine, etc.). Or it may be any of a large number of medicines that have been tried, with varying success for this purpose: they include bethanacol, amantadine, yohimbine, and others.

Viagra, Cialis, or Levitra can also be useful, primarily for men, but sometimes for women as well. These medicines work by blocking phosphodiasterase-5, or PDE5, an enzyme which breaks down a chemical that induces erections. Viagra and related medicines prolong physical arousal, often for hours. For another person I was treating, Paul, sexual functioning was worsened by his "performance anxiety" in bed. Viagra removed anxiety from the equation of sexuality: certain that he would have an erection throughout the sexual experience, he could focus more on his partner. Viagra doesn't directly improve the ability to have an orgasm but can work more indirectly for people who have this SSRI side effect, by increasing physical arousal. Among women who have sexual dysfunction related to SSRIs, although these medicines may be somewhat helpful, they are probably less effective. Testosterone has been shown to help some women; others are helped by the addition of bupropion, buspirone, or bethenacol, or by switching to another antidepressant (such as bupropion or mirtazapine). Other drugs currently are in development to help women with sexual dysfunction, although the first such agent, flibanserin, recently failed to receive approval from the Food and Drug Administration.

expose her unborn baby to unknown risks? What are the risks to a man who is taking these medicines—do they affect his fertility, could they have a negative effect on his sperm? (This was one of Mark's concerns when he and Susan and I met.)

These dilemmas are part and parcel of the New Neuropsychiatry. As I see it, they are signs of its success.

It is *because* New Neuropsychiatry treatments can be so successful that these issues are raised. If you're so depressed that you hardly care if you live, sex is the last thing on your mind. Only when you're well do you become upset if your antidepressant has sexual side effects. Only if you're feeling pretty good, if you have the psychological reserves needed to have children, if you're feeling competent and optimistic—only then must you face the uncomfortable dilemma of whether or not to keep taking Prozac during pregnancy and afterward.

If you follow newspaper headlines, the treatment of disorder appears to involve a painful trade-off. Take your Prozac or Zoloft, and your depression will likely improve. But your sex life could go downhill. The dark rumors about sexual side effects of the SSRIs were confirmed a few years after the medicines' introduction, when in the early 1990s it became clear that SSRIs could interfere with the ability to have an orgasm. Viagra soon came along, perhaps slightly mitigating things, but leaving many people feeling like captives of the pharmaceutical industry. And, from the narrow view, there often is a trade-off. SSRIs indeed can have sexual side effects. And Viagra (and other similar medicines like Cialis or Levitra) often improve sexual functioning, at least in men.

But the New Neuropsychiatry takes a broader view. It is not just Prozac versus Viagra. The disorders themselves have to be included in the picture. In a broader view, the newer model of psychiatry has led us toward new views of sexuality, toward understanding the effects of disorders, and of treatment, on sexuality, and then to issues of pregnancy, childbirth, and the postpartum period

For Mark Maple, the pharmacology solution was not complicated. The SSRI was both improving his libido (because he was no longer depressed) and worsening his sex life (because it made orgasm more difficult). Probably the orgasm problem resulted from "pushing" his serotonin system too hard with his current dose of Prozac 80 mg/day, affecting the balance between serotonin and norepinephrine. His feeling of emotional flatness and blahness probably resulted from the same imbalance. Or possibly from a build-up of breakdown products of Prozac, which can stay in the body for several months (Prozac has a much longer "half-life" than other SSRIs). Fairly minor medication changes probably could help. Options included adding Wellbutrin (which works on dopamine and norepinephrine), switching to a shorter half-life SSRI like Celexa or Zoloft, or switching to a medicine that affects both norepinephrine and serotonin in a more balanced way (an SNRI), such as Effexor, Cymbalta, or Pristiq. It would also be possible to add any of a large number of other medicines, like Viagra. Viagra (sildenafil) wouldn't directly affect his orgasm problem but often seems to indirectly help this problem by increasing arousal.

After a brief discussion, Mark and I opted to start by keeping the Prozac at the same dose and adding a small dose of Wellbutrin SR 100 mg/day. If that didn't work, we would consider increasing it to as much as 450 mg/day. And if that didn't work, there were a lot of other choices.

Then Came Babies

At times these days, many years into the New Neuropsychiatry revolution, my office was looking like an obstetrician's waiting room (and on other occasions, like a pediatrician's office!). Many of my female patients, it seemed, were pregnant, or talking about having babies, or pushing their strollers through the waiting room, or walking in with toddlers in tow. And the discussion that I was having with Hannah was an almost-daily one.

For Hannah, the issue was this: having had severe panic and depression for so many years, she had never considered the possibility of having children as being realistic. Now that she was feeling good, it seemed like a possibility, indeed seemed compelling. Why not have a child? Life was opening up for her. At the age of 38, she felt the need to make up her mind fairly quickly.

Hannah's question was: *should* she? Could she handle motherhood? Over several sessions she had discussed these concerns. She thought she could, but how could she be sure? What if the panic attacks returned? More immediately, how could she possibly get through pregnancy? If she did become pregnant, should she stay on the medicine? Or should she come off it, and risk going into panic and depression again? Clearly the SSRI medication was a big factor in getting her to the point that she was *ready* to have a child. During her many years of disorder, Hannah had felt entirely unable to shoulder such responsibilities. Motherhood still seemed like a big deal, but at least it was possible. But if she did keep taking the medicine, wouldn't it be dangerous to expose her baby to something that might be dangerous?

"I've read all the materials you gave me, I looked on the Web, I talked to my OB and to the pediatrician. And I still don't know what to do."

Not long afterward, Allen and his fiancée Donna also wanted to meet with me. Only a year after meeting, they were planning to get married. They too were thinking of having children—though not right away. The issues were slightly different for them, because Allen was not taking medication for his panic disorder. But Donna was worried about the degree to which Allen's anxiety might be genetic and what risks their children might face. Allen also wondered how to protect his child or children from having panic disorder, which had affected so many areas of his life. They were wondering whether maybe they should consider adoption instead.

"It clearly does run in my family," Allen said. "My sister has panic attacks, my mother does too—she used to always keep me home from school as a kid,

Pregnancy, Childbirth, and After

Out of concern for their baby's development in the womb, many women wonder about taking medications during pregnancy and after their babies are born. If you are facing this situation, there are several options for treating depression during pregnancy, which include

- ► Stopping medications throughout pregnancy
- ► Stopping medications in the early phase of pregnancy and restarting them later in pregnancy, when the baby's organs are more developed and possibly would be less affected by medications
- ► Restarting medications after childbirth
- ► Trying various forms of psychotherapy or nonmedication therapy (such as treatment with a light box)

After raising these issues, I would encourage you and your partner to discuss treatment alternatives with your mental health or medical providers. Would it be better to try to come off medication while trying to conceive or after you know you are pregnant? If you need to take medication during pregnancy, which medications are the least worrisome? (For instance, lithium has long been avoided during pregnancy, because it was thought to cause an increased risk of abnormalities in the fetus's heart valves, Ebstein's anomaly, but recent research suggests that this risk is very low. Nevertheless, many psychopharmacologists still take a woman with bipolar illness off lithium during pregnancy and substitute a low dose of antipsychotic medication such as haloperidol or risperidone). Also, there may be certain choices to make: if a woman is taking both a benzodiazepine (like Xanax or Ativan) and an SSRI, it is clearly better to get rid of the benzodiazepine first, because benzodiazepines are associated with known fetal abnormalities and the SSRIs are thought to be relatively safe.

If your plan is to stop medication, the question comes up of when it is best to stop. Recently there has been a recommendation that it might be advisable to gradually discontinue SSRI medicine about seven to ten days before the baby's birth, to decrease withdrawal symptoms in the newborn baby. Of course, it is not always possible to stop medication because of the risk of disorder returning—Hannah (who you meet in this chapter) is an example of this. Research has suggested that some particular medications may be riskier (benzodiazepines, barbiturates), or less risky (SSRIs, neuroleptics). Among the antidepressants, there are more data about Prozac and Zoloft, and less about Wellbutrin, Celexa, and Luvox.

Of course, many substances in our environment may carry risk, so that psychotropic meds aren't the only (or even the highest) risk that a woman faces as she contemplates pregnancy. Our world is full of innumerable toxins, including household chemicals, cosmetics, food additives, all of which may carry risk. Managing risk is the key, not eliminating it.

Beyond the issue of whether to take medication during pregnancy, it is important to plan for the time after the baby is born. The risk of depression returning is greater after the baby is born than it is during pregnancy—perhaps not surprising, given the dramatic shifts in hormones that follow childbirth, and the stresses of having a baby and the months of disrupted sleep that are part of the package. Thus I discuss with people I am treating how we can plan for these early months, to provide additional help at home, especially in the first several weeks, which can decrease the risk of depression. And then, should the woman become depressed anyway, what to do.

What about breast-feeding? If you need to be taking antidepressants, is breast-feeding safe for the baby? Most of the psychotropic medications are excreted in breast milk (and thus could be transferred to the baby), but most studies show that the risk to the baby is fairly low. Still, some women will decide not to take that risk, and will choose to bottle feed instead.

What about just "toughing it out"—deciding not to get treatment for postpartum depression? No doubt many women decide to do this. However, the risk of untreated depression is significant. Untreated depression in the mother can cause problems for her baby's emotional development; sometimes, as can be seen in the headlines, untreated depression can have very serious and even fatal consequences.

In a broader medical context, many women with a variety of illnesses are successfully managed through pregnancy, childbirth, and the postpartum period. In general, most women with depression can go on to have uneventful pregnancies, deliveries, and healthy babies, and have rewarding experiences of motherhood. Thus the goal of the New Neuropsychiatrist during this time is to help the person through a successful experience of pregnancy, childbirth, and parenting, and, like any doctor, to work with both the woman and her partner to help them make the best possible decision and to achieve the best possible outcome.

because she had attacks when she was alone, she wanted me with her. And now . . ."

There was a pause.

"I know I want to break the cycle. I want my kids to be free, not held back."

Such conversations tend to be similar, variations on a theme. By now, I have had this conversation dozens of times; each time a little bit different, based on the person's history and treatment response, on particular worries and concerns. The decisions made differ for each couple, but the goal is the same—achieving the best outcome.

The obvious question during pregnancy is whether medicine needs to be continued, whether the medication is an antidepressant or a mood stabilizer, or some other class. Drugs vary in their risk. For instance, the relative risk of the different SSRI medications, Prozac and Paxil and Zoloft, is relatively similar. There is, on the one hand, more information available about Prozac (which generally indicates a benign effect on pregnancy); on the other hand, Zoloft and Paxil might be preferable for the woman who plans to come off medication when she gets pregnant, because they are cleared from the body more quickly. Some classes of drugs are known to be toxic to the fetus—both psychotropic medications such as the benzodiazepines (Ativan, Valium, Xanax, Klonopin, etc.) and nonpsychiatric medications (such as the acne medicine Accutane, the antibiotic tetracycline, or the antiseizure medicine Dilantin).

There are other chemicals to consider as well: Think of what we can call the "psychopharmacology of everyday life"—substances such as alcohol, cocaine, and tobacco, and so on, which may be riskier than any SSRI medication. Not to mention cosmetics, hair dyes, household cleaners, and other compounds that we live with.

Beyond that, there is the risk of untreated psychiatric illness during pregnancy: most obviously, untreated bipolar illness may have a bad course during pregnancy, but untreated depression as well (although depression may improve during the months of pregnancy)—especially if the woman has a history of severe depression, including suicidal or self-destructive behavior.

And of course *after* childbirth, clearly there is evidence that depression is bad for mothering abilities—a mother who has persistent depression is likely to have difficulty meeting her own needs, much less those of her baby. Untreated postpartum depression can have catastrophic results.

So it is a matter of weighing one kind of risk against another.

Like Hannah, Marietta (see Chapter 5) had had an excellent response to Celexa, which had made her depression largely a thing of the past and also made her much less sensitive to rejection and other setbacks. Marietta had married Victor a few years into her remission, and they were soon considering whether to have a baby. Like Hannah, Marietta worried about the risks of taking SSRI medications during pregnancy. Unlike Hannah, Marietta was adamant that she wanted to be off Celexa during pregnancy.

Over the past decade, we have learned a lot about the possible risks of SSRI medications in early, middle, and late pregnancy. And about the risks of breast-feeding when mothers are taking SSRIs. And so on. Specialists have begun developing strategies to manage disorders during these periods

About the issue Mark had raised—whether SSRI medicine would affect his sperm—less was known. "There are only one or two papers on the subject, and those are animal studies. We don't know everything," I said. But so far there hadn't been any red flags. Mark could certainly consider going off Prozac for several months—but he would have to keep in mind that it would take at least eight to ten weeks for the medicine to clear out of his body. Mark thought about it for about a millisecond. "No way. It just wouldn't fly!" So he opted to stay on the medicine.

One Other Issue: Genes

"If we decide to have a baby," said Allen. "We want to know, what is the risk that he or she would have panic disorder?" Because he wasn't taking medicine, it wasn't a question of whether there was exposure to SSRIs. It was a question of passing genes that might cause the disorder on to his children. Donna also had many relatives who suffered significantly from depression and anxiety disorders, so maybe she also had genes for these disorders. This too is a common question these days for the New Neuropsychiatrist. There are genes associated with panic disorder, or depression, or bipolar illness, or obsessive-compulsive disorder, as well as schizophrenia.

Panic disorder, for instance, often runs in families. About 2 percent of the general population has panic disorder, whereas 25 percent of the relatives of a person who has panic disorder have it. Among twins, if one twin has panic disorder, the chance is 11 percent that a fraternal twin (who shares 50% of the twin's genes) will have it. It is 24 percent among identical twins, who share 100 percent of genes. What conclusion do we draw from that? One could say, "Oh my God, a 25 percent risk—more than 12 times higher than that of the average person." Allen and Donna chose to look at it as "a 75 percent chance that our baby won't get panic disorder." And even if their child did develop panic disorder, Allen and Donna felt that they already knew techniques for coping with—and even recovering from—such a condition.

However, as New Neuropsychiatrists will point out, we *all* have genes that predispose us to various diseases, whether heart disease, cancer, or psychiatric illnesses, and it is important to put the risk of a particular psychiatric illness in the context of various risks, medical and otherwise, which may be present.

It was still fairly abstract to Allen and Donna, because they had just started living together and weren't married yet, but it was a question they wanted to start thinking through now, rather than waiting until Donna was pregnant.

Marietta and Victor

Marietta was adamant about wanting to be off Celexa during pregnancy. She had clearly done her homework and made up her mind. When she and Victor and I met, all she wanted to know was, "How soon before we start trying should I go off the medicine?"

We talked about this for a while, but I also tried to broaden the discussion, so she and Victor could address some of the issues that were likely to come up. For instance, how quickly to come off medication? What to do if she felt depressed again during pregnancy? Should she get back into therapy during pregnancy; might that help her stay out of depression. Should she stay off medication after the baby was born? What about breast-feeding, in the event that she ended up back on medication?

Hannah and Jorge

Hannah brought Jorge to her next session a few weeks later. Hannah's situation differed from Marietta's in some crucial ways. Hannah's depression was more severe than Marietta's. Marietta had been able to function reasonably well even when depressed, whereas Hannah's anxiety and depression symptoms had been long-standing, severe, and unrelenting. In her entire adult life, the only time Hannah had any significant period without symptoms was after starting medication. She was convinced that her symptoms would come roaring back if she stopped taking the Zoloft.

It is understandable to want to protect your baby from exposure to any unnecessary risks, including medications. When we began to talk about it that day, it became clear that Hannah was adamant about the necessity of continuing medicine—the way a diabetic person might need insulin.

"My question," she said, "Is whether it is safe for me to be pregnant on these meds, or whether I should give up on the idea of ever having biological children."

Given her family history, what were the odds that her baby could turn out normal? What if Zoloft had some effect on her baby's brain? Could she ever forgive herself?

So we discussed the scientific literature on genes and depression and on studies of the psychological and intellectual development of children exposed in utero to SSRI medications. Up to now, these kids seemed to be turning out normal. But who could know the long-term risks? Hannah wanted more information.

A month or so later, Hannah and Jorge were back. They had seen a genetic counselor to discuss their concerns about passing on depression genes to their child. And they had seen a specialist in the treatment of depression during pregnancy for a consultation. "It was all worth it, because it gave us a chance to think things through." Ultimately, after all their research and discussions, they had decided to go ahead: they did want to have a family. In their view, the risks seemed manageable. In the scheme of things, a higher genetic risk of developing mood and anxiety disorder, and the apparently small risks from SSRI medicine, seemed worth taking.

"We're thinking about being parents, how we can create a good environment so our child won't have as much risk for getting these problems." Hannah's own childhood had been marked by terrible stresses, especially her parents' marital and financial problems. Jorge's childhood had been no picnic either. "Those are excellent things to think about," I said.

As to immediate issues, we discussed possible medication changes, in that there was more data with Prozac than Zoloft during pregnancy and thereafter. Hannah decided to stay on Zoloft. And Marietta decided to taper off Celexa.

Each of them was soon pregnant, Hannah within a number of weeks of stopping birth control, Marietta after about three months. And Mark's wife, Susan, was pregnant within a month after they married.

The New Neuropsychiatrist is generally optimistic about having babies. People who have significant mood and anxiety disorders—even with strong family histories of postpartum depression—can be helped through the childbirth process. There is usually a way to do it, to get through pregnancy and childbirth while minimizing the risks of depression. And on top of this, there are ways to have a healthy baby. The numerous happy couples wandering through my waiting room (and those of thousands of other New Neuropsychiatrists) could not possibly be a coincidence: they no doubt reflect the growing success of our treatments.

So, for Marietta and Victor, for Hannah and Jorge, for Susan and Mark, and for Allen and Donna, treatment contributed to the development of each of their relationships in ways that I could not have possibly predicted. But *unpredictable* change, as we have seen, is key to successful New Neuropsychiatry treatments. Organic changes are often—perhaps usually—unpredictable. One common pathway, a humbling yet exhilarating one, is through the assumption of the complexities of parenthood.

Marietta

Marietta continued doing well off medicine until she was about seven months into pregnancy. Despite her cognitive therapy sessions, she felt increasingly moody and agitated and had difficulty sleeping.

She increased therapy sessions to twice, and then three times, a week. She was determined to try to stay off medication. Her obstetrician was concerned that Marietta wasn't eating enough or gaining enough weight, and gave her some nutritional supplements. Marietta kept to a strict regimen of getting enough sleep and exercise. She even bought a light box to try some home phototherapy, a treatment used for seasonal affective disorder. It was a struggle, but she was able to get through the pregnancy without medication.

One evening I got a call from Victor. "Things are getting a little exciting here," he said. He was at the hospital, and Marietta was in labor. "I didn't know if we'd make it here in time! Her water broke, she was having contractions about every three minutes, and I couldn't get hold of the car service!"

"But you're there now?"

"Yeah! And everything's OK. They figure she has about twenty, thirty minutes before we go into delivery."

"Well, keep me posted," I said.

"Yeah, gotta go!"

I had a feeling that everything would be all right.

Then, five days after baby Beatrice was born—healthy, squealing, at seven pounds, two ounces, already with wisps of curly red hair—Marietta had a sudden and severe drop in mood. She called me. All the old symptoms, she could feel them starting to roar back. She couldn't stop crying. She had frightening, irrational thoughts about hurting the baby. After a long talk, we decided that it was best if she returned to the Celexa.

Immediately she had to make a decision about breast-feeding, because there is evidence that the SSRIs may be excreted in breast milk and that the baby might, theoretically at least, be exposed to the medicine. We discussed pros and cons of checking levels of Celexa in her breast milk samples, even the possibility of taking blood samples from the baby. Marietta and Victor asked the pediatrician about the risks.

In the pediatrician's opinion, Celexa wasn't much of a risk because breast-fed babies so rarely get a significant level of SSRI medicine in their blood. So Marietta went ahead with breast-feeding and baby Beatrice showed no evidence of any bad effects. She had some irritability, true, but there was no way to tell if it was anything more than colic. Overall Beatrice was an easy baby, calm, with a good temperament. Or, as Victor put it, "A miracle child!"

Marietta continued on her Celexa over the next year, during which time, as I could see when she brought Beatrice with her, as far as anyone could tell they were both doing fine.

Hannah

Hannah felt good—scared, but happy. Actually, having made the decision, and being pregnant, she felt wonderful. Perhaps a surge of hormones or perhaps from knowing that she was indeed able to move forward to have the type of life she had always dreamed of, that she had feared she would never achieve. It was a wonderful time for Hannah.

Hannah stayed on Zoloft throughout what ended up being an uneventful pregnancy. There was some return of symptoms when she was about thirty-five weeks pregnant—requiring an increase in her Zoloft dose. This is not an uncommon effect when in the last few months of pregnancy, when there is often a lot of weight gain and water retention, diluting the SSRI.

I will never forget the way Hannah looked late in pregnancy, her face utterly radiant. Her belly enormous, she moved slowly, having difficulty walking into my office because her hips hurt, but she was glowing with excitement.

Hannah called me from the hospital the morning after her baby daughter, Julia, was born. She was exhausted: labor had lasted more than twenty-four hours and she had eventually been given a C-section.

"I'm doing okay," she said. "Mostly just uncomfortable. But I can't believe I have such a beautiful baby!"

After considering all the possible issues, she opted not to breast-feed.

She and Jorge hired a baby nurse for the first week after she returned home to take some of the stress off. After Julia was a few days old, Hannah started to have more side effects from the Zoloft (because the mother loses so much weight after childbirth, "enough" medicine may quickly become too much), so I told her to decrease the dose.

Baby Julia did well also. She seemed a bit jittery for her first week of life, but it was hard to tell if this was related to her exposure to the Zoloft or not. In any case, the pediatrician who followed her for her first five years of life felt that Julia was normal in every way that he could determine.

Hannah came in when Julia was about a month old. She had her in a Snuggli, curled peacefully against her.

"How are you feeling?" I said.

"Pretty good, consider that I'm not sleeping much." She felt "capable, not overwhelmed by anxiety." She had a "great feeling of being able to be there emotionally" for her baby. Indeed, disorder had not been banished, but it had been managed.

The Larger View

Mark brought Susan to one of his visits when she was five months pregnant, and he called me from the hospital after their baby, Caleb, was born. After which, nearly every visit he showed me baby pictures, pictures of Susan holding Caleb, pictures of the three of them: as if to continually remind both himself and me of the reality that life had finally delivered happiness to him. Allen and Donna had a healthy baby girl about two years after they got married, having gone through two cycles of in vitro fertilization.

From the narrow view, one could see each of these pregnancies as tales of managing disorder, making decisions, and minimizing risks. We followed a process of collaborative decision making, sharing knowledge, and weighing risks and benefits in a way that is essential to the New Neuropsychiatry.

In a larger view, these were the stories of couples who had moved from the quagmire of disorder and into recovery—back to the trajectory of normal life. Hannah for sure—her life had been transformed. Marietta and Victor. Allen and Donna. And Mark and Susan. They had all returned from the exile of disorder. After periods of suffering, self-absorption, and withdrawal, they had returned to the fold of normal human life. It was wonderful to observe.

This is the most gratifying part of a doctor's job: being able to help people move from disorder to a brand-new lease on life.

One other thought came to me one day when my waiting room was full of pregnant women and infants and toddlers and strollers: the neurobiological changes of becoming parents, and whether this too may facilitate brain recovery. With all its stresses, parenthood appears to enhance the sprouting of integrative fibers that connect the prefrontal cortex, the hippocampus, the anterior cingulate of the cortex, and other centers of the brain. In a wide range of animal species (including ducks and chickens and rats and rabbits), pregnancy induces brain reorganization, a process switched on by hormones including oxytocin.

While the precise chemical mechanism hasn't been delineated in humans (it is thought to involve a different hormone, vasopressin), I could only speculate about what I saw almost weekly with Hannah and Marietta—and from my discussions with Mark and Allen as well. At almost every visit, I observed new personality aspects, new capabilities coming to the fore. It was hard not to imagine that these changes involved a powerful process of brain reorganization, with the activation of chemical switches, and the sprouting of new neuronal connections.

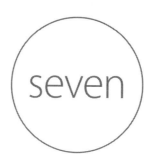

seven

Mapping the Route

From the Low Road to the High Road

"Should I kill myself today?"

ALL WAS NOT WELL in the waiting room. Just ask Lynette Linden. Especially the day that Cindy emerged with her twins, smiling and chatting with the receptionist and with other people in the lobby before she began wrestling them into the double stroller. Just one week earlier, Lynette had arrived while Hannah and Jorge were leaving my office and spending a long time putting on their coats and deciding where to go for lunch. Then—as today—Lynette observed every move.

"So, why is *she* here?" Lynette spoke as soon as the door shut behind Cindy. "She doesn't need treatment; she obviously doesn't have any problems. Just look at me, I think about suicide every day. After all these medicines, after all these years, and I'm still depressed. I'm never going to get better!"

Not that I could tell her anything about Cindy, but Lynette wouldn't have heard my response, anyway. She was too miserable. Lynette was new to my practice, but not new to psychiatric treatment. Did Lynette feel disappointed by the New Neuropsychiatry? Betrayed would be more accurate. Lynette had major depression with melancholia (symptoms including an inability to find pleasure in positive things combined with physical agitation, insomnia with early morning wakening, and feelings of guilt) that was recurrent and thus far was treatment-resistant. Such seeming inability to recover from an illness is called "refractory," because the disorder or disease seems to be stubbornly clinging to the person who has it.

She had first come to see me three months earlier, desperate to find some way out of the emotional quagmire that had enveloped her for more than twenty-five years. Her longtime psychiatrist, having exhausted his repertoire, was more than happy for me to try my hand.

So I had juggled her meds. After a few changes, Lynette was indeed somewhat better, less troubled by agitation, frequent waking, startle reactions, and continual feelings of hopelessness. But she was still not well. Many symptoms remained, albeit in a muted form.

Every day she asked the question, "Why should I live?"

Plus—here was the rub—even if we were able to get Lynette Linden to feel less anxious and depressed (not a sure thing, given that she had a history of numerous failed trials), she still was convinced that she had "missed the boat" in life. Lynette was 47 years old, so it was unlikely that she would ever have a biological child. Her career was stuck, and her family was scattered and had never been close. Worst of all, Lynette was alone; she was sure she'd never find somebody to love.

Lynette had first come for treatment when the SSRIs were brand new. The new medications had filled her with unaccustomed optimism. Could these miracle drugs lift her from a state of misery and fear? Could they help her achieve her dreams of running her own business, being happily married, and having three kids? That was many medications ago; now she would be glad to have a week without constant urges to overdose on alcohol and prescription drugs.

I wish that I could say Lynette was an atypical patient in my office these days, but the reality is, she isn't. There are many Lynettes. Even though New Neuropsychiatry treatments are more effective than ever, there are people who don't respond completely to them. Some have temporary improvement that slips away; others find that nothing gives much relief.

In some strange way, the mood and anxiety disorders themselves appear to be evolving along with efforts to treat them. Studies such as the STAR*D study of depression suggest that perhaps one-third of patients are now treatment resistant, as defined by lack of response to a full dose of an antidepressant medication. Like Mark Maple, Lynette initially had a terrific response to SSRI medicine, and after a few months of 20 mg/day of fluoxetine (Prozac), she had become calmer, happier, and more energetic—and was able to go back to school in computer sciences after a decade of waitressing. She got engaged, then married. Two or three months later, thinking she was "cured," she stopped her medicine. But the anxiety and depression returned. Her doctor restarted the SSRI. Lynette didn't get the same oomph, even though they increased the dose from 20 milligrams to 40, then finally all the way up to 80 milligrams per day. After each increase, she felt better for a while, but then symptoms would begin to return. He had then added Wellbutrin, a dopamine-enhancing drug, in an attempt to boost the SSRI medicine's effect, and again Lynette felt better for a short time. Shortly after her divorce was finalized, following three years of marriage, her agitation and sleeplessness returned yet again.

It was a series of battles, with victories that were hard-won yet temporary. Year after year, Lynette Linden and her doctor fought valiantly to regain the same familiar terrain, to find an elusive stable zone. Eventually, she decided to change doctors.

So here we were, after umpteen treatments, and Lynette was no better. Actually, on close examination Lynette *was* better—she definitely couldn't see going back to life before medicine and therapy. But she was not well. Plus, so much time had passed that Lynette was convinced that she would never make up for what had been lost.

Who could argue with the accuracy of Lynette's observation in the waiting room? Truly, something was different about Cindy and Allen and Mark, and my other patients who had achieved good outcomes relatively quickly. But what was it? And why hadn't Lynette responded? Most important, was there any way for her to obtain the same benefits that Cindy was obviously enjoying?

When All Else Fails

Paolo Omicron was another disappointed veteran of the New Neuropsychiatry. Like Lynette, he came to his first office visit clutching a list of all the medicines that had not worked. (Ironically, Paolo would have envied Lynette for her brief respites from depression: at least she experienced a few months of happiness! Lynette had tried perhaps six or eight medicines, whereas Paolo had tried more than two dozen with no success.)

Referred by a friend of his and a former patient of mine, Paolo trudged into my office one rainy March afternoon. He was 38 and had just lost his job in the film industry. He was married to a former graphic designer, had two kids to support, and the IRS was after him for unpaid taxes.

"Nothing works for me!" It was like a challenge for a duel. "I think I'm immune to drugs!" Currently he took four medications (Paxil 40 milligrams a day and Xanax, from 6 to 8 milligrams a day, as well as several pills a day of Restoril and Ativan)—impressive doses, yet ineffective against his disorder.

Medicines *ought* to help Paolo, but each night at 3 or 4 a.m. he would jolt awake, agitated and anxious, and all he could do was channel surf or browse the Web. His stomach continually churned, his hands were clammy, he couldn't concentrate, and nothing, absolutely nothing, gave him pleasure. Classic symptoms of major depression, chronic and severe.

Not only had medicine failed Paolo, but so had two attempts at cognitive-behavioral therapy, an approach that should have helped. He'd had good therapists, too, who knew what they were doing. In despair, he had even walked onto the Brooklyn Bridge more than once, just to "scout things out."

I must have looked alarmed at hearing this, because he quickly added, "Not that I would jump. I've never done anything to hurt myself. But it's there. It's a way out when I can't take things anymore."

Everywhere I looked, in my first meeting with Paolo, every corner of his life I peeked under, every question about his health or interests, seemed to uncover deeper reservoirs of misery. And indeed, after twenty or thirty minutes, I began to feel more than a little discouraged.

Haves and Have-Nots

Like it or not, in the New Neuropsychiatry, our world has become divided into haves and have-nots. The "haves" are those people, perhaps two-thirds of those with disorders, who are lucky enough to respond to treatment, achieve remission, and who may even proceed into the abovementioned state of post-disorder and work toward recovery. In New Neuropsychiatry, they could be referred to as being on the High Road. The "have-nots," unluckily, don't move on so easily. They engage in New Neuropsychiatry treatment—they take their medications faithfully and attend therapy just as regularly, they struggle just as much to get their stress levels down and their circadian rhythms reregulated. Yet their efforts go for naught. As Lynette so perceptively put it, "I'm at war with my brain!" Let's say that they are on the Low Road, not in recovery.

In thinking about the problem of treatment resistance, it is crucial to realize that the High Road and the Low Road are not just metaphors: research is also showing that they reflect different patterns of brain activity.

For people on the High Road, treatment response—the move from disorder into remission—appears to involve a process of brain repair, the activation of brain-healing compounds such as brain-derived neurotrophic factor, as I have discussed in Chapters 5 and 6. Furthermore, on the High Road, success reinforces its own trajectory. For example, the calmed-down brain makes it more possible for a person to get into and maintain good relationships. For Mark and Cindy, therapy and medicine worked to calm their jangled brain circuits. Once their brains were working better, their love relationships improved. And good interpersonal relationships have their *own* healing power in the brain!

As we've seen in Chapter 6, the High Road thus appears to be *literally* a higher road. We believe that it involves activation of pathways in the higher brain and normalization of activity of the prefrontal cortex and the anterior cingulate—the areas of planning and problem solving, of emotional and cognitive integration—and the ventral tegmental area, which releases dopamine to the pleasure center of the brain. By higher brain, I mean the parts of the brain involved with thinking as opposed to reacting. In other words, the process of responding to treatment in itself not only reduces anxiety and depression but also allows people to come up with better solutions to life's problems and to take more joy from their day-to-day existence.

The Low Road also winds through the brain, involving overactivation of lower brain centers, the parts that react to perceived threats and that are the most active during fight or flight. Treatment nonresponders appear to live in a chronic state of limbic activation, in which their lower brain centers call the shots, causing fear, sadness, pain, and guilt. Daily life is dominated by discharges of fear chemicals from the amygdala. When the amygdala rules, the adrenal glands (perched atop the kidneys) actually grow in size, and shoot out high levels of steroid hormones. The hippocampus shrinks; the medial prefrontal cortex and cingulate—the brain's integrative centers—become relatively less active, unlike on the High Road. Other parts of the brain likely have to work overtime to make up for these deficits, leading to exhaustion and discouragement. Worse, for some people the only things that relieve feelings of distress may themselves cause further problems. Compulsive eating can make a person feel better temporarily, as may compulsive shopping, or sex, or gambling—or large amounts of alcohol or marijuana. Compulsive behaviors *do* temporarily calm the brain—but at the expense of you as a person.

So, I could not disagree with Lynette or Paolo and could not attribute their observations to the excessive pessimism of the depressed. Lynette and Paolo rightly observed themselves as stuck in a quagmire of suffering. Whereas with the High Road the brain appears to be regenerating and reconnecting again, with the Low Road, there is the risk of disorder settling into the lower brain, strengthening its hold. Over time, anxiety and fear can become givens. Extreme avoidance and withdrawal can become the norm. Even medical problems can worsen—because, as we have discussed, depression is bad for the body, not just the mind. In the worst case scenario, disorder not only remains: it threatens to become disability.

For a New Neuropsychiatrist, the fundamental question is: why do some people not respond to treatments? To date, we have only the broadest clues of what factors—biological, psychological, behavioral, and genetic—explain this. Beyond that, is it possible to help people to escape from the Low Road, even after years of ineffective treatment, after years of suffering? If so, how? What can work? This is the challenge.

If you have a refractory disorder, the question is personal: *can* you get better? If so, how? What will work for you? How can current knowledge from research and practice help this recovery process occur? What can you do to help yourself?

Hope versus Gullibility

Twenty-five years ago, in the waning days of the Old Psychiatry, one of my favorite residency supervisors used to tell patients who had not gotten better, "We'll keep trying. Don't give up. There are new treatments coming out all the time."

As a young doctor-in-training, I thought this advice seemed at best dubious, even self-serving. Why not just level with patients and tell them the truth, however harsh? "You're not getting better. There's nothing more we can do for you."

Options in Treatment-Resistant Depression

If you have tried one—or maybe several—types of medications and are still stuck in a disordered state, you might be wondering what your options are. Psychopharmacologists have vastly greater choices than our predecessors of twenty-five or thirty years ago. There are now so many medications that few people can honestly say, "I've taken everything," almost no single doctor can know them all. Strattera, lamotrigine, pregabalin, new nonamphetamine stimulants—the *Physician's Desk Reference* (PDR) is stuffed with intriguing new medications. Many people with depression who got little benefit from SSRIs do respond well to agents such as Wellbutrin or Remeron or to dual-mechanism antidepressants like venlafaxine or duloxetine or desvenlafaxine. Recent studies of nonresponders (e.g., at Massachusetts General Hospital, Columbia, and other leading research centers) show that most depressed or anxious people, no matter how treatment resistant, *will* eventually respond to treatment—after the second, third or fourth trial of medication. Basic pharmacological principles work for the vast majority of people: give enough medicine for enough time and most disorders will respond.

Some researchers have developed flowcharts to guide doctors through this maze. John Rush, MD, a psychiatry professor at the University of Texas, and his colleagues developed the Texas Medication Algorithm Project (TMAP), which includes a multistep guide for treatment of resistant depression. Sometimes this requires higher doses of medicine, or adding more medications, but sometimes it means cutting out extraneous medications and adding new therapy approaches instead. Few people go through to the last phase without improvement. In the TMAP and other similar approaches, if several trials of single medicines don't work, then combinations of two antidepressants are often tried. Other medicines can be added to antidepressants—lithium, thyroid hormone, buspirone, amphetamines, or modafanil. Recently, the "atypical" antipsychotic medicines Abilify, Seroquel, and Zyprexa have been shown to help treatment-resistant depression.

In some situations, with appropriate discussion of potential risks and benefits, and close monitoring, the dose of medicine can be increased above the usual PDR-recommended range—for instance, some people respond to doses of Celexa or Prozac over 100 mg/day, whereas the PDR recommended maximum doses are 60 mg/day and 80 mg/day respectively. When side effects get in the way of treatment response, dosage can be adjusted; if a medicine can't be changed, other medications can be used to treat side effects (Inderal for tremor, Viagra or Cialis for sexual side effects, etc.). Sometimes combined medicine and psychotherapy may help lead to better outcome. Both individual and group therapy can be helpful, as well as self-help programs such as Freedom from Fear (www.freedomfromfear .org) or the Mood Disorders Support Group (www.mdsg.org).

Beyond the various medication options, we have unconventional choices. We can use enhancements of omega-3 fatty acids, which have been shown to be helpful for mood stabilization. Phototherapy—exposure to bright lights that mimic the sun—is a treatment that can help seasonal affective disorder.

In some instances, hospitalization may be necessary. Brain stimulation treatments, including modified forms of electroconvulsive treatment, or ECT, as well as newer approaches like transcranial magnetic stimulation, or TMS, have also been shown to be helpful. Helen Mayberg, MD, PhD, has even shown that implanting electrodes in the brain for deep brain stimulation can help severe treatment-resistant depression.

There are also a wide range of new medications currently in development that work by radically different mechanisms. They include

► *Glutamate blockers*: Glutamate is a neurotransmitter that, in small doses, helps the brain by sending out signals that aid in memory and learning. When the level of glutamate is too high, it can kill brain neurons. So blocking it is hoped to keep such damage from occurring and possibly restore the brain to earlier functions. (See the discussion on Cindy and glutamate in Chapter 6.)

► *GABA agonists*: GABA—gamma-aminobutyric acid—is a one of the main neurotransmitters of the brain. Many antianxiety and anticonvulsive medications, such as barbiturates, are "agonists" of it; that is, they increase the amount of it available in the body. Researchers are always looking for new applications of these drugs.

► *CRF receptor blockers*: CRF—corticotropin-releasing factor—is a hormone released in times of stress. It is well known that such stress hormones affect both physical and mental well-being. Blocking CRF could be helpful in reducing the effects of stress on the body.

► *NK1 antagonists*: Substance P is a short-chain peptide that plays an essential role in transmission of pain impulses. Neurokinin antagonists block NK1, which is the brain's main receptor for Substance P, and have been shown to have antidepressant activity.

continued on page 68

> - *Melatonin agonists*: Melatonin is a hormone secreted by the pineal gland that regulates the sleep-wake cycle. Drugs that increase the activity of melatonin receptors and also interact with the serotonin system through the $5HT2_C$ receptor, appear to have antidepressant effects and are currently under study.
> - *Cannabinoid receptor blockers*: The body's cannabanoid system, particularly the cannabanoid type 1, or CB1, receptor, has been discovered involved in memory and emotion, as well as motivation, pain sensation, and hormone secretion. Drugs that block this system have been demonstrated to decrease appetite, craving for cigarettes, and possibly to have mood effects, though the one drug studied most to date, rimonabant, helped with weight loss but actually made depression worse! However, other drugs in this class might be antidepressants.
>
> It is likely that in a few years we will have significantly wider options. Some new medicines emerge from FDA approval processes, and others are spillovers from other medical specialties, especially from neurology, where it seems as if practically every new anticonvulsant medication finds a place in psychiatry. And who knows? Things that we haven't even thought of yet may provide another breakthrough in aiding people in treating disorders.

Now, more than two decades later, there is a new generation of treatment-resistance and psychiatrists are hard-pressed to give answers to relieve suffering. There is a crucial difference now, however. In the Old Psychiatry, "hope" was like a Hail Mary pass in the final seconds of the Rose Bowl when you are down by a touchdown with the ball on your ten-yard line. Sure, you *might* connect, it isn't impossible that you can win. Just highly unlikely. With the New Neuropsychiatry, the hope of helping you recover is increasingly based on knowledge. We have better data on treatment-resistant depression. We have more treatment options. And we have learned about the underlying biology of depressive illness and recovery. As time passes, as our research advances, we are certain to learn much more.

It is also becoming increasingly clear that there are ways you can avoid being set on the Low Road for a lifetime, ways you can interrupt the pathway to chronicity. Some of them are simple, reflecting rules from Pharmacology 101, and the importance of returning to basic principles:

- Get full treatment of your disorder.

- Get your symptoms under full control.

- Stay on medication (or in psychotherapy) long enough to go into remission: take enough medicine for a long enough period of time.

- Make whatever possible lifestyle changes to further reregulate your systems.

Current research confirms these points. As simple as they may seem, these suggestions are hardly trivial. As William Carlos Williams wrote in "Asphodel, that Greeny Flower,"

> It is difficult
> to get the news from poems,
>   yet men die miserably every day
>   for lack
> of what is found there.

The same in a sense is true for the New Neuropsychiatry.

Many so-called treatment-resistant cases are actually cases in which a person took an inadequate dose of medicine or quit treatment way too early. But what about when someone *did* take enough medicine for enough time? Paolo and Lynette certainly had done so. Then a fuller reassessment may be indicated, and we may need to think more broadly about how to use the key principles of the New Neuropsychiatry to achieve a response. Treatment resistance is clearly complicated—and we are just beginning to understand that genetic and other factors may be involved.

These days, we think of disorder as a state of the brain with overactivation of particular brain centers, pathways, genes, neurochemicals, and so on and underactivation of others. If a treatment-resistant disorder is an especially persistent and destructive example of these abnormal patterns, then it stands to reason that there must be things that maintain this abnormal state. These can include, put broadly, how you live your life, including thoughts and behavior patterns. Some people are at more risk for developing treatment resistance based on their genes, as we have seen. You can't do much to select

Possible Genetic Reasons for Lack of Response to Treatment

Why do some people seem not to respond as easily to medication as others do? Why do some people succumb to life stresses that others might shrug off? Intriguing New Neuropsychiatry research suggests a number of other common reasons for lack of response to antidepressant and antianxiety treatments and for other questions that have perplexed psychiatrists for decades. Here are just a few of them.

An entire field of pharmacogenetics is emerging, which has already provided insights into possible reasons for nonresponse. Nonresponse may occur because your liver metabolizes antidepressants quickly, causing very low blood levels despite normal doses. Conversely, slow metabolism may cause very high blood levels, and increased side effects with normal doses. The liver's ability to metabolize drugs, through its P450 enzymes, varies greatly from one individual to the next. P450 liver enzyme tests are now available to evaluate the activity of an individual person's drug-metaboliz-ing enzymes, thought they are not yet widely used in practice.

Genes may determine one's likeliness of responding to a given antide-pressant, as well as one's resilience—one's ability to cope with life stress. The brain chemical serotonin is inactivated by being transported into brain cells by what is called the serotonin transporter, or the 5HT-T system. The 5HT-T system can be slightly different between one person and another, based on their genes. Avshalom Caspi and colleagues' study of this system showed that people who have certain types of the serotonin transporter gene (a variant with a "short arm") had more depression and suicidality than people who had two copies of the long arm transporter. So, depending on

new genes at this point; you are stuck with what you inherited from your parents.

But you *can* work to change your thoughts, attitudes, behavior patterns, social interactions, levels of activity, physical health, use of substances, and so on. This will allow you to turn *on* healthier genes and turn *off* genes that are less healthy. Behavior changes the expression and activation of genes in your brain and the levels of various hormones, neurotransmitters, and brain growth factors, as well as the level of activity of different brain centers. If Low Road circuits are dominant and you are trying to reactivate High Road circuits, whether you have genes for the transporter with a short arm, long arm, or one of each, your reactions to life stress can vary greatly.

Other studies show that disorders may be more diverse than we usually think. Genetic studies show that there is no single gene for depression or for the anxiety disorders and that a variety of gene types, which affect very different parts of the brain, may be associated with a higher risk of developing depression. Thus, an antidepressant that works for one person may not work for another because the underlying biology of their disorders may differ. For one person, an SSRI may help to get the hypothalamic-pituitary-adrenocortical (HPAC) stress-response system back in order, and the subsequent growth of new cells in the dentate gyrus of the hippocampus may allow for relief of cognitive symptoms. For another person, the same medicine may have a very different effect on their brain. Similarly, for some people, gene types might explain why psychotherapy works well, or not at all.

Finally, there may be subtle effects of different medicines on different parts of the brain. New data suggest that the SSRIs have powerful effects on the hippocampus, but less impact on the prefrontal cortex. They cause almost no regrowth in that area. In contrast, mood stabilizers, such as the mineral lithium and the anticonvulsant mood stabilizers (such as Depakote)—do cause regrowth in the prefrontal cortex. Perhaps, depending on your type of depression, this explains why an SSRI alone won't do it for you, no matter high the dose. Perhaps another class of medicine must be added: maybe a touch of Depakote or lithium will lead to remission.

your involvement in changing thought and behavior patterns is essential. This explains why so much of my work with Lynette and Paolo involved changes in their activities, behaviors, and patterns of thinking. Psychotherapy is particularly helpful for many cases of treatment-resistant disorders, and so are exercise, learning, socialization, and nutrition—all of these can be seen as ways to break the dominance of Low Road circuits and to open the closed loop of failed thought patterns and emotions.

Treatment resistance requires pulling out all the stops, considering all possible tools and options, and making a concerted effort to get unstuck.

206 Heal Your Brain

All Hands on Deck

So what can be done? If your problems seem to resist treatment, what will help? Is it possible to move from the Low Road to the High Road and to find your stable zone? What could I do with Paolo and Lynette to help them out of the quagmire? Would it be possible to help them get back onto the High Road and heading toward recovery?

The key to getting out of the quagmire is "you" and "me" and "them." "You" the patient, "me" the doctor, and "them" being your family and friends. Getting out of the quagmire is more difficult than beginning treatment, because many prior efforts—often by good doctors and therapists—have already failed. Sure, sometimes it is as simple as making the right diagnosis or adding a new medication. But even if there is a diagnostic or medication breakthrough (as happened with both Lynette and Paolo, as you will see below), getting out of the quagmire is still going to involve a campaign—an ongoing process of hard collaboration. No matter how much a new medicine might help, it will just be the first step.

At this point it is essential to put everything on the table. Knowing what has failed is not enough, however. What is more important is knowing what has been partially successful. Putting together several approaches that each helped a little, or helped temporarily, can be the key to escape from the Low Road.

It is essential to look over the map of your life.

Reviewing the Map

On a practical level, I ask people whose disorder is treatment resistant to bring in a detailed flowchart, to include all the therapy approaches they have had, medication types and doses, benefits and side effects, and to graph major life issues at different times. Beyond that, a flowchart of their life, with milestones, events, moves, losses, and accomplishments.

What do I look for as I review these maps? I seek clues to disorder, hints of what might perpetuate their trajectory on the Low Road, and suggestions of shortcuts upward—as in the children's game Chutes and Ladders—to the High Road.

Lynette

Lynette Linden brought in a timeline drawn across four taped-together sheets of letterhead. Before the age of 21, she had been a happy and gregarious person. Then came a cruel blow. A stranger broke into her off-campus apartment, held a knife to her throat, and threatened to kill her. She had gone to the student health services and to the police, reported the rape, and even moved to a new part of town. She fell into a depression, and her friends convinced her to go to the university counseling services, where she received a few sessions of psychotherapy but soon dropped out.

Over time, she fell into a habit of eating compulsively to "feel better" (mostly donuts and cookies and other carbs) and gained twenty-five, then thirty, then forty pounds. To lose weight, she began exercising regularly, even obsessively—whether running at the gym or, more recently, on a treadmill at home. In her late 20s, she started medicine, which initially was helpful.

She graphed it all out: her initial good responses to medicine, which then—time after time—petered out. Things took a turn for the worse when she was in her late 30s, when she was accosted near her apartment, pulled into a park, and robbed. She got away without physical injury but was again traumatized. Her timeline showed increasing cycles of misery and isolation, and her gradual decline into a joyless life of fearfulness and isolation. These days, she rarely left her apartment except to go to work, to visit her elderly grandfather, or to go to an appointment.

Why didn't the New Neuropsychiatric treatments help Lynette? I had to think of every possibility. If medicines weren't helpful, why would Lynette even have had an initial response? Beyond that, once she *did* feel better, why didn't the response stick? When I had first heard Lynette's story, I wondered whether her liver was the culprit. Some people are "fast metabolizers" of SSRI medication and may need whopping doses. But as she talked, as we reviewed her timeline and life history, the situation became clear. Her previous doctor and I had been treating her for depression and binge eating disorder, but she had a complicating condition—posttraumatic stress disorder (PTSD)—which was set off by the rape nearly twenty-five years ago and worsened by the second attack fifteen years later.

No matter what we did with medication, her brain still seemed to be stuck in a disordered, traumatized state, her amygdala firing, causing startle reactions and intense fear of any close human contact. In talking to Lynette, it became clear that, other than seeing her work colleagues, doctors, and grandfather, she was incredibly isolated. There were almost no other people in her life—following her various traumas, she had lost touch with most friends from childhood. Though she was once active in her community, after the second attack Lynette had ended all nonwork socializing. The fact is, her life *was* depressing. Not surprisingly, given her confinement and isolation.

How could we activate a recovery process for Lynette? The therapy she'd had in the past hadn't helped much. She probably needed an approach more specific for the treatment of PTSD, namely, exposure therapy. Some medication changes might be useful. Whereas increasing her SSRI dose just made Lynette more anxious and agitated, perhaps by decreasing the dose I could find the lowest amount needed to prevent her from becoming depressed. And perhaps I could add a second medicine to help with her anxiety and binge eating, Topamax, an anticonvulsant that also has antianxiety and antibingeing effects. To get off the Low Road, Lynette would need to find room for people. Calming her amygdala circuits with medicine wasn't going to be enough.

This was not what Lynette wanted to hear: she clearly wanted a new miracle drug. And she expressed more than a little dismay when I began to ask her, How could you bring more people into your life?

Our plan? Referring her for exposure therapy for PTSD and to a therapy group for rape survivors. I could help her find a therapist who specialized in this condition, who could help her to tolerate exposure exercises, including eventually going back to the places where the attacks had occurred. On the medication front, I recommended making the changes mentioned above. Given Lynette's preoccupation with suicide, it is important to note that mood stabilizers have been shown to decrease suicidal ideas and behaviors (if Topamax didn't stop these ideas, we could always try lithium, which has been shown to have antisuicide effects). Then there was the issue of physical activity, always key for people who have treatment-resistant disorders. It was great that Lynette already liked to exercise, but wouldn't it make more sense for her to exercise with other people? Getting her to go to the gym several times a week would be pointless unless there was something she enjoyed there. Were there any sports that she liked?

Put on the spot, Lynette flushed. I could tell that she was accustomed to her routines and that it irked her to think of changing. But now she allowed a glimpse of a smile.

"Volleyball," she said. "I used to play in college." She had been co-captain of her college intramural team many years ago. Dubious, Lynette agreed to the medication changes. She agreed to the referral for exposure therapy and (reluctantly) to check out the rape survivors group. She even agreed to go to the local gym "once" to look over the volleyball situation. She was willing to give these approaches a try "for a few months," though her expectations were low.

The way that I began to know that Lynette's new plan was working was that a month later, on her own initiative, she came in to session with a new roadmap of her life—looking ahead, not backward. Nothing complicated: it was the volleyball schedule for the coming season. For volleyball nights, she had arranged with a cousin to check up on her grandfather. With the medication changes, she was feeling better and had nearly stopped bingeing on carbs. But she'd been at this point enough times before that she refused to get her hopes up. Curiously though, she hadn't thought of suicide in weeks.

Paolo

Paolo's life map was an Excel spreadsheet, recording his "miserable so-called existence" over the past decade. He too had plenty of pills. Whereas Lynnette's doctor tended to change from one medicine to another, Paolo's doctor merely bumped up the doses of Xanax and Paxil and Ativan and Restoril—so much that Paolo had become "out of it"—lethargic and overweight. His concentration was zilch—maybe from the high doses of sedatives or from hippocampal damage thanks to chronic stress. On his timeline, it was clear that ever since the Xanax dose was increased above 3 or 4 milligrams a day, a strange thing had happened. Instead of being calmed, Paolo found himself living life from one Xanax to the next—riding a roller-coaster, sedated one moment, agitated the next. Now he was so knocked out that he had nearly fallen asleep a few times while driving—yet, paradoxically, was so anxious that he could never relax. At night, he clenched his jaw, grinding his teeth, and had even cracked two molars because of this incredible tension. Underneath Paolo's lethargy, he was deeply depressed and agitated. Clearly his amygdala was still calling the shots!

Paolo's case reflects a common situation: the poor treatment response of patients who have anxious depression. In the STAR*D study, many of the more than 30 percent of patients who did not respond to any of the study's four levels of treatment had anxious depression. Something might be different about people who have these conditions, and various treatments have been shown to help.

The question was how would we get Paolo off of his roller coaster, out of his seemingly inexorable downward cycle?

It seemed clear to me on going through his timeline that Paolo's depression had never been brought into remission. His "vegetative symptoms" of sleep disturbance, poor concentration, increased appetite, and so on, had never been controlled. His doctor had been fooled by the anxiety symptoms and had given him only modest antidepressant dosages while loading on the antianxiety meds. But in my view, Paolo's anxiety symptoms were only one component of a severe melancholic depression, which had never fully responded to treatment.

We decided to pick one antianxiety medicine (Klonopin, which is long-acting and unlikely to lead to addiction) and to gradually eliminate the Xanaxes and Ativans and Restorils, his host of other antianxiety meds. We would switch to one of the serotonin-norepinephrine reuptake inhibitors (SNRIs) and gradually increase the dose. Why an SNRI? This class of medicine works on two transmitter systems, both serotonin and norepinephrine, and is highly potent—and has been shown to help people who haven't responded to SSRIs alone. For Paolo, this was to mean the SNRI medicine Cymbalta up to 120 mg/day. This required checking his blood pressure on a regular basis, because high doses of SNRIs can cause hypertension.

My solution was not just a matter of changing medications. That was necessary but hardly sufficient. For, one thing had to be taken into account: the thing that was generating all these symptoms—his extreme anxiety and agitation. In recent years, Paolo's conscious mental life was dominated by a stream of continual negative thoughts. Similar to Allen (who also had intrusive negative thoughts), Paolo was convinced that he was worthless, a "loser," and that he would never get better, he would never get anywhere in life. For the past two years, such thoughts were almost continuous. Beyond that, though, Paolo had severe *physical* agitation: you could say that his depression lived in his body. His stomach, his back, his neck, his head, his jaw—he experienced stress and fear throughout his body, which in turn increased his hopelessness and depression. These symptoms just confirmed that he was "falling apart."

Paolo needed to gain control of his mind and his body. Was there some way for him to diminish this torrent of self-criticism, and to calm his body's stressed-out condition?

Adding even more medications seemed unlikely to do the job, indeed, was likely to be counterproductive. Instead, I suggested that Paolo could benefit from physical and mental approaches to help him to increase self-regulation and self-calming. There was no guarantee these approaches would help, but it didn't seem that there was much risk to trying them. Yoga, meditation, exercise—he needed to find something visceral, something intense.

Over the next several sessions, Paolo came back with one book after another, with printouts from WebMD and the Mayo Clinic Web site and online book reviews.

"What about mindfulness?" he asked me one day.

Mindfulness is a meditation-based form of stress reduction derived from Buddhism and yoga. It uses meditation exercises to create a heightened awareness of the present moment and experiences. Studied since the late 1970s by Dr. Jon Kabat-Zinn and colleagues at the University of Massachusetts Stress Reduction Clinic, it can be a powerful way for depressed people to calm their overactive minds.

I taught Paolo diaphragmatic breathing (for more on this, see Chapter 3), and brought his wife, Stella, in as well, both to educate her about depression and to encourage her to push Paolo to get involved in a yoga or meditation class at their local health club. But clearly that wasn't going to be enough: so I referred Paolo to a local cognitive-behavioral therapy institute for mindfulness training and cognitive therapy.

And then, we waited. Paolo saw his CBT therapist for about twenty weekly sessions, faithfully kept his "thought logs" and practiced mindfulness exercises, and then went back for regular check-ups. He and Stella went to a weeklong mindfulness retreat, which helped them master and practice mindfulness techniques.

Over the next several months, I was privileged to observe the awakening of Paolo. There were some tense moments as the Xanax cleared from his system, as he felt a rush of "rebound" anxiety. I got a number of weekend and late-night phone calls. And yet, only one month into treatment, he noted that his concentration was improving and that he was no longer procrastinating on important projects at work. Though fearful that the SNRI medicine would lead to more side effects, Paolo was relieved when his appetite decreased and his sexual dysfunction improved as well. He religiously practiced mindfulness exercises twice a day. He wasn't a fan of yoga classes, but many years ago having been on a high school swim team, he decided to try swimming again. Swimming, he said, gave him the same meditative effect as yoga.

Increasing Resilience

In their 2004 book *The Peace of Mind Prescription*, Dennis Charney and Charles Nemeroff talk about the crucial topic of resilience—how people can deal positively with stressful events and thrive despite various threats and challenges. They review the broad range of research on this topic and suggest strategies by which people can increase their resilience to better cope with stress. These are particularly relevant for people who have treatment-resistant depression and anxiety disorders. According to Charney and Nemeroff, resilience has four components, or "pillars": (1) physical resilience; (2) psychological resilience; (3) one's social world; and (4) one's set of external supports.

Physical resilience: Charney and Nemeroff say that, "regardless of age or physical condition, people can improve their resilience by taking simple steps such as eating well, exercising, getting enough sleep, and avoiding excessive use of alcohol and other recreational drugs. Aerobic exercise, for instance, reduces cortisol, raises testosterone, improves insulin function, and alters a variety of brain chemicals in ways that improve mood."

Psychological resilience is related to two key factors: appraisal and the sturdiness of one's world view. The concept of appraisal struck home for a man I was treating named Paolo when he read the book, particularly the sentence, "Generally speaking, adverse events can be viewed as either threats or challenges." A situation that is viewed as a threat, "elicits fear, apprehension, anxiety, and defensiveness." In contrast, "Situations viewed as challenges . . . have quite different hormonal and emotional qualities. Challenge implies the possibility for growth or gain, and the emotions surrounding a challenge are often positive." These include senses of excitement and eagerness to face a new situation. "The hormones release by an appraisal of challenge include growth factors, insulin, and other compounds that promote cell repair, trigger relaxation responses, and stimulate efficient energy use." Paolo particularly related to one paragraph of *The Peace of Mind Prescription*, in which the authors note that people who see life stresses as threats (rather than challenges) "will erode their resilience by constantly engaging defensive bodily responses, which are biologically taxing." Effective coping can thus be enhanced by learning to turn threats into challenges.

In the *social world,* having at least one confiding relationship and working to develop a network of friends and family are key to resilience.

Finally, adequate *external supports* (including money, education, food, clothing, and shelter) are essential. (These days one should also add health insurance, disability insurance, and savings for retirement to Charney and Nemeroff's list.)

Becoming more resilient, in Charney and Nemeroff's view, includes several key factors, all of which are relevant to treatment-resistant disorders:
- Treating medical and psychological illnesses
- Treating substance abuse and addiction problems
- Exercising and eating right (including physical toughening and tempering through exercise)
- Taking time off
- Developing or preserving at least one confiding relationship
- Challenging one's self
- Looking for meaning through involvement in a cause larger than yourself
  I would add a fifth pillar, so to speak, to Charney and Nemeroff's list: *learning*. Learning new things—both about oneself (including about one's disorder) and about the world—seems likely to increase resilience. Learning about disorders clearly helps people to recover more easily, as any number of the people discussed in this book illustrate. Learning new things also is associated with better brain function over a lifetime and better health—and may help increase brain connections and possibly enhance brain recovery.

On one occasion he brought in a book by Dennis S. Charney, Charles B. Nemeroff, with Stephen Braun, *The Peace of Mind Prescription*, which he had found on the Internet and which he had evidently read closely, to judge from the enormous number of yellow Post-Its and underlined passages throughout.

"I think it's a problem of appraisal," he said to me.

"What do you mean?" I asked.

"Whenever I see something that is difficult, I see it as a stress, something that can hurt me, rather than as a challenge."

"And?"

"Well, in the book, they say that that sets off a whole range of different responses, which is exactly like what happens to me. That a threat causes a release of bad chemicals, and a challenge causes a release of good chemicals."

He had decided that swimming was going to be his way of trying to change threats into challenges, to try to teach his body to become calm again. And to increase his level of resilience.

Paolo began to swim regularly at the local Y. At first he could swim only two or three laps without collapsing in wheezes, but gradually his endurance improved, and by the end of the summer he was swimming more than two miles a day. He found studies on the Web about research on rats that showed that exercise increased neurogenesis in their brains, that its effect was additive to the effects of antidepressants. Between Paolo's jokes about being my laboratory rat, he reported that his stomach stopped cramping and churning for the first time in nearly a decade. And the Brooklyn Bridge? Paolo "forgot" to walk near it, the idea of suicide becoming increasingly irrelevant as he reawakened from his prolonged limbo.

The Man Who Went to the Birds

Treatment resistance is complicated. Clearly, it often involves more than simple disturbances of serotonin, norepinephrine, or other brain chemicals, and just as clearly, successful treatment generally involves more than just adjusting medications. Often, thoughts and behavior patterns play a key role in maintaining a disorder that seems resistant to treatment—especially the enduring and pervasive ways of thinking and acting that we think of as personality, or personality style.

Kenneth was a prime example of the importance of personality style affecting response to treatment. He was a 66-year-old widower who had sunk into a state of severe and chronic depression following the death of his wife.

"Nothing will help," Kenneth firmly stated the first time we met, adding emphatically "I already tried that"—whatever "that" I might have suggested—"it didn't work."

This was basically correct, I realized, in reviewing his history: No matter what medicine Kenneth took, nothing helped, not even full doses of Effexor XR, one of the most powerful antidepressants. His doctor had put him on more than a dozen different medicines; typically, Kenneth took them for a few weeks, maybe a month, then stopped, convinced they were worthless. That was just the beginning: therapy had been even more of a failure.

How could a New Neuropsychiatrist help Kenneth? At first I had no clue.

Apparently, Kenneth had been successful for most of his life but had gone downhill when his forceful and personable wife, Velma, had died five years earlier. They had met as teenagers and had never been apart. Once she was gone, depression took over his life. He had never been an easy person—in fact he had never been close to his kids and had few friends, but now he became truly impossible: demanding, critical, nagging, dependent, indecisive, clinging, and suspicious—both afraid of being alone and impossible to be with. Though it was clear to his sons and their wives how much he was suffering, they also found him more insufferable than ever and had finally given up on him.

What could be done?

In reviewing Kenneth's life map, I tried to be guardedly optimistic. Kenneth was obviously in a state of grief and depression from having lost Velma—and enraged that she could have "left" him when she died. No doubt he had always been demanding and difficult—but most likely these traits became exaggerated as a result of his clinical depression. I had to remind myself of a New Neuropsychiatry truth—that personality traits worsened by mood disorders usually *improve* once the depression is adequately treated.

This was going to be a challenge. First, finding medications and therapy approaches to help Kenneth out of his depression. Beyond that, helping Kenneth find some way to rebuild his High Road brain—or, to be honest, to build it to begin with. Because, as I got to know him, it became clear that ever since his highly stressful childhood with minimal parenting, he had always struggled in life, depending heavily on his late wife, Velma. *She* had been his higher brain! First off, Kenneth needed to back off from his kids, to stop calling them night and day, and to find other social contacts, something to give his life meaning. However difficult, Kenneth had to leave his kids alone.

After careful review of his previous medication treatments, it was clear to me (as an intrepid New Neuropsychiatrist) that medication had been *partially* helpful. On Effexor XR, on Prozac, on Paxil, Kenneth grudgingly admitted that sleep was "a touch" better; his concentration was "maybe not so bad." Possibly he had felt more energetic, and on a few days, even his mood was "not exactly terrible—maybe a little bit lifted." His previous doctors heard Kenneth's vociferous complaints about each medicine and apparently conceded defeat time after time, quickly switching to another medication, only to conclude that that one was no good either. Had his doctors just given up too soon, before fanning the embers of response by increasing dosage? Before trying supplementation with a second medication? Or just by persuading him to wait for further benefits?

Kenneth's transformation occurred in slow motion. With an antidepressant and a low dose of an atypical antipsychotic medication (several have been shown to help treatment-resistant depression), Kenneth gradually began to emerge from hopelessness. He reluctantly attended a bereavement group at his local Y—which, as he told it, consisted of widows berating their late husbands and mothers mourning children who died tragically young. Kenneth quickly fled this group—but rather than merely returning to his Barcalounger and his *New York Times* crossword puzzle, he became involved in a volunteer program for retired executives who helped underprivileged children.

"It's okay," he said—high praise from Kenneth. "At least we're not yammering. We're doing something."

Volunteering allowed Kenneth to back off from his family. As painful as it was, he gave his sons space. After months of self-imposed isolation, Kenneth was astonished to receive a phone call from Steffi, one of his daughters-in-law, asking if he would feed their twin parrots while she and his son were on vacation. "What, they can't pay someone to do it?" Kenneth asked. But he dropped by their apartment each day to feed the birds—that vacation and the next one as well. Feeding the birds was the sum total of his contact for months. Gradually, over a year or more, his depression lifted and even went into remission. Over that time Kenneth developed a relationship with his daughter-in-law. It was low-key, even cool. He struggled to hold back, to not appear overly needy. Over time, Steffi opened up to Kenneth, talking about work problems, issues with her parents. After the birth of their second child, Kenneth was surprised and gratified when they asked him to lead the baby's naming ceremony.

In watching Kenneth's life come back together—or more accurately, come together—I observed the disappearance of a cranky curmudgeon and the emergence of a thoughtful, kind, and interesting (though quirky) person—the late repair of a personality that had been damaged by ongoing depression.

Patricia

Then there was a woman I will call Patricia. Patricia came for her consultation with a large round hatbox of pills: Zoloft, Zyprexa, Ativan, Neurontin, plus St. John's wort, ginkgo biloba, ginseng, valerian, and melatonin. In all, there were eighteen drugs, herbs, and supplements, a virtual pharmacy of despair.

A tall, thin, blonde who still looked like the model she had once been—and who now worked as a paralegal in a midtown firm—Patricia was outwardly stunning. In reality, her life was chaos. Beyond dreadful mood and poor sleep, Patricia also had a pattern of bingeing on high-carb foods, not unlike Lynette. But there was one crucial difference: whereas Lynette often *thought* of suicide but had never done anything injurious, Patricia had hurt herself numerous times. Often when upset, Patricia would cut her wrists or abdomen with a razor blade. Twice she had taken serious overdoses, ending up in emergency rooms having her stomach pumped. These things were particularly likely to happen when she was ending relationships with men. Men were often initially attracted to Patricia only to flee when they found out how unstable she was.

Patricia's roadmap showed a difficult course. She had attempted suicide first in her late teens and again after her college boyfriend cheated on her. Since then, there had been more cutting and overdoses, a pattern of clinging to nasty guys. Her relationships had become increasingly chaotic, her suicide attempts more frequent and severe. Reviewing Patricia's map, I saw that personality—patterns of thought and behavior—played a key role in her suffering. Personality and biological depression, each worsened the course of the other. Treatment that focused only on treating Patricia's depression was doomed to failure.

The New Neuropsychiatry has a healthy respect for "personality"—when personality is thought of as sustained patterns of behavior, thinking, and ways of relating with other people. Clearly, personality can affect the outcome of treatment. Thirty years ago, in the days of the Old Psychiatry, we used to think of personality as "just" psychological. New Neuropsychiatry research shows that personality *isn't* just psychological. Personality is as driven by and determined by biology, by your genes, and by your brain chemistry as any mood or anxiety disorder. Repeated patterns of thinking and behaving and relating to other people are etched into the brain's circuitry.

Patricia clearly had borderline personality disorder (BPD)—a condition characterized by (as the DSM-IV puts it) a "pervasive pattern of instability of mood, interpersonal relationships and self image, beginning by early adulthood." Intense and unstable relationships; impulsive sexual activity, substance abuse, and binge eating; mood swings from high to low within a few hours; and frequent suicidal ideas or acts—Patricia had them all. Recently, fascinating MRI research studies have shown that people who have BPD have abnormal patterns of brain activity. Specifically, in BPD the amygdala, the center of their fear system, is set off by seeing *any* face, friendly, neutral, or unfriendly; whereas in people who do not have BPD, only threatening faces cause the amygdala to fire.

Threats everywhere, hyperawareness of rejection, intense neediness—Patricia fit many of these patterns. She frantically tried to avoid being alone at nights and on weekends. She was continually afraid that she would be abandoned by her boyfriends—which often became self-fulfilling prophecies.

While Patricia had some symptoms of depression, there was no need for her huge box of pills. A single SSRI should be sufficient.

The rest of the plan for Patricia? I would recommend that she find someone who practiced dialectical behavioral therapy. Also known as DBT, this approach was developed by researcher Marsha Linehan, PhD, specifically for BPD. Though Patricia had been in therapy for almost ten years, it was "insight-oriented" therapy with a psychologist who rarely spoke other than to make comments about her dreams—and hadn't led to much improvement.

DBT is a prime example of New Neuropsychiatry therapies. It is highly structured and specifically designed for the treatment of a particular disorder—in this case, borderline personality. It uses a combination of behavioral and cognitive approaches to decrease self-injury and suicidal behaviors, such as cutting and overdoses, often found with people who have these disorders.

Unlike Patricia's long-time therapist, her new DBT therapist, Dr. Chan, began by using practical methods to help her suppress her self-mutilating behaviors. Dr. Chan helped her find other types of behavior as alternatives to cutting herself and to avoid situations that would trigger her self-injuring impulses. DBT typically combines once-a-week individual psychotherapy sessions with once-a-week "skills training" groups. Group members learn new skills to regulate emotions and tolerate painful feelings and to find better ways to interact with other people. Dr. Chan gave her cell phone number to Patricia, so that if Patricia felt suicidal, she could contact her. "Aren't you afraid you're going to get calls all day and all night?" I asked. Dr. Chan assured me that this rarely happened, and she was sure that once things calmed down with Patricia, she would rarely be called.

Dr. Chan's first priority was helping Patricia bring the self-mutilation under control (at which point it is crucial for patients to keep diaries of their behavior and responses). The second stage was to increase her ability to experience emotions, both positive and negative, *without acting*. Third was to work on increasing her self-respect and on achieving her individual goals. And, finally, the last stage was to help Patricia to deal with common types of emotional quandaries faced by individuals with BPD: feeling incomplete, feeling disconnected from others, a lack of joy and meaning in life. It even focused on helping her to increase her feelings of spirituality.

Patricia Gets Better

Patricia struggled to get involved in treatment, missing sessions and complaining bitterly that Dr. Chan was "too bossy." But over time, she stopped cutting. She became less compulsive about buying and spending and did less bingeing on food. She began to quote a variety of Dr. Chan's aphorisms to me: "Resistance can become strength." "Boring can be good." "Fear can make you stronger and more resilient." She had always been unable to contain herself when upset and had been forced to act. Now she became able to wait until the storms of feeling subsided.

After two years, Patricia became involved in a relationship with Henry, an attorney at another law firm. At first the relationship seemed likely to go the way of her other ones—intense and passionate at first, then disappointing and extremely tumultuous. When Henry briefly started dating another woman, all hell broke loose. Patricia became distraught, overwhelmed by urges to cut. But with Dr. Chan's help, Patricia stuck it out and worked on "not cutting" and then on "staying in there" with Henry. It was difficult for her to resist the urge to phone him at any hour of day and night, but her DBT lessons came in handy. Eventually, to my surprise, Patricia and Henry got back together. Over several months their relationship became more serious, they got engaged, and about a year later, they married. She and Henry moved to the South, and I lost touch with her.

Recently, Patricia came back into town for a visit. She was had just had her second child and was doing well. She was more or less on the High Road. Like many other people who have BPD, successful treatment led to an improvement in the core symptoms of her disorders—both her personality disorder and her mood disorder.

"I have my hands full taking care of my house and working part-time and being a mom," she told me. She had read extensively about her condition, becoming somewhat of an expert on BPD and its treatment. "Is there such a thing as 'a recovering borderline'?" she asked. "That's what I think I am."

She took one or two 50-milligram pills of Zoloft a day—a modest dose, but enough to "take the edge off" her despair. While she occasionally felt an urge to cut, she was usually able to resist. And when she struggled with feelings of abandonment—when Henry was on an extended business trip halfway around the world—she was able to use DBT principles to calm herself.

Good Complexity

Particularly when we encounter people who have treatment-resistant disorders, the New Neuropsychiatrist is respectful of the power of thought and behavior patterns and of the complex way in which they weave into a person's personality and can influence the outcome of disorder. Not everything is immediately reducible to a handful of neurotransmitters; the maps and schemas of the mind are immensely powerful. This is the secret power of the New Neuropsychiatry: the ability to address persistent thought and behavior patterns as a way out of the quagmire of the Low Road.

The path to recovery is different for each person. The goal, though, is to find stability, then gradually to reintroduce complexity into a world that has been reduced to a terrible simplicity of suffering. Neuropsychiatry theorist Dr. Daniel Siegel talks about how "complexity theory" applies to the personality. Complexity theory is "a mathematical derived collection of principles governing the behavior of physiochemical systems, such as groups of molecules or patterns of clouds." In his view, as discussed in Chapter 6, complexity is the desired outcome of treatment, coming between the extremes of what he describes as rigidity and repression and chaos. Escape from the quagmire, the defeat of the tyrannical amygdala, requires a search for "good" complexity in life. This is what Kenneth and Patricia and Paolo and Lynette would each embody in different pathways to recovery. And for each of them, achieving complexity required activating the higher brain—both to help in taming the lower brain and in reengaging them in the satisfactions of life.

Paolo Emerges from the Quagmire

Over time, Paolo too emerged from his quagmire of major depression and oversedation. With medicine (Cymbalta and Remeron), mindfulness, and exercise, Paolo's mood and sleep finally came back to normal and his agitation faded. He cleared his desk at work and began buying new clothes to replace his worn and baggy outfits. In any case, he needed a new wardrobe, having lost almost twenty pounds, mostly thanks to regular swimming.

Swimming changed the shape of Paolo's body—and the patterns of his mind. When he came to sessions, he would describe his progress in mastering flip-turns and in implementing the Australian pattern of breathing every third stroke. A swimmer myself, I would appreciate the deep sense of calm that one could achieve by swimming lap after lap, the meditative rhythms of moving through the water. And I could appreciate that this was not just intense exercise: it also had the effects of increasing his serotonin and norepinephrine and testosterone levels, decreasing his cortisol, and boosting his neurotrophic chemicals.

Paolo became calm, alert, relaxed, attentive. For the first time in years, he could sleep through the buzzing of his alarm clock without medication; he no longer felt close to dozing off when stuck in traffic jams. Once Xanax and Restoril and Ativan had been eliminated, Paolo's concentration improved markedly and his short-term memory came back on line.

It was gratifying to watch Paolo as he began to get his life back in order. "Do you know how much I owe the IRS?" he asked me one visit. "I haven't filed my returns in six years!" (Actually, because his income had been so low, the IRS owed him a refund for at least two of those years). He began paying overdue bills and did a massive housecleaning, throwing out years worth of accumulation.

Lynette Finds her "Stable Zone"

Lynette went through the rigors of exposure therapy for PTSD, including confronting intense memories of her traumatic experiences and returning to the places where she had been attacked and doing desensitization exercises. She also faithfully attended a rape survivor's group for nearly a year. But the biggest change in her life was volleyball. Volleyball was the perfect game for Lynette—team-oriented, aggressive yet ultimately silly.

She started going out for beers after games with her team members and got to know Timothy, one of the other league coordinators. At first he annoyed her because he was constantly teasing her, like some eighth-grade kid.

"Maybe he likes you," I said.

"Are you kidding?" she responded, but then she conceded, "Well, maybe."

Gradually he began to show a romantic interest in her, which was terrifying to her and caused the reemergence of urges to flee. Luckily, Timothy was also in therapy and was patient with the feelings she was experiencing. A local businessman who owned a picture-framing store, Timothy was divorced, with joint custody of his teenage daughter. He was involved with his church and active in Alcoholics Anonymous, having been sober for more than a decade. At first Lynette didn't think he was her type. She gradually began to realize that, despite their differences, they were well matched.

Lynette's life got more complicated in a hurry once she met Timothy's daughter, and there were no shortage of crises and family dramas as Lynette and Timothy began to spend more time together. One spring, her grandfather had a stroke and was moved to a skilled nursing facility; Lynette was both devastated and relieved. Shortly afterward, she decided to move in with Timothy. Before her new treatment, she would have been shaken by such events and was always bracing for catastrophe.

"This is real life," I would tell her. "You can handle it. You're doing great."

"That's true," she would admit, "It's not exactly what I imagined, but it's pretty good."

She and Tim even began to talk about moving to the suburbs, then one visit she sprung the news: they had bought a house!

"Okay, I admit it," Lynette said one visit. "I don't think of suicide every day any more."

"That's so difficult to admit?"

"It felt like such a part of myself. 'I'm Lynette, should I kill myself?' And now I spend all my time at the design center, looking at floor tiles for our kitchen. And . . ."

"And what?"

"I'm having fun." She laughed. "The design center. Who would have imagined? So who has time to think about suicide?"

Enigmas of Nonresponse

The stories I've told in this chapter are ones of triumph over entrenched disorders, of cases in which recovery emerged from the thoughtful application of New Neuropsychiatry principles. However, not every case has a happy outcome, despite the best efforts of doctors, therapists, and patients. Sometimes this is for obvious reasons, but other times it is a mystery. Every psychiatrist knows of patients who seemed inevitably destined to commit suicide, no matter what interventions might be tried, and of people who have sunk back into depression despite the best treatments.

Recently the *New York Times* told the story of Steven Schnipper, a 56-year-old award-winning designer, who worked at prominent positions, including as executive director of design at Estee Lauder. In "A Life on the Decline, and Then the 'Why?'" the *Times* reporter describes how Schnipper's life went slowly awry in his 50s, apparently as a result of severe depression: he lost one job after another, developed severe financial difficulties, withdrew from his family and friends, and despite being in psychotherapy and taking antidepressant medications, ended up committing suicide. In explaining Uncle Steven's suicide to his four-year-old son, his brother Scott was able to say only that his brother had died "from a disease called depression."

Indeed, depression, especially treatment-resistant depression, can be a progressive and insidious illness. Paolo Omicron experienced the severity of this condition. After more than a decade of remission, his depression came back with a vengeance. It began after his wife became seriously ill—with multiple sclerosis—requiring huge financial and personal costs. It worsened when he required abdominal surgery and was unable to swim for several months. Not going to the pool seemed the least of his troubles at the time, but the return of his depression dated from that period. The crucial blow was when Paolo was diagnosed with Parkinson disease at the relatively young age of 50. All of these stresses overwhelmed Paolo, and he became profoundly depressed again. Despite numerous medication changes and intensive therapy, despite consultations with other doctors and even an inpatient stay, he has achieved only a few weeks or months of well-being, a tenuous state of existence. Indeed, he has emerged from his state of profound depression, but these days he cannot count on feeling good for any extended period of time. As far as I can tell, we've done everything right—and yet his disorder seems to overwhelm all of our current treatments. At present, possible choices include electroconvulsive treatment or other brain stimulation treatment—and if that does not work, possibly the implantation of electrodes for a course of deep brain stimulation. There are still other options to try, but it is hard to for him and his family to remain optimistic.

Think Forward

If you struggle with an ongoing disorder, perhaps these stories in general inspire some hope; and if you are early in the course of a disorder, these are cautionary tales. Surely you would want to avoid becoming as severely entrenched in disorder as Paolo or Lynette or Kenneth. Luckily, as I mentioned before, it is clear that there *are* ways to avoid becoming chronic. Some are simple medical truths: Get a full trial of treatment, get your symptoms under control initially, and then stay on medications (or in therapy) long enough to get solidly into a phase of recovery.

Beyond that, as we have seen in this chapter, New Neuropsychiatrists have an emerging understanding that there are ways to get out of the quagmire, to move out of chronicity, recurrence, and toward recovery.

I talked earlier (in Chapter 6) about the "stable zone." The concept was developed in treating bipolar disorder, describing the brain levels of glutamate as affected by lithium. I think it applies to all the disorders we've explored in this book, whether it might be depression or OCD or panic or bipolar disorder. Therapists need to work with you to do whatever it takes to get to a stable zone, whether it means starting therapy, adjusting the dose of medication, using several medicines together, combining medicine and therapy, or looking more broadly at how you live your life—and using all the tools that New Neuropsychiatry has at its disposal.

Even after Lynette and Kenneth and Patricia were well into recovery, we often returned to the map, retracing our steps, and to rethink where to go and how to get there. And equally important, how to *stay* there! (Or with Paolo, we searched the map for clues how to get back to that happier place). But even if we were tracing over the same increasingly tattered sheets of paper, we were actually looking at a different map. Initially, for each of them, the map was a closed loop, a hopeless portrayal of limbo. Once they were on the High Road, though, their map began to look forward, toward the future rather than the past.

Eventually I came to realize that we were looking at a map of their minds. Once it had been a map of the Low Road, with fear on one side and despair on the other and with chaos continually hovering overhead. When they first drew it, they had mapped the world from the Low Road, a world of limbo in which the limbic system rules. Now it had become a map of the High Road, a complex integrated system including left and right brain, associatively linking past and present, detail and narrative, mind and body. It was a recasting of the story of their lives and, perhaps, a remodeling of their brains. And such a remapping can also happen for you.

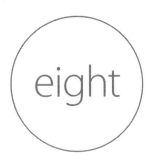

eight

Returning Home
Staying Well

A Renewed You

ABOUT 9 A.M. SATURDAY, after a busy week of work, you wake up feeling pretty good. Quite good, in fact. You had a decent night of sleep, and you have a busy weekend ahead: household stuff, your kid's soccer game, socializing with some friends, a few hours of preparation for an out-of-town meeting next week.

Overall, things are going well these days. You're feeling good, the family is fine, and the dark days, they're long gone. Occasionally there is a twinge of suffering, like a bad back acting up again—after stress at the job, at the change of season, or during a hard business trip. But overall, life is back in order. As much as you can expect these days, that is, with the world being the way it is.

In terms of the story of your life, the phase of disorder is moving into the past tense. "I went through a rough patch, a difficult time because of X, Y and Z." Or perhaps, as often happens, you hardly recall the details of the episode, it has largely faded from your awareness.

You get out of bed. You're starving, you need some coffee and breakfast. Then you will be ready to face the day.

At the table, there they are, next to your vitamins: the antidepressant meds.

The Safety Center

Columbia scientist Michael Rogan, PhD, and colleagues, including Nobel Prize–winning Eric Kandel, have investigated the powerful impact of the brain's safety system. Behaviorists like Ivan Pavlov and B. F. Skinner have long focused on danger—linking punishment with a signal, typically a musical tone or chord. Rogan has devised ingenious mouse experiments. In these studies, a mouse is put in a cage whose floor is electrically wired to deliver mild shocks. When shocked, a mouse responds by freezing, by hunkering to the floor, and by remaining motionless. If a sound, a tone, is played repeatedly just before the shock occurs, after a certain number of repetitions, the mouse learns to associate the tone with the shock. And if the tone alone is played (even without the shock being delivered), as any Psychology 101 student knows, the mouse will freeze, anticipating the worst. Neuroscientists have shown, not surprisingly, that this model involves activation of the brain's fear center, anchored in the amygdala—which can be confirmed by brain imaging studies (the amygdala and related areas light up, demonstrating increased blood flow). In such states, certain genes are turned on, increasing the brain's production of fear chemicals.

Rogan and Kandel brilliantly asked: What if you condition the animal by playing a different tone when there is *not* going to be a shock? Not surprisingly, the animal soon learns that it is safe when this particular tone is sounded—and this tone becomes a clarion call that "all is clear." Conditioned *safety*, not conditioned fear. And the mouse moves freely around its cage, confident that it won't be shocked. This "all clear" signal is processed by a different part of the brain—rather than by the amygdala, it passes through a "safety center"—centered in the dorsal striatum and connected to parts of the brain that are, as Rogan puts it, "dedicated to the processing of reward, reward contingencies, or positive affective states." And during these signals of safety, various other genes are turned on, which produce more of the brain chemicals (most likely including the chemical dopamine) to propagate a sense of safety—and even happiness.

One more remarkable aspect of this: how these signals affect the mouse's travel patterns. Normally when kept in a cage, a mouse will scurry along its edges. Even in the wild, it does not like wide-open spaces, where it would be vulnerable to predators such as owls or foxes. So it will hug the wall of the cage, running around the perimeter—only occasionally quickly running through the middle of the cage. In nature, such quick forays are probably rewarded with food, increasing the animal's chance of survival, despite the risk of being eaten. As mentioned before, when shocked electrically (or when warned by a tone that a shock might occur), the animal won't even do this much traveling—it will hunker down, staying nearly immobile, anticipating the worst.

What happens when the animal gets the "all clear" signal? Something very different. The animal now runs into the *middle* of the cage and stays there, basking in its sense of freedom and safety. It actually *avoids* the usually safer edges of the cage, preferring to spend most of its time in the usually forbidden open spaces.

Human analogies of this naturally come to mind—postgame celebrations at a football game, recess period at elementary school, armistice celebrations after war ends. The universal signals of safety are broadcast—often a tone or sound!—and humans, like our murine cousins, congregate in usually forbidden zones.

Even more interesting, many types of psychotherapy have traditionally emphasized the importance of safety, particularly for treatment of people who have been traumatized. In posttraumatic stress disorder (PTSD), therapists commonly tell patients, "You are safe here." Especially in group therapy for survivors of rape and other assaults: the group is a "safe place" to discuss painful events. Alcoholics Anonymous meetings too are refuges of safety in which people are encouraged (but not required) to speak—and when they feel comfortable and safe, then they often do speak. More broadly, the psychotherapist's office is in itself a safe place in which to explore feelings, to venture forth freely.

Recently, Daniela Pollak, PhD, another Columbia researcher, has studied a behavioral approach for "learned safety" in mice. She found that learning safety increases neurogenesis in the dentate gyrus of the hippocampus and turns down the activity of certain transmitters in the amygdala, norepinephrine and dopamine. Interestingly, these effects are similar, but not identical, to the effects of antidepressant medicines.

Is it possible that humans, in recovering from psychiatric disorders, also have a reactivation of the safety centers in our brains? It is a big leap to go from mice to humans, but this question can be investigated by research studies. And if so, therapies and medicines could be developed to more specifically enhance the appropriate activity of our safety centers!

What do I need this stuff for? How long do I have to take these? (Or: how long do I need to see the therapist?) Haven't I done enough?

It's kind of like the bookend of the times when you were suffering so much. Back then you were looking everywhere for help, trying to figure out what was wrong and how to get better.

Now, feeling better, you're ready to call it quits with treatment. But is that a good idea? You're going to have to talk to your doctor, your therapist, your spouse, maybe some friends. Maybe you'll take a look at the Web too, looking up "stopping antidepressants," "risk of getting depressed again," or the like.

You have reached the end of treatment—the final stage of the New Neuropsychiatry. At the beginning of treatment, there was a flood of information about medications, therapists, and a whole host of other things, far too much to think about, and all too many choices. This phase is confusing too—for different reasons, though, from the beginning of treatment. Now, everyone has an opinion, sure, but it's hard to find good information, to know who is right.

So, welcome to this new phase. After many years of ignorance, research studies have just begun to illuminate the ending of treatment. We know a lot less than we would like to. And some of the information we've gotten is not very pleasant—for instance, about the chances of having further episodes, whether of depression or for panic disorder.

But it's better to have that information, even if the truth is unpleasant, so you can plan for the future, right? Otherwise, what is there to do but keep taking the meds forever—or stopping them on your own, at the risk of walking off a cliff?

Another decision point—how will you make up your mind?

A Flight into Health

"Did I tell you about my trip?" asked Hannah Wrenn Ramos.

It had been several months since we had last met, so at first I didn't recall whether Hannah had mentioned that she might be traveling that summer. At that point, several years into treatment, we were meeting only every two or three months for what amounted to little more than checkups, during which we chatted about recent events and her photography exhibits and her kids—now Julia had a younger brother, Jordan—and I would refill her prescriptions. Hannah had cut back on visits to her therapist, too, seeing her only occasionally.

"Well, it was my first plane ride, and I went with Jorge and the kids to Mexico." She was speaking almost off-handedly, and it took me a few moments to put her words together.

I realized that she was telling me about the first plane ride in her life.

"It was great!" she was saying, "It was incredible to see the turquoise water along the coastline, all the white sand beaches." Excitedly, she went on, describing how they rented scooters, how they went snorkeling and visited ruins, how she photographed everything.

Hannah flying to Mexico? Given her lifelong—and all-consuming—fears of traveling, I never imagined she could leave the New York area, much less the continental United States.

How had she done it? Hannah described how she had strategized with herself to get through the plane ride: taking an extra half-pill of Klonopin the night before and another one just before getting on the plane. And—following the model her therapist had sketched—how she struggled against images of catastrophe as the plane sat on the runway, vigorously working at "thought-transforming." Once they were aloft, she had felt euphoric. After all, Hannah's entire life, her family's life, was based on the fear of leaving home. Her mother had never in all her 77 years been on an airplane.

"If I feel the panic rising, I've learned that it's less bad if I just let it wash over me. It's only if I try to hold it back, to stop it, that it really gets terrible."

Now, post-Mexico, it was clear to Hannah that her all-consuming anxieties had stopped other forms of exploration as well, interfering with her ability to leave home from her middle school days onward, blocking many improvements in her life. Now that Hannah had successfully flown to Mexico, she could see few limits to what else she might do.

At a certain point in successful New Neuropsychiatry treatments, it is not unusual, I find, for patients to take a trip. Not a harried business trip, some overnighter to Des Moines or South Carolina, and not a weekend to fulfill an obligation to see Mom back at the homestead. Instead, they book a trip they've always yearned for, but that something has prevented them from taking.

This was the case for Mark Maple, who went to Italy with Susan and their baby, Caleb, to celebrate their second wedding anniversary. And for Cindy, who took off with her husband, Roland (but without kids), for a week of hiking in New England. And Allen, who took Donna to a resort in the Southwest for her birthday. Perhaps for you, too, as your recovery continues, a trip is in store. Perhaps you take off for Europe or for the Cape or California for a long-awaited respite from quotidian life. You deserve it—your spouse agrees—it's been a long time since you've felt so good. This is a good way to take a much-needed break. Or if a trip to your dream location is not possible right now, you can get out of your routine to a local museum or nature preserve. Something that awakens your sense of adventure can do wonders to restore body and soul—and the higher brain.

In a sense, such trips are a manifestation of recovery, of the ebbing away of disorder with successful New Neuropsychiatry treatment. In the midst of disorder, when chaos reigns, escape may beckon, but such travels are generally miserable, making a mockery of the concept of escape. More often in disorder, the deranged maps of the agitated brain make withdrawal essential, make it necessary to hunker down in your apartment or house, sometimes to literally hide under the covers, and hence the mere prospect of travel becomes dizzying and miserable, utterly impossible. When you have entered the stable zone, though, such long-yearned-for adventures become possible, and often irresistible.

All of this makes me think about some remarkable new neuroscience research. For a long time, neuroscientists have focused on the brain's fear center—the amygdala, about which I have written so much in this book. In panic disorder, in PTSD, and most likely in depression as well, this system is hyperactive, hypersensitive—and all-too-easily sent into "red alert" mode.

Recent research has shown that the brain *also* has what might be called a "safety center." Focused around the dorsal striatum (a subcortical area of the brain that includes the caudate nucleus and the putamen and that is involved with movement and in executive function, as well as with reward systems) this center communicates a sense of safety, of security. If the amygdala sends off air raid sirens, and tells an organism to dive for safety, the dorsal striatum rings out "all clear!" Laboratory animals can be conditioned for danger, but they can also be conditioned for safety. Is it possible that when humans are in the process of recovery, eventually there is a healing of safety circuits in the brain? And is that healing related to your feeling of overall well-being once your disorder has resolved?

While in the throes of their disorder, people hunker down in fear, immobilized like the electrically shocked mice. And even afterward, after disorder fades, many times they stay in one place, still fearing the worst. Only after a profound and prolonged remission do some people—like Hannah and Mark and Cindy and Allen—begin to roam freely. Is it possible that the dorsal striatal system, the safety circuitry, is slower to respond to treatment than the amygdala and hippocampus, slower to recover? That eventually in recovery it again kicks in? And that once it again sends an appropriate "all clear!" siren, the world once more becomes safer to explore? Currently—though it can be investigated by researchers—this is just speculation.

Though she planned and executed it largely on her own, Hannah's trip to Mexico was a culmination of years of New Neuropsychiatry work—week after week of hard work in sessions with her therapist, and many psychopharmacology visits with me, in which we struggled to find the right combination of medications to bring her devastating symptoms under control.

As Hannah told me, she was feeling healed, feeling "whole." As she put it, "I'm a regular person now." Her trip resulted from—and further strengthened—a new sense of confidence. Indeed, she had largely achieved her goals.

But on a more practical level, was Hannah's treatment over? Should she quit therapy? And should she consider coming off medication? Or would that be a recipe for disaster?

Then there was Mark Maple.

He had just come back from a month in Italy with his family. They had had a great time just relaxing and enjoying being together. It was their first real break in years.

"I feel just plain good," Mark said, leaning back on the sofa in my consulting room, looking relaxed, even happy. He had put on a few pounds since getting married and had an expression that I could best describe as marital contentment.

"I was thinking about how different a place I'm in now," Mark began, "compared with when I first saw you." Basically, there was no more checking behavior; a dramatic drop in his previously all-consuming anxiety; an ability to focus wholly on his job and his family without a constant barrage of intrusive thoughts. "And it wasn't just the SSRI," he said, "it was the way the medicine put a floor under me, so I could work in therapy on all the issues that had been bottled up inside me for years."

There was a pause: I think I knew where he was headed.

"So, if I hear what you're saying," I said, "It sounds like you feel treatment is over. And you're thinking of coming off medicine."

Mark burst into laughter. "No, no way! Please, don't even mention that! I have nightmares where I worry for some reason they've stopped manufacturing SSRIs. I mean, I don't think I need to be in therapy forever. I don't want to come off SSRIs, ever."

Surprisingly, Marietta had similar feelings.

"I'm wondering . . ." She paused.

"What?" I said.

"Do I really have to come off medicine?"

I remembered how much of a struggle it had been when Marietta first started SSRI medication, how frightened she was of side effects, and how she didn't want to take it at all. And how reluctantly she agreed to restart the Celexa after her baby, Beatrice, was born, but only on the condition that we take her off of it as soon as possible.

This issue had come up before, last spring—a vague discussion about how she could (and perhaps should) stop taking Celexa at some point: after all, she had been doing so well; her depression had faded away, and things had settled down in her life. But now she and Victor were considering having a second child—this gave the question more urgency. If Marietta *was* going to have another baby, there was no reason for her to expose the child to medicine unless absolutely necessary. And yet Marietta was hesitant.

This is a not uncommon paradox in New Neuropsychiatry treatment. Early on, patients often ask their doctors, "How long do I have to stay on this stuff?" and "How soon can I get off of it?" Later, when they are firmly ensconced in the stable zone, they're more likely to protest, "Why do I have to stop? Can't I wait?"

"What?" Marietta said. "You look like you're about to say something."

"I was just remembering how when you started Celexa, you made me promise to take you off as soon as possible. Now you're telling me just the opposite. I'm a bit confused."

She laughed. "Well, why rock the boat?"

You

Perhaps you too have mixed feelings. Now, firmly ensconced in recovery, you are ready to contemplate ending treatment, but you are not sure whether to shake things up or not. You feel better, stable again, confident, strong. You have your life back, so why risk losing all your gains? No longer do you awaken at night overwhelmed by dread. You are working hard and productively, you take satisfaction from your marriage and kids or from your friendships, your involvement in community affairs. You even feel playful at times, relaxed. You can have fun. Your trip, your "flight into health" was a validation of your recovery.

So, even though you can end treatment, should you? What are the risks, the benefits? The pros and cons?

What should you do?

If your case involves having a single episode of depression, notable for its severity and acuity but fully responding to treatment—you definitely fall into the camp of people who can stop taking medicine.

But it may be that things were worse for you—in that there were more episodes in your past, or worse symptoms, and perhaps you have a sinking sense that it won't exactly be easy to quit. So you may fall on the other side: the side of those who need medication (and perhaps psychotherapy as well) like a person who has diabetes needs insulin. As a way to preserve health. To make life livable.

Where do you fit?

Can We Stop?

As we have seen in this book, New Neuropsychiatry treatments often increasingly provide full responses and lead the way toward remission and recovery. Increasingly, we can say that your episode of disorder is "over" and can discuss finishing treatment. In a way, Hannah's treatment was complete: her plane ride was a confirmation that the struggle with disorder had been won. Sure, she would continue with skirmishes, mopping-up operations. One part of me *wanted* Hannah to be well enough to stop treatment. I wanted our work together—the half-dozen years of medication treatment, the prescriptions, the panicky phone calls, the therapy, all that—to have been enough to liberate her from her disorder.

It all came back to the map. Hannah had remapped her brain. So had Mark and Allen and Cindy, and so had Marietta—and so, perhaps, have you. Over

Do I Need to Keep Taking Medicine?

When is it safe to stop taking medication and who can stop doing so safely? The answer to these questions depends on the severity of the disorder you have and on the frequency of your symptoms. Research conducted over the past twenty years or so gives us some guidelines to answer these questions. But before you make the decision to stop taking your medications, consult your psychiatrist, doctor, or mental health practitioner. We wouldn't want you to undo all the psychological gains you have made—and all the healing you have done to your brain!

It takes at least six to twelve months of treatment to bring a disorder firmly under control (we used to think that three or four months was enough). And now we have some good studies—true, many fewer than the thousands of efficacy studies—but still, a few dozen good studies on the benefits of continuing treatment and on the consequences of stopping treatment.

In the late 1980s, Ellen Frank and David Kupfer, researchers at the University of Pittsburgh, coordinated a large study of people with highly recurrent depression, looking at the benefits of continued antidepressant and psychotherapy treatment and at the risks of stopping treatment. Published in 1990, this study concluded that people who had had three or more previous episodes of depression required ongoing—probably lifetime—treatment with antidepressant medicine. If they stopped medication treatment, they almost invariably got depressed again; but if they continued medication, they almost always stayed well. The continued benefit of medicine was found three years after their episode of depression, and five years

several years, as Hannah faithfully took her medication and struggled with making changes in therapy, we had seen that lasting changes could occur. Sometimes slowly, and other times by quantum leaps, Hannah had built on these changes, and her life had continued to improve, so that her current situation was almost unimaginably better than life before treatment.

Would these changes "stick" if she stopped treatment?

In his 1996 book *The Emotional Brain*, neuroscientist Joseph LeDoux says, "Therapy is just another way of creating synaptic potentiation in brain pathways that control the amygdala. The amygdala's emotional memories . . . are indelibly burned into its circuits. The best we can hope to do is to regulate their expression. And the way we do this is by getting the cortex to control the amygdala." What this means for you is that a combination of therapy and later as well. On the plus side, such findings (and those of similar studies) suggest that disorder can be kept under control with continued treatment. On the minus side, it is clear that people who have more severe illness—either worse symptoms or more frequent episodes—aren't as successful in coming off medication or stopping therapy as those who have had only one or two episodes of depression, or whose depression was not so severe. Some people, like it or not, will require lifetime treatment.

We have numerous other studies as well. Lifetime medication treatment has clearly been shown to be necessary disorders such as schizophrenia or manic-depressive illness (also known as bipolar disorder). For less severe disorders, the story is somewhat different. For each major type of mood and anxiety disorder (panic disorder, OCD, major depression, and so on) we now have several studies showing how ongoing treatment for two or more years can keep symptoms at bay. Experts have developed treatment roadmaps that can give guidance for when lifetime treatment is needed, and when it is unnecessary.

The point is this: unlike Old Psychiatry practitioners a few decades back, New Neuropsychiatrists *do* have data about both continuing treatment and about stopping treatment and can start to give people rational advice about when it is—or isn't—safe to stop medicine or therapy. Though there are not as yet strong data about how best to end treatment, there are reasonable suggestions about how to ease the transition off of medications. And it is now possible to at least begin to quantify the risk that disorder will return.

medication can allow you to restore order out of chaos, to replace knee-jerk reactions with thoughtful responses. It can in fact heal your brain.

Well, Hannah had gotten her cortex to control her amygdala, thanks to medication and her work in psychotherapy. As LeDoux puts it in another book, *The Synaptic Self*, "Psychotherapy is fundamentally a learning process for its patients, and as such is a way to rewire the brain." If treatment has worked, your cortex (higher brain) is now in reasonably firm control of your amygdala (lower brain). The fear responses no longer rule your life.

But, the question is, how often does this rewiring require *ongoing* treatment in order to work? Are the new circuits, the new more-adaptive connections, permanent? Or will they require continuous input from medicine or therapy to persist?

In brief, this is what we know: If you have had a single episode of depression or a year or two of panic attacks, you most likely can stop treatment—it appears that your brain can recover. However, if you've had several (i.e., three or more) episodes of depression or a number of years of obsessive-compulsive disorder, the odds are that you need treatment for a long time—probably indefinitely. The anxiety and mood circuits of the brain are easy to break and hard to fix. Extended periods of disorder, or repeated episodes, seem to scar the brain. Yet briefer but more extreme experiences, severe trauma like rape or an airplane crash, can also cause permanent changes. Even the apparent resurgence of the hippocampus and the dorsal striatum and other brain centers with our New Neuropsychiatry treatments are not yet able to entirely undo these injuries.

At the same time, there is a great deal of variation from one person to the next. What is true for one person may not apply to another. Understandably, many people will want to test themselves—who wants to accept the possibility that they may need treatment for a lifetime?

Furthermore, there are many gray zones, in which it is not clear how the guidelines may apply. What if you've had *two* episodes of depression? The guidelines suggest one year of treatment for people with one episode, lifetime treatment for those with three or more. With two, you are somewhere in the middle. What if you've had three episodes but they came twenty years apart, at ages 15, 35, and 55—is ongoing treatment necessary? After all, your next episode may not come until you're well into your 70s.

With Hannah, my hunch was that—underneath the SSRI—her amygdala had not quieted down. Weeks, even months, would pass without any symptoms; then, a deadline at work, her kids coming down with a bad flu—and the panic would return. Not full-force—instead, like lightning flashing on the horizon or an echo of distant thunder. But panic and fear nonetheless. Furthermore, Hannah had had these symptoms for more than twenty years. True, in getting better, Hannah had most likely grown other pathways from her cortex and her dorsal striatum (the safety center) and other higher brain centers, which allowed her to ignore, circumvent, or otherwise overpower her amygdala's shrill warnings. But the signals, the burnt-in pathways of overactivity, alas, appeared to remain.

So if she stopped medicine, the risk was that the old map would rise up again, the old pathways would become reactivated. Her disorder might return.

As Hannah and I discussed this issue on that rainy April afternoon, it became clear that her question had been more theoretical than real. She felt all too insecure in her improvement; she was just testing the waters. And yet, what if, three or four years from now, she wanted to come off Zoloft and Klonopin, even in defiance of the odds? As a New Neuropsychiatrist who is reasonably aware of the scientific literature and who has seen many hundreds of patients, how would I advise her?

For the Foreseeable Future

Some disorders just won't go away. With current treatments, you are going to have it for many years, perhaps for a lifetime. This does not mean being doomed to a life of misery, though. The challenge becomes how to have the best possible life despite having such a disorder. Similar to Hannah, Mark, and Cindy also were likely to need treatment for the foreseeable future, given the treatments that we currently have available in the New Neuropsychiatry. Likewise, virtually all of the people with disorders that seemed to be treatment resistant who I discussed in Chapter 7: Kenneth, Patricia, Lynette, Paolo.

Often this means a paring away of treatment to the essentials, to the minimum amount of medicine or therapy needed. A full dose of SSRI medication is usually still required to keep panic disorder or depression under control, but maybe remission can be maintained with a smaller number of medicines or your regimen can be optimized to minimize side effects. Therapy may be cut back to once or twice a month rather than every week, or, sometimes, completely ended. And you can make plans with your doctor: if an episode appears to be returning, what should you do?

If you can keep such a chronic disorder under control, if you can get into *and* stay in your own "stable zone," then life can be good. Eventually, if all goes right, disorder can recede into the background, and you may almost forget it is there. Disorder is not entirely a negative experience, either. Perhaps disorder may have tempered, even strengthened, you, as Mark and Allen were to contend. Perhaps the experience of having survived this type of scarcely visible adversity will give you a better understanding of the human condition, more insight and a deeper sense of empathy.

Mark Moves On

Mark Maple openly admitted that he needed to take Prozac forever. How did he know this? One visit, Mark confessed that he had tried on his own to come off medication.

"I experimented several times this past summer," he told me, "but I realized I just couldn't." Even when he tried tapering the medicine slowly, symptoms had started coming back. Though he knew how to interrupt the checking behavior and obsessive thoughts, Mark quickly concluded that it would take most of his waking energy to do so. These obsessions were so intense, so unremitting—as days passed, the urges to check, to count, to call would rise up, and Mark would be overcome by an almost déjà-vu feeling that "I've been here before."

(Indeed, I wondered if he might be one of those people whose disorder results from a genetic twist—perhaps a deficiency in production of glutamate, a neurotransmitter that can turn off the activity of the primary cells of the lateral amygdala.)

Over the next several months, Mark and I were able to pare his treatment down to the essentials. He gradually stopped Klonopin, an antianxiety medicine—tapering from 3 milligrams a day down to 2, then 1, then 0.5 milligrams a day, and he phased out Trazodone, which had been helping him sleep. We even put him on a new preparation of Prozac, "Prozac Weekly," a slowly absorbed formulation that needs to be taken only once per week. This seemed to work okay, but Mark often forgot to take it, so he decided to just take two 40 mg tablets of Prozac every morning—what he called "vitamin P"—along with his multivitamins and blood pressure medicine. Mark stretched out the time between visits to Liz. "I like Liz a lot," Mark would say, "but I don't need to see her anymore."

Eventually Mark's disorder was indeed on the "back burner." He decided to get his Prozac refills from his primary care doctor, who also provided his cholesterol and blood pressure medications. Although his treatment was technically "interminable," as far as need for specifically *psychiatric* treatment, Mark's case was over. What Mark still had—like his high blood pressure—was a problem that could be treated by his GP. A lifetime condition, but one that could fade into the background of his life.

More than that, more interesting than the specifics of adjusting his medicines and therapy, were the realities of Mark's new life. Unending treatment clearly didn't mean he was stuck in a quagmire; quite the opposite. Susan and Mark had moved into their new apartment downtown, a place that at least for the moment had enough room for their two children. It wasn't just a matter of being in a relationship and being a father.

Liz, his therapist, pointed out some subtle ways in which Mark changed after entering remission. Freed from his agonizing symptoms, Mark had finally been able to have the kind of insight he had sought unsuccessfully for so many years of psychoanalysis—he could identify day-to-day origins of his surges of anxiety and fear. When checking and worrying had dominated every waking moment, Mark had been emotionally withdrawn from Susan. Now, able to step back from his urges and compulsions, he indeed had developed what Liz called "self-observing ego"—he could see the effects of these obsessions on his relationship with Susan. Plus, he could take responsibility for his behavior, and act more maturely.

Over the years, Mark's black moods and furious obsessions had become part of his "self," a seemingly essential part of "Markness." Now Mark's depression and obsessions began to seem weird to him, alien, not-himself. For years, all-consuming anxiety had made Mark unable to be emotionally intimate; he would brood, withdraw, would often storm out of the house, needing to "be alone." Now Mark began to open up emotionally to others, in particular to his wife. He was better able to understand Susan's needs—and to try to provide what she needed rather than withdrawing emotionally. According to Susan, he had also become more physically affectionate.

The biggest change of all came when Mark finally felt ready to become a father—not once but twice. A few years after ending treatment, Mark e-mailed me some photos: he and Susan in a city park, the kids in a sandbox behind them. And another one of their apartment, crowded with the kids' toys and dolls and electronics, even a colorful plastic slide. A happy family, as far as I could tell, hardly different from any other.

Cindy Decides

Cindy was doing well. She had finished her dissertation, was completing a postdoc fellowship and applying for jobs. After all the couples therapy, she and Roland had settled into a fairly happy marriage. Now they faced the hectic issues of normal life, of a two-career couple in early twenty-first-century

When You No Longer Need Medication

You have talked to your psychiatrist or other mental health provider, and you agree that it is time to consider stopping taking your medications. Just like eliminating any other substance that your body has adjusted to taking on a daily basis, there are ways to increase the chance of a smooth landing when coming off psychiatric medications.

► *Gradually taper off medicine.* A gradual tapering off of medicine is generally believed to be better than stopping abruptly, and some studies have borne this out. At the very least, a slow taper will avoid "rebound" side effects such as jitteriness, insomnia, dizziness, and the like. It is also more likely to give time for your own brain to crank up the production of necessary neurotransmitters such as serotonin and norepinephrine.

► *Maintain body rhythms.* It also makes sense to pay attention to maintaining your body's rhythms, especially the circadian rhythms of sleep-wake cycles. Disorder is, after all, a condition of dysregulation of all sorts of mind-body rhythms. Now that you are in remission, keeping reregulated makes sense.

► *Normalize your sleep.* I always tell people to do this at this phase—which often, given our society's current frenetic lifestyles, takes a concerted effort. This is particularly true for bipolar disorder, also known as manic-depressive illness. For whatever reason, for many people worsening of bipolar disorder is set off by disrupted sleep, and often maintaining sleep can prevent new episodes. (University of Pittsburgh researcher Ellen Frank, PhD, developed a treatment for bipolar disorder, social rhythms therapy, to provide guidelines to regularize behavioral rhythms.) This probably holds true for many people who have depression and anxiety disorders as well. Knowing, for instance, that several nights of insomnia have been a warning sign for return of depression in the past, it might be possible to head off an episode by taking sleep medication for a number of nights.

► *Minimize depressants and stimulants.* Watching your intake of alcohol and caffeine and nicotine makes sense, and of course so does entirely avoiding substances of abuse like marijuana or cocaine.

► *Reduce stress.* It also makes sense to "destress" your life to the degree possible—to make long-awaited and deferred life changes first, and make sure you are well settled into a new order of things long before stopping treatment! It obviously doesn't make sense to stop anti-depressant medicine or therapy in the midst of a job change, a divorce, a family crisis, or a legal case.

► *Reach out to others.* During the period of tapering off medicine, it also makes sense to use your social networks, to do your best to connect meaningfully to people you care about.

► *Exercise body and spirit.* Keep using your body to your advantage—to continue your "mindfulness exercises," or yoga classes, or meditation rituals. These may make a powerful difference. Regular exercise too. Even spirituality, prayer and other devotions may protect against the return the symptoms of a disorder.

► *Explore therapy.* Psychotherapy may be a way to make tapering off medicine go more smoothly. Many studies have shown that particular types of psychotherapy, especially cognitive-behavioral therapy (CBT) and interpersonal therapy (IPT), can help prevent depression from returning during the time that medication is being discontinued.

► *Make a plan.* Contingency planning, including planning for managing work stresses, travel, illness, can be a lifesaver. It is useful to have a plan in case of variations from your routine, such as travel to different time zones, illness, and other challenges. This can include a few nights use of sleep medication, or a return to relaxation and breathing exercises, or even a few psychotherapy "booster sessions," and may help to relieve symptoms before they can contribute to the return of a full-blown disorder.

America. She and Roland were buying a new house in the far reaches of the suburbs. They had gotten a dog, bought a second car. I was sure that their new neighbors would never have a clue know how she and Roland had suffered.

She couldn't stop medicine entirely: her bipolar II disorder required life-long treatment. But was this a good time to simplify her medications? Perhaps to end therapy? It was hard to imagine a peaceful, low-stress time in Cindy's life any time soon! But she had already started the process. Perhaps a year ago, she had started "forgetting" to take her Zoloft several days a week, without any adverse effects. So I told her to stop it. For a while she had kept on taking the occasional half-pill of Risperdal to help with sleep, but one weekend she ran out, and slept just fine. She had gained some weight on lithium, and also complained of shakiness, so a few months ago I had switched her to Lamictal 200 mg/day, an anticonvulsant that has mood-stabilizing properties. By this point, she was taking only the Lamictal, of which we now dropped the dose from 200 to 150 mg/day. She also had an old bottle of Valium at home, but she couldn't recall the last time she'd taken one of them.

Lamictal 150 milligrams a day—less than a sixth of a gram, perhaps one-five-hundredth of an ounce! That tiny amount of a potent chemical had been—and would continue to be—key to her recovery. Now, seven years later, Cindy's remission has held. Will sees her from time to time for therapy "boosters," I see her every three or four months for medication refills, and she is still doing fine.

Terminable Treatments

If you can stop treatment, what is the best way to do so? Is there anything you can do to prevent the old pathways from lighting up again, from short-circuiting all your gains? After all, you have struggled so hard to get into a "stable zone" of recovery, to undo all the damage in your life. How can you maximize your chances of staying there without treatment? New Neuropsychiatrists have some practical knowledge about how to do so but much less firm data than we would like. Pragmatically, these are things that may allow the "new map" to stay in command as you ease out of treatment, that may protect you in some way from a resurgence of the old map of disorder.

Among the patients I have described, who seems likely to be able to stop treatment? Marietta, who had had one episode of depression—she most likely could stop medicine. Especially now that she was considering getting pregnant again (she would have to be followed carefully after her second child was born, because of the risk that she might become depressed again). And Allen Johnson—Allen could almost certainly stop treatment. Having never taken medicine made things easier at this point. Allen had "gotten" the essence of CBT—having gone to sessions and support groups, having done his homework exercises and read innumerable articles and books. And having practiced breathing and muscle relaxation exercises until he could practically do them in his sleep. He could treat himself; so why should he see a therapist anymore?

Another candidate is Warner, a 43-year-old man, who had slid into an episode of major depression after he was laid off from his job. He was drawn into a lawsuit involving his old company, which consumed more than a year of his life. Required to testify against his friends and former coworkers, Warner had become severely depressed, his DSM-IV diagnosis being "major depression, single episode, severe." After the lawsuit ended, he remained immobilized, unable to resuscitate his career. Warner started cognitive therapy, but only partially improved, so antidepressant medicine, Zoloft 150 mg/day, was added. Then Warner got better. He was gradually able to start networking, find a new job, and extricate his family from its financial bind. Soon things were back on track, and after about a year he felt ready to stop the medicine. Warner continued his cognitive therapy sessions while stopping the medicine, because he read that this could protect against depression coming back. Warner's doctor began gradually decreasing his antidepressant by 25 milligrams every few weeks. There were a few moments of anxiety as his sleep temporarily worsened, and he became irritable for a few days, but eventually Warner settled in for a smooth landing. He saw his therapist for a few months afterward, then stopped that treatment as well.

Marietta Has Another Baby

Marietta had some apprehensions about her decision to try for a second child at the "advanced" age of 41. But once we determined that she should try to come off medicine, she plunged ahead, tapering down on the Celexa dose 5 or 10 milligrams at a time.

How to prevent herself from getting depressed again? Again we went through all the possible options, including cognitive therapy, exercise classes, even using a light box—the kind of device used for seasonal affective disorder, and in the end, Marietta decided to just go back and see her old therapist twice a week. Plus, she kept trying to minimize her stress, to the extent possible for the mother of a 2-year-old. She cut back on her work schedule, refusing to travel except when absolutely necessary, and made efforts to get as much sleep as possible, to exercise regularly, and to eat well (which she tended not to do).

Despite a fair amount of anxiety, Marietta's pregnancy and delivery went well. She felt overwhelmed on returning home a few days after her daughter Anna's birth, and found herself crying for the better part of a day. What was going on? Was this the usual "blues"? Or was it something else, perhaps a return of postpartum depression?

It was tough to decide. Marietta felt agitated, tearful, overwhelmed, and all that—but she fell asleep when Anna was resting and hadn't lost her appetite. "I'm down, but I'm not depressed," she said. I wasn't sure. Perhaps she should go on meds for a little while. But three low days didn't make a major depression.

So we decided to wait and see—and a few days later, her mood began to lift. It was not necessary to restart the Celexa this time, but she agreed to check in every month or so for the time being.

"I'll certainly let you know if anything changes," she said.

And there we were. Marietta kept in contact with me over the following months; when Anna was about five months old, Marietta even put herself back onto Celexa for a few weeks, but then she felt the depression lifting and "forgot" to keep taking it. And nothing bad happened. She continued doing fine off medication.

Allen Unpacks

For Allen Johnson, ending treatment meant tapering down therapy. Rather than coming for weekly cognitive-behavioral sessions, he had gradually cut them back to once per two weeks, then once a month. He kept doing his relaxation and breathing exercises, finding them especially useful as sleep aids, and kept running regularly.

Even though we were meeting infrequently, it was clear that things were still improving. Travel was no longer news; cohabitation was. When they got engaged, Donna moved in with Allen in his apartment in the city. It was an enormous change. Not only did he have to accommodate her things, rearranging closets and medicine cabinets, he had to move in himself! Allen had lived in the apartment for years without ever really unpacking. He finally unpacked the many boxes that he had brought into his apartment a decade earlier. He even hung pictures on the walls.

About the time he and Donna got engaged, Allen had started contacting old friends again through Facebook, classmates from grad school and college, buddies he had lost touch with. Then he joined Facebook groups for his high school, even his primary school. Over time these new contacts with old friends became part of his recovery. He would compare where his life stood to these friends—for instance, his best friend from high school, who had been married for a decade, had two children and owned his own house. Allen would be reminded of where he stood: "still single, still renting, unsure if I'm ready to get married." Why did he do it? Despite his lost years, it gave him confirmation that he was coming back. After years of being socially withdrawn, he was finally looking forward to seeing his old friends again.

After he and Donna had a child, I saw him a few times. His life was going fine, with nothing in the way of panic. Treatment was no longer necessary.

Life Goes On

At times one can even see a protective effect of having recovered from a disorder.

Take the events of 9/11/2001. On that Tuesday morning a little before 9 a.m., when the first plane hit the World Trade Center, Mark was on his way to a conference in midtown Manhattan. Susan was somewhere downtown—perhaps still at their apartment, perhaps at her office, or somewhere in between.

It was the kind of disaster that Mark had dreaded for many years. For a long time Mark had irrationally feared something bad would happen to Susan, hence his innumerable efforts to reach her by phone, his urges to check up on her to prevent disaster—all in all, as if 9/11 had already been under way.

In the confusion of that morning, Mark struggled to keep his head. He found refuge in a hotel lobby and dialed Susan on her cell phone. Of course, the lines were jammed, or the networks were down. There was not even a dial tone. So Mark began walking. He hiked several miles downtown, battling against the thousands of people who were fleeing the burning towers—until finally he arrived back home at their smoke-filled apartment, where his kids were safe with their babysitter, who herself was terrified. There were hours of chaos and uncertainty, the skies filled with smoke and dust, endless hours during which Mark had no idea where Susan was, because cell phones and beepers and voice mail systems were out of commission. Mark stayed with his kids and the babysitter, putting wet towels against the window frames in a vain effort to keep the dark billowing clouds of smoke out.

Eventually, Mark found out that Susan had gone to stay at a friend's apartment, that she was safe, that everything was okay. Despite Mark's history of vast worries about Susan, he coped remarkably well in the aftermath of 9/11. Once he found Susan, Mark did not need to keep obsessively checking up on her. He knew she was safe. He felt almost calm, he told me, stable, secure.

"With all the psychotherapy and medication I've had," Mark told me, "I feel like I'm protected."

Allen Johnson also checked in with me after those events. He too had been downtown that day. The dust and smoke set off asthma attacks, but he was able to control them by using inhalers and without going to the emergency room. He too described feeling protected by his knowledge of panic. He was practiced at self-calming, at meditation and mindfulness and breathing exercises, so that in the midst of all that was going on he had been able to induce a sense of rationality, even tranquility.

Mark and Allen observed many of their co-workers developing disorders from 9/11-related trauma in weeks afterward, including, as Mark put it, "very strong people who would never have considered seeing a psychiatrist, who never would have otherwise gotten a disorder." Many of them became severely depressed or developed flashbacks and phobias. "In a way," Mark added, "this is what I've been preparing for my whole life, so when it actually happened, it was almost a relief."

Time after time in the months after 9/11, I heard similar statements from patients: "I'm doing so much better than my co-workers who have never had a mental symptom," and "I see them dropping around me, I'm coping much better."

The Future

Clearly the New Neuropsychiatry has not yet reached the phase of being able to cure all disorders, despite the best intentions. This shows a crucial need: a need for more research, more effective treatments, and especially for a better understanding of basic neurobiology of disorders. With more knowledge of the basic mechanisms of psychiatric disorders, maybe one day they can be prevented from happening or treated so effectively that they go away indefinitely, so that so many people won't need ongoing treatment.

And who knows what the future will bring? Francis S. Collins, director of the National Institutes of Health, proposed that we are entering a period of "personalized medicine" in which treatment can be tailored to individual needs of each person who has an illness. One can easily imagine how this might apply to the New Neuropsychiatry. Perhaps someone in the future who has a mood or anxiety disorder will undergo a battery of neuropsychological testing and an MRI scan to look at brain anatomy, functioning, and connectivity and at the levels of various brain chemicals. A swab of cells from your cheek or a blood sample could be put onto a gene chip to determine which medicines will work for you and which are not worth trying, and perhaps even what type of psychotherapy might work for you. And it is easy to imagine that such a workup could discover exactly which of your specific brain pathways are off-kilter, perhaps pinpointing exactly which one of the three major prefrontal cortex behavioral circuits are out of whack and where they went awry. And your doctor will be able to provide a medicine, probably just one dose, to improve the functioning of that system alone! Or some focused type of psychotherapy.

Who knows? Maybe it will happen, and if it does, then it's likely that our current New Neuropsychiatry treatments will look simple-minded at best, especially because they require such a huge amount of effort for a fairly modest amount of benefit. But the New Neuropsychiatry is where we are for now.

In the years following the events of 9/11, we appear to have entered a new period of extreme global stress, economic, political, and in a sense psychological. It may be a new paradigm of life in the twenty-first century—the way in which extraordinary mental and psychological experiences become ordinary, because of the vastness of global events and the interconnectedness of all humanity through technology. Just as depression has surged in a global epidemic, so too may trauma, and the psychological consequences such as posttraumatic stress disorder, which may affect hundreds of thousands of people directly, and many millions more indirectly. In such a world, the concepts of resilience become ever more relevant, especially because people who have mood and anxiety disorders can be more vulnerable to such stresses; or, as Mark and Allen's experiences suggest, may learn to protect themselves even against conditions of extreme stress.

The question being, how to find safety within one's own brain in an unsafe world, and how to thrive amid uncertainty and even chaos.

You Postdisorder

Now that you are postdisorder, are you still feeling weakened, are you still struggling to deal with day-to-day problems? Or has suffering with (and through) your disorder tempered you, giving you greater compassion and understanding and perhaps even strengthening you against adversity?

When you were caught up in the throes of disorder, at many times you felt your life was over. Now, at the end of the trip, it is possible that things look entirely different. Life is just beginning, and it looks pretty good.

In any case, you (and I) have reached an ending. Ahead we see an open road, perilous but remarkable.

So, working with your doctor, you decide it is time to end your treatment. You decrease the dose by half a pill every two weeks. Perhaps you feel something while the medicine starts going out of your system—some restless nights, a brief dip in mood. You even stop the taper for a while at your doctor's suggestion, and wait a month or so before starting to decrease the dose again.

You mean to keep your sleep schedule regular, but travel and work interfere, and there's not much you can do when you're on the road. Once you're back home, though, you do your best to get back on schedule. You make time to exercise regularly, which seems to help your mood. And to keep your coffee and alcohol consumption to a minimum—it's hard to tell if that makes any difference or not, though.

Finally, you're off medicine. You stopped seeing your therapist a while back and now your doctor suggests a follow-up visit a few months from now.

So far, no symptoms. So far, so good.

And that, knock wood, will be it.

Acknowledgments

I WOULD LIKE TO thank my friends and colleagues at Columbia University Department of Psychiatry, who have provided the rich intellectual, clinical, and academic environment in which it has been possible to think broadly and to synthesize work from an extremely wide range of research as well as diverse settings of clinical care.

On a day to day basis, I experience this scientific creativity in work with my friends and colleagues in the Depression Evaluation Service, including Drs. Patrick J. McGrath, Jonathan W. Stewart, Deborah Deliyannides, and Judith Rabkin, and other project staff including Sarah Black, Sarai Batchelder, Donna O'Shea, and Vito Agosti. The Depression Evaluation Service is part of the Division of Clinical Therapeutics, which spans the mood disorders, eating disorders, anxiety disorders, impulse control disorders, and neuroinflammatory disorders, in a way that facilitates creative thinking about these conditions and their treatment, particularly in view of our growing understanding of underlying neural mechanisms. The director of Clinical Therapeutics, Dr. Timothy Walsh, plays a key role in facilitating creative new thinking across traditional disciplines. We are part of the Columbia University Department of Psychiatry, an enormous department with over 1,200 faculty members, with researchers in everything from epidemiology to policy research to modern psychoanalysis to genetics to cognitive neuroscience to molecular therapeutics, and that provides psychiatric care in a vast range of clinical settings. Columbia Psychiatry and the New York State Psychiatric Institute, where many of its programs are based, epitomize the best of the New Neuropsychiatry. I am grateful to its directors, including the current Chairman Dr. Jeffrey Lieberman and his predecessors particularly Dr. John Oldham, for providing me opportunities to grow within this department over the past decade.

Other colleagues at Columbia Psychiatry and the New York State Psychiatric Institute who have been particularly helpful in the development of ideas for this book include Drs. Bradley Peterson for neuroimaging, Gerald Bruder for psychophysiology, Andrew Skodol for personality disorders, and Holly Lisanby on brain stimulation treatments. I have had many stimulating discussions with Drs. John Markowitz and Carlos Blanco on topics related to psychotherapy, as well as with Barbara Stanley, who works on borderline personality disorder. Dr. Rita Charon, who runs the Program in Narrative Medicine at the Columbia University College of Physicians and Surgeons, has helped to develop my understanding of the importance of narrative in medical and psychiatric treatment. David Lane, the peerless librarian at New York State Psychiatric Institute, has always able to locate relevant citations, no matter how obscure, on an almost instantaneous basis.

I am equally appreciative to many former colleagues at Beth Israel Medical Center where I worked for over 15 years. Though less rarified than Columbia, Beth Israel had the advantage of being immersed in the realities of life on the Lower East Side of New York, with an amazing ranging of people, cultures, and disorders. Arnold Winston, Beth Israel's director of psychiatry, encouraged his faculty to think creatively in developing new clinical and research programs in psychotherapy and medication treatment, which got me started in early studies of the treatment of chronic depression. I had many productive discussions with my Beth Israel colleagues, including Henry Pinsker, Lisa Samstag, Richard Rosenthal, and Philip Yanowitch. Similarly, in private practice I have had many fruitful interactions with psychotherapists including Liz Halstead, Paulette Landesman, Judith Maidenbaum, Marcia Blank, Jordana Skurka, Neill Cohen, and Ron Aviram.

I owe a particular degree of gratitude to my family, to my wife, Lisa, for her patience, support, and good humor over the many years that this book required, and to our kids Sarah, Ben, and Jason who often raised interesting New Neuropsychiatry questions without even knowing it. My sister Kathryn Hellerstein has provided encouragement, advice, and support as this book has gradually taken shape. My parents Drs. Mary and Herman K. Hellerstein established an environment of broad intellectual excitement, creativity, and endless questioning of the status quo for their six children, one that has served me in particularly good stead while writing this book. Not entirely incidentally, it was just over 20 years ago that my father's trade book *Healing Your Heart: Reversing Heart Disease without Drugs or Surgery*, was published; no doubt *Heal Your Brain* has some similar themes to Dad's book.

I am grateful to the MacDowell Colony in Peterborough, New Hampshire, for providing me an ideal setting to bring this project to completion in the spring of 2009. At the Johns Hopkins University Press, I particularly thank acquisitions editor Wendy Harris and staff editor Michele Callaghan who helped bring coherence and consistency to a large and complex manuscript. I would especially give thanks to Cindy Hyden for reviewing earlier versions of the manuscript and suggesting thoughtful revisions.

Lastly, I owe profound thanks to my patients who have provided so much insight over more than two decades in a variety of hospital, clinic, research, and office settings. The dialogues of the New Neuropsychiatry have been inspired by many dialogues with inquisitive and creative people who are seeking treatment for their own depression or anxiety disorders.

Notes

Introduction

p. 1, *the eminent psychiatrist Jack Gorman:* Gorman, J. *The New Psychiatry.*

p. 2, *Columbia University Department of Psychiatry:* www.columbiapsychiatry.org and www.nyspi.org (I am the editor of these Web sites). For Columbia Department of Psychiatry grand rounds, see www.columbiapsychiatry.org/grand_rounds.

p. 2, *"hyperactivity of area 25, the subgenual anterior cingulate":* Mayberg, Defining neuro-circuits in depression; Mayberg, Modulating dysfunctional limbic-cortical circuits in depression; Mayberg, Brannan, Tekell, et al., Regional metabolic effects of fluoxetine in major depression; Mayberg, Lozano, Voon, et al., Deep brain stimulation for treatment-resistant depression.

p. 2, *prairie voles:* Insel and Young, Neurobiology of attachment; Winslow, Hastings, Carter, Harbaugh, and Insel, Central vasopressin in pair bonding in monogamous prairie voles.

p. 2, *memories in aplysia:* Kandel, Molecular biology of memory storage.

p. 3, *My father, Herman K. Hellerstein, MD:* Hellerstein with Snyder, *A Matter of Heart.*

p. 4, *first wave of neuropsychiatry, which emerged in the late nineteenth century:* Insel and Quirion, Psychiatry as a clinical neuroscience discipline; Martin, Integration of neurology, psychiatry and neuroscience; Sabshin, Turning points in twentieth-century American psychiatry; Yudofsky and Hales, Neuropsychiatry and the future of psychiatry and neurology.

p. 4, *we have begun to understand how our treatments can slow or stop the process of injury to these parts of the brain and can even, perhaps, begin to repair some of them:* Gage, F.H. Brain, repair yourself.

p. 5, *hippocampus—the brain's learning and memory center—is key:* A review of MRI studies by Videbech and Ravnkilde showed that the volume of the hippocampus is decreased about 10 percent in people who have major depression compared with healthy individuals.

Burgess, Maguire, and O'Keefe, Human hippocampus and spatial and episodic memory; Dranovsky and Hen, Hippocampal neurogenesis; Malberg, Implications of adult hippocampus neurogenesis in antidepressant action; Malberg, Amelia, Nestler, and Duman, Chronic antidepressant treatment increases neurogenesis in adult rat hippocampus; Santarelli, Saxe, Gross, et al., Requirement of hippocampal neurogenesis for the behavioral effects of antidepressants; Videbech and Ravnkilde, Hippocampal volume and depression.

p. 6, *study of London cab drivers:* Maguire, Burgess, Donnett, et al., Knowing where and getting there; Maguire, Gadian, Johnsrude, et al., Structural change in the hippocampi of taxi drivers.

p. 6, *new brain cells* do *appear during adult life in certain parts of the brain:* Dranovsky and Hen, Hippocampal neurogeneses; Gould, Reeves, Graziano, et al., Neurogenesis in the neocortex of adult primates; Jacobs, van Praag, and Gage, Adult neurogenesis and psychiatry; Jacobs, van Praag, and Gage, Depression and the birth and death of brain cells; Malberg, Implications of adult hippocampus neurogenesis in antidepressant action; Santarelli, Saxe, Gross, et al., Requirement of hippocampal neurogenesis for the behavioral effects of antidepressants.

p. 7, *stories (or, as my colleagues might put it, "narratives") are essential to the New Neuropsychiatry:* Habermas and Bluck, Getting a life; Williams, Barnhofer, Crane, et al., Autobiographical memory specificity and emotional disorder.

p. 9, *suicide rates, which after a century of increase have dropped significantly since the introduction of SSRIs:* Jick, Kaye, and Jick, Antidepressants and the risk of suicidal behaviors; Erlangsen, A., Canudas-Romo, V., and Conwell, Y. Increased use of antidepressants and decreasing suicide rates: a population-based study using Danish register data

p. 9, *"safety centers" in the brains of mice:* Pollak, Monje, Zuckerman, Denny, Drew, and Kandel, Animal model of a behavioral intervention for depression; Rogan, Leon, Perez, and Kandel, Neural signatures for safety and danger in the amygdala and striatum of the mouse.

Chapter 1. Disorder

p. 15 sidebar, *Depression in the United States:* Cross-National Collaborative Group, Changing rate of major depression; Kessler, Berglund, Olga Demler, et al., Epidemiology of major depression; Olfson, Marcus, Druss, Elinson, Tanielian, and Pincus, National trends in the outpatient treatment of depression.

p. 16, *such profound states of disorder are bad for your brain—and for your body:* Belmaker and Agam, Major depressive disorder; Hendrie, Albert, Butters, et al., NIH cognitive and emotional health project; Higgins, Is depression neurochemical or neurodegenerative?; Mann, Medical management of depression; Nestler, Barrot, DiLeone, et al., Neurobiology of depression; Sapolsky, Stress is bad for your brain; Stout and Musselman, Depression and cardiovascular disease.

p. 16, *how common, and how devastating, mental disorders can be:* Cross-National Collaborative Group, Changing rate of major depression; Kessler, Berglund, Olga Demler, et al., Epidemiology of major depression; Olfson, Marcus, Druss, Elinson, Tanielian, and Pincus, National trends in the outpatient treatment of depression.

p. 18, *innumerable new drugs have entered the marketplace:* Albers, *Handbook of Psychiatric Drugs*; Gorman, *Essential Guide to Psychiatric Drugs*; Holden, Future brightening for depression treatments.

p. 22 sidebar, *Brain Functioning in Depression:* Thanks to Dr. Gerald Bruder, at the New York State Psychiatric Institute, who helped to clarify a complex and confusing body of research studies.

p. 24, *depression includes serious dysregulation of body rhythms:* Belmaker and Agam, Major depressive disorder; Nestler, Barrot, DiLeone, et al., Neurobiology of depression.

p. 24, *body and mind are interconnected in depression:* Gillespie and Nemeroff, Early life stress and depression; Mann, Medical management of depression; Nestler, Barrot, DiLeone, et al., Neurobiology of depression.

p. 30, *I have a postpartum depression:* Donahue Jennings, Ross, Popper, and Elmore, Thoughts of harming infants in depressed and nondepressed mothers; Wisner, Parry, and Piontek, Postpartum depression; Yonkers, Treatment of women suffering from depression who are either pregnant or breastfeeding.

p. 30, *Dr. Ivan's Depression Central Web site:* Dr. Ivan Goldberg, a psychopharmacologist in New York, runs a Web site at: www.psycom.net/depression.central.html. Other sites with useful information about depression include www.nimh.nih.gov/health/topics/depression/index.shtml and www.mayoclinic.com/health/depression/DS00175.

Chapter 2. The Evaluation

p. 37, *fear as a symptom of abnormal brain function:* LeDoux, *The Emotional Brain*; LeDoux, *Synaptic Self*; Lydiard, Break the "fear circuit" in resistant panic disorder; Stein, Neurobiology of panic disorder.

p. 38 sidebar, *The DSM:* The various versions of the *The Diagnostic and Statistical Manual of Mental Disorders* (DSM) include DSM-III (1980), which was published the year I began residency training, DSM-IV (1994), and a minor revision, DSM-IV-TR (1994); the DSM-5 is in preparation, with publication anticipated in May 2013. American Psychiatric Association, *Diagnostic and Statistical Manual of Mental Disorders*, 3rd edition; American Psychiatric Association, *Diagnostic and Statistical*

Manual of Mental Disorders, 4th edition; American Psychiatric Association, *Diagnostic and Statistical Manual of Mental Disorders*, 4th edition, text revision.

p. 39, *mood disorders so often coexist with anxiety disorders such as panic disorder and OCD:* Kessler, DuPont, Berglund, and Wittchen, Impairment in pure and comorbid generalized anxiety disorder and major depression.

p. 41, *By narrative, we mean the story of what is happening in your life:* The ability to tell a story about one's own life usually develops during adolescence, as described by Habermas and Bluck's paper. Psychiatric disorders can cause disturbances in the ability to tell such stories; conditions such as borderline personality disorder impair the ability to tell a coherent life narrative; and depression interferes with the ability to recall and recount the events of one's life.
Habermas and Bluck, Getting a life; Williams, Barnhofer, Crane, et al., Autobiographical memory specificity and emotional disorder.

p. 42, *Checking out the Body's Systems:* Sadock and Sadock, *Kaplan and Sadock's Comprehensive Textbook of Psychiatry*, pages 652-788 and 789-823.

p. 43, *these exquisitely sensitive fear circuits were driving Mark's behavior:* Davis, Neural circuitry of anxiety and stress disorders; Davis, Neurobiology of fear responses.

p. 45, *most common postpartum reaction is depression:* Donahue Jennings, Ross, Popper, et al., Thoughts of harming infants in depressed and nondepressed mothers; Wisner, Parry, and Piontek, Postpartum depression; Yonkers, Treatment of women suffering from depression who are either pregnant or breastfeeding.

p. 46, *It Runs in the Family:* Freedman, Long-term effects of early genetic influence on behavior; Gillespie and Nemeroff, Early life stress and depression.

p. 50 sidebar, *Medical Factors:* Sadock and Sadock, *Kaplan and Sadock's Comprehensive Textbook of Psychiatry*, pages 1765-1887.

p. 54, *it connects nearly all parts of the brain:* Azmitia and Whitaker-Azmitia, Cell biology and maturation of the serotonergic system; Grove, Coplan, and Hollander, Neuroanatomy of 5-HT dysregulation and panic disorder.

p. 56 sidebar, *The Rising Incidence of Depression:* For general information, see Andrade, Caraveo-Anduaga, Berglund, et al., Epidemiology of major depressive episodes; Cross-National Collaborative Group, Changing rate of major depression; Kessler, Berglund, Olga Demler, et al., Epidemiology of major depression; Olfson, Marcus, Druss, Elinson, Tanielian, and Pincus, National trends in the outpatient treatment of depression; Weissman, Bland, Canino, et al., Cross-national epidemiology of major depression and bipolar disorder.

p. 56, sidebar, *For decades (until the SSRIs were introduced):* Erlangsen, Canudas-Romo, and Conwell. Increased use of antidepressants and decreasing suicide rates: a population-based study using Danish register data.

p. 57 sidebar, *our stress response systems are tied together:* Grove, Coplan, and Hollander, Neuroanatomy of 5-HT dysregulation and panic disorder; McEwen, Neurobiology of stress; Nestler, Barrot, DiLeone, et al., Neurobiology of depression; Sen, Duman, and Sanacora, Serum brain-derived neurotrophic factor, depression and antidepressant medications.

p. 58 sidebar, *Different Disorders Need Different Medications:* Hales and Yudofsky, *Essentials of Clinical Psychiatry.*

Chapter 3. The Treatments

p. 64, *In working with people who have panic disorder . . . beautiful linkage between mind and body:* Charney and Drevets, Neurobiological basis of anxiety disorders; Davis, Neural circuitry of anxiety and stress disorder; Davis, Neurobiology of fear responses; Grove, Coplan, and Hollander, Neuroanatomy of 5-HT dysregulation and panic disorder; McEwen, Neurobiology of stress; Stein, Neurobiology of panic disorder.

p. 72. sidebar, *Take a Deep Breath and Control Your Anxiety:* Barlow, *Clinical Handbook of Psychological Disorders;* Barlow and Craske, *Mastery of your Anxiety and Panic;* Barlow and Cerny, *Psychological Treatment of Panic;* Borkovec and Costello, Efficacy of applied relaxation and cognitive-behavioral therapy in the treatment of generalized anxiety disorder; Bourne, C. *The Anxiety and Phobia Workbook;* Conrad and Roth, Muscle relaxation therapy for anxiety disorders; Jacobson, *Progressive Relaxation.*

p. 74, *Mark's initial problem was posttraumatic stress disorder (PTSD):* American Psychiatric Association, *Diagnostic and Statistical Manual of Mental Disorders,* 4th edition; Davidson, Stein, Shalev, and Yehuda, Posttraumatic stress disorder; Hull, Neuroimaging findings in posttraumatic stress disorder; Schiraldi, *Post-Traumatic Stress Disorder Sourcebook.*

p. 84, *STAR*D long-term study of depression:* Rush, Trivedi, Wisniewski, et al., Acute and longer-term outcomes in depressed outpatients.

p. 87, *Despite the benefits of single treatments, there are many situations in which it makes sense to start treatment with a combined approach:* Bauer, Whybrow, Angst, et al., World Federation of Societies of Biological Psychiatry guidelines for biological treatment of unipolar depressive disorders; Jindal and Thase, Integration of care; Thase, When are psychotherapy and pharmacotherapy combinations the treatment of choice for major depressive disorder?

p. 88, *psychotherapy called CBASP (a type of cognitive therapy):* Keller, McCullough, Klein, et al. A comparison of nefazodone, the cognitive behavioral-analysis system of psychotherapy, and their combination for the treatment of chronic depression.

p. 90, *Regular physical exercise may specifically help to repair the brain injury . . . by increasing the levels of the neurotrophic factors:* Convit, Wolf, Tarshish, and de Leon, Reduced glucose tolerance is associated with poor memory performance and hippocampal atrophy among normal elderly; Dunn, Trivedi, Kampert, Clark, and Chambliss, DOSE study; Erickson and Kramer, Aerobic exercise effects on cognitive and neural plasticity in older adults; Koehl, Meerlo, Gonzales, et al., Exercise-induced hippocampal cell proliferation requires beta endorphin; Mather, Rodriguez, Guthrie, McHarg, Reid, and McMurdo, Effects of exercise on depressive symptoms in older adults; Pereira, Huddleston, Brickman, et al., In vivo correlate of exercise-induced neurogenesis in the adult dentate gyrus; Russo-Neustadt, Beardy, Huang, and Cotman, Physical activity and antidepressant treatment; Trivedi, Greer, Grannemann, Chambliss, and Jordan, Exercise as an augmentation strategy for treatment of major depression; van Praag, Shubert, Zhao, and Gage, Exercise enhances learning and hippocampal neurogenesis in aged mice.

Chapter 4. On the Road

p. 105, *maybe the medicine is making her suicidal?* Cipriani, Geddes, Furukawa, and Barbui, Metareview on short-term effectiveness and safety of antidepressants for depression; Gunnell, Saperia, and Ashby, Selective serotonin reuptake inhibitors and suicide in adults; Jick, Kaye, and Jick, Antidepressants and the risk of suicidal behaviors; Khan, Khan, Kolts, and Brown, Suicide rates in clinical trials of SSRIs, other antidepressants, and placebo; Simon, Savarino, Operskalski, and Wang, Suicide risk during antidepressant treatment.

p. 107, *symptoms of bipolar II disorder:* Only in recent years has bipolar II disorder has begun to be studied seriously. While it is clear that bipolar II disorder is often missed in evaluating depression, it is not yet clear how best to manage the depression that occurs in this disorder and whether the use of antidepressants without mood stabilizers helps or worsens its course.
Bowden, Strategies to reduce misdiagnosis of bipolar depression; Ghaemi, Boiman, and Goodwin, Diagnosing bipolar disorder and the effect of antidepressants; Hirschfeld, Lewis, and Vornik, Perceptions and impact of bipolar disorder; MacQueen and Young, Bipolar II disorder; Suppes and Dennehy, Evidence-based long-term treatment of bipolar II disorder; Yatham, Diagnosis and management of patients with bipolar II disorder.

p. 108, *They* weren't *insights; they were "intrusive thoughts"!* Baer, *Imp of the Mind*; Donaldson and Lam, Rumination, mood and social problem-solving in major depression; Lyubomirsky and Nolen-Hoeksema, Effects of self-focused rumination on negative thinking and interpersonal problem solving.

p. 111, *some hyperactive circuits in his brain:* Mayberg, Defining neurocircuits in depression.

p. 116, *trying to retrain his fear systems:* LeDoux, *Emotional Brain*; LeDoux, *Synaptic Self*; McEwen, Neurobiology of stress.

p. 117, *Scientists believe that the brain's structure actually becomes pared down to deal with severe crises:* Viamontes and Beitman, Neural substrates of psychotherapeutic change, parts I and II.

p. 118, *how he could be remapping his brain by his travels:* In infancy, childhood, and adolescence, the brain undergoes much remodeling. How much do brains continue to change in adult life? And are humans different from other mammals, such as mice, which may have more brain plasticity throughout life? Van Praag and colleagues did an interesting study demonstrating that even in "aged mice" neurogenesis still occurs!

See van Praag, Shubert, Zhao, and Gage, Exercise enhances learning and hippocampal neurogenessis in aged mice. See also p. 122, "hippocampus of cab drivers" below.

p. 119, *second stage in the New Neuropsychiatry is remission:* Israel, Remission in depression; Nierenberg, Petersen, and Alpert, Prevention of relapse and recurrence in depression; Nierenberg and Wright, Evolution of remission as the new standard in treatment of depression; Shulman, Response versus remission in the treatment of depression; Thase, Evaluating antidepressant therapies; van Rhoads and Gelenberg, Treating depression to remission; Zimmerman, Posternak, and Chelminski, Implications of using different cut-offs on symptom severity scales to define remission from depression.

p. 122, *hippocampus of cab drivers enlarges to allow them to store a detailed mental map:* The hippocampus is key to a range of brain functions, including spatial and episodic memory. It has been clearly shown to shrink in depression. Studies show how the brain can be remapped by learning and practice, whether taxi-driving or juggling. Antidepressant medication and exercise also cause neurogenesis in the hippocampus.
Burgess, Maguire, and O'Keefe, Human hippocampus and spatial and episodic memory; Draganski, Gaser, Busch, Schuierer, Bogdahn, and May, Neuroplasticity; Maguire, Gadian, Johnsrude, et al., Navigation-related structural change in the hippocampi of taxi drivers; Sheline, Neuroimaging studies of mood disorder effects on the brain; Sheline, Wang, Gado, et al., Hippocampal atrophy in recurrent major depression.

p. 122, *studies show that* all *antidepressant and mood stabilizer medications appear to specifically cause neurogenesis in this part of the brain!* Conversely, medicines that do not cause neurogenesis in the hippocampus are not effective as antidepressants.
Dranovsky and Hen, Hippocampal neurogenesis; Malberg, Implications of adult hippocampus neurogenesis in antidepressant action; Manji, Moore, and Chen, Clinical and preclinical evidence for the neurotrophic effects of mood stabilizers; Manji, Quiroz, and Gould, Cellular resistance and neuroplasticity in mood disorders; Pakpan, Lithium and valproate may provide neurotrophic and neuroprotective effects; Santarelli, Saxe, Gross, et al., Requirement of hippocampal neurogenesis for the behavioral effects of antidepressants.

Chapter 5. A New Vista

p. 127, *Thomas Frodl and colleagues:* Frodl, Koutsouleris, Bottlender, et al. Depression-related variation in brain morphology.

p. 128 sidebar, *Changing Definitions of Response, Remission, and Recovery:* Different research groups often define these terms somewhat differently. For instance, one group may define remission as a score of 7 or less on the Hamilton Depression Rating Scale, while another group may require a score of 4 or less. Depending on what the magic number is, there will be more or fewer people who can be considered to "remit" with treatment. Regardless of the exact cut-off, psychiatrists have realized that remission is the new goal of treatment. Remission is more likely than purely responding to treatment to give patients back their lives.

Israel, Remission in depression; Nierenberg, Petersen, and Alpert, Prevention of relapse and recurrence in depression; Nierenberg and Wright, Evolution of remission as the new standard in treatment of depression; Shulman, Response versus remission in the treatment of depression; Thase, Evaluating antidepressant therapies; van Rhoads and Gelenberg, Treating depression to remission; Zimmerman, Posternak, and Chelminski, Implications of using different cut-offs on symptom severity scales to define remission from depression.

p. 130, *Lewis Judd found that such people stayed well:* Judd, Akiskal, Maser, et al., Major depressive disorder; Judd, Paulus, Schettler, et al., Does incomplete recovery from first lifetime major depressive episode herald a chronic course of illness?

p. 130, *best way is by using rating scales:* For instance, our research group, the Depression Evaluation Service at New York State and the Columbia Department of Psychiatry, has the Quick Inventory of Depressive Symptomatology (QIDS), a self-rating scale of depression. See http://asp.cumc.columbia.edu/depression/survey/index.asp. 16-item Quick Inventory of Depressive Symptomatology (QIDS), Clinician Rating (QIDS-C), and Self-report (QIDS-SR): Rush, Trivedi, Ibrahim, et al. The Hamilton Depression Rating Scale: Hamilton, A rating scale for depression. The Beck Depression Inventory: Beck, Ward, Mendelson, et al. An inventory for measuring depression. The Montgomery Asberg Depression Rating Scale: Montgomery and Asberg, A new depression scale designed to be sensitive to change.

p. 132, *She became involved with Weight Watchers:* See www.weightwatchers.com; in particular, their Weight Watchers online program.

p. 135, *Y-BOCS (the Yale-Brown Obsessive-Compulsive Scale):* www.cnsforum.com/streamfile.aspx?filename=YBOCS.pdf&path=pdf; Kim, Dysken, Kuskowski, Yale-Brown Obsessive-Compulsive Scale.

p. 136, *psychotherapy should focus on here-and-now solutions:* Thase, When are psychotherapy and pharmacotherapy combinations the treatment of choice for major depressive disorder?

p. 138, *In recent years, we have learned about the mirror neurons:* Rizzolatti and Craighero, Mirror-neuron system.

p. 139, *Research suggests that remission is accompanied by changes in the brain:* For instance, Gervasoni et al. found that brain-derived neurotrophic factor increases when depression goes into remission, a finding that has been confirmed by other researchers. However, Mayberg found that part of the brain, the rostral cingulate, remains hyperactive during remission, suggesting that the brain has to work to prevent reactivation of the depression circuits.

Gervasoni, Aubry, Bondolfi, et al., Partial normalization of serum brain-derived neurotrophic factor in remitted patients after a major depressive episode; Mayberg, Defining neurocircuits in depression.

p. 139, *a surge of brain-derived neurotrophic factor:* Gervasoni, Aubry, Bondolfi, et al., Partial normalization of serum brain-derived neurotrophic factor in remitted patients after a major depressive episode.

p. 141 sidebar, *Medical students, for instance, have measureable growth in gray matter:* Draganski, Gaser, Kempermann, et al., Temporal and spatial dynamics of brain structure changes during extensive learning.

p. 141, *posttraumatic stress disorder . . . often irreversibly changes the brain in some ways:* Hull, Neuroimaging findings in posttraumatic stress disorder.

p. 145, *Long ago, Sigmund Freud underlined the distinction between depression and grief:* Freud, Mourning and melancholia.

p. 147, *A second issue was what psychiatric researcher Dr. Robert Cloninger, of Washington University in St. Louis, called "harm avoidance":* Harm avoidance refers to a reluctance to do activities of daily life (such as setting up business-related meetings, calling a person you are interested in for a date, etc.) because of a concern for a possible negative outcome. Harm avoidance is often elevated in people who have depression and anxiety disorders, and it affects their ability to function well in daily life, including work performance and social activities.
Cloninger, Tridimensional Personality Questionnaire; Cloninger, Svrakic, and Przybeck, Psychobiological model of temperament and character.

p. 147, *These kinds of thought patterns . . . probably result from the brain changes of chronic stress:* Viamontes and Beitman, Neural substrates of psychotherapeutic change, parts I and II.

p. 150, *how a person's disorder affected his or her established patterns of thought and behavior, what could also be called personality:* Over time, depression (and other conditions, such as anxiety disorders) has a negative impact on personality and social relationships. Chronic but not short-term depression often causes changes in personality, including elevated harm avoidance, as described above. Also, many studies have shown that having both a personality disorder *and* major depression makes it more difficult to recover from depression. Antidepressant medication treatment actually decreases personality problems and has been shown to improve social functioning. Black and Sheline, Personality disorder scores improve with effective pharmacotherapy of depression; Grilo, Shea, Skodol, et al., Two-year prospective naturalistic study of remission from major depressive disorder as a function of personality disorder comorbidity; Hellerstein, Kocsis, Chapman, et al., Double-blind comparison of sertraline, imipramine, and placebo in the treatment of dysthymia; Mulder, Personality pathology and treatment outcome in major depression; Pilkonis and Frank, Personality pathology in recurrent depression.

p. 151, *Conquering Negative Thoughts:* Cognitive therapy, pioneered by Aaron Beck and Albert Ellis, has focused to a great extent on challenging and correcting excessively negative thoughts.
Beck, Emery, and Greenberg, *Anxiety Disorders and Phobias*; Beck, Rush, Shaw, et al., *Cognitive Therapy of Depression*.

See also Baer, *Imp of the Mind*; Donaldson and Lam, Rumination, mood and social problem-solving in major depression; Lyubomirsky and Nolen-Hoeksema, Effects of self-focused rumination on negative thinking and interpersonal problem solving.

p. 152 sidebar, *Cognitive-Behavioral Therapy:* Cognitive-behavioral therapy was pioneered by Albert Ellis, who developed rational emotive therapy, and Aaron Beck, the founder of cognitive therapy.

Beck, Emery, and Greenberg, *Anxiety Disorders and Phobias*; Beck, Rush, Shaw, and Emery, *Cognitive Therapy of Depression*; Ellis and Dryden, *Practice of Rational Emotive Behavior Therapy*; Ellis and Harper, *Guide to Rational Living*.

p. 152 sidebar, *break the hold of the amygdala's fear system:* Johnstone, van Reekum, et al., Failure to regulate; Lydiard, Break the "fear circuit" in resistant panic disorder.

p. 152 sidebar, *MRI studies have shown that cognitive-behavioral therapy:* Goldapple, Segal, Garson, et al., Modulation of cortical-limbic pathways in major depression.

p. 153, *Ryan had a high level of harm avoidance:* Avoidance may be a key factor that maintains depression. People who have depression often avoid difficult situations and problems, and as a result these problems can worsen over time, leading to a vicious cycle in which depression also worsens. In recent years, a therapy approach called behavioral activation (BA) has been developed to actively reverse these avoidance patterns in people who have depression, using activity scheduling as a powerful tool to change behavior. BA therapists view negative thoughts and rumination as a type of avoidance behavior. In contrast to cognitive therapists, who focus on changing such negative thoughts first and then changing behavior, BA therapists focus on changing behavior first, with the belief that after behavior becomes more adaptive, one's mood, thoughts, and feelings will naturally improve. Studies have shown that BA is as effective as medication or cognitive therapy in treating depression.

Addis and Martell, *Overcoming Depression One Step at a Time*; Martell, Addis, and Jacobson, *Depression in Context*. See also the information on harm avoidance for page 23 above.

p. 154, *what psychiatrists call "rejection sensitivity":* Rejection sensitivity is one of the key symptoms of "atypical depression," which also often include excessive sleep, lethargy, weight gain, and a feeling of leaden weight in one's limbs. Atypical depression has been shown to respond to MAO inhibitor antidepressant medications, though currently SSRI medications are the first choice of most doctors.

Downey and Feldman, Implications of rejection sensitivity for intimate relationships; Quitkin, Depression with atypical features.

p. 157, *My guess is that this reflects problems in the vestiges of poor functioning of the subgenual prefrontal cortex:* Drevets, Price, Simpson, et al. Subgenual prefrontal cortex abnormalities in mood disorders.

Chapter 6. Moving Forward

p. 165, *Being postdisorder:* A number of years ago, Dr. John Markowitz wrote a paper describing how people who have dysthymia, or chronic depression, often enter a new state after responding to medication, which he described as a "postdysthymic" state. One could broaden that term to a wider range of conditions by describing a "postdisorder" state that can be encountered once a person's disorder has been in remission for a significant period of time (i.e., several months to years). Markowitz, Psychotherapy of the post-dysthymic patient.

p. 167, *process of reengagement in life:* Li, Ma, Li, et al., Prefrontal white matter abnormalities in young adult with major depressive disorder ; Siegel, *Developing Mind*; Siegel, Interpersonal neurobiology approach to psychotherapy; Siegel, Toward an interpersonal neurobiology of the developing mind.

p. 167, *So our brains' sexual neurotransmitter:* The specific transmitter that governs attachment varies by species. For a discussion of this issue, see Hiller, Speculations on the links between feelings, emotions and sexual behaviour.

p. 170, *committee of the American College of Neuropsychopharmacology . . . defined recovery:* Rush, Kraemer, Sackeim, et al., Report by the ACNP Task Force on response and remission in major depressive disorder.

p. 175, *When I saw Cindy in those days, I kept thinking about glutamate:* Dixon and Hokin, Lithium acutely inhibits and chronically upregulates and stabilizes glutamate uptake.

p. 175, *Staying in remission is an ongoing process and challenge:* This can involve adding psychotherapy approaches such as cognitive behavioral therapy (Fava et al., Hollon et al., Teasdale et al.), or making medication changes, as seen in the STAR*D study. Fava, Rafanelli, Grandi, Conti, and Belluardo, Prevention of recurrent depression with cognitive behavioral therapy; Fava, Ruini, Rafanelli, et al., Six-year outcome of cognitive behavioral therapy for prevention of recurrent depression; Geddes, Carney, Davies, et al., Relapse prevention with antidepressant drug treatment in depressive disorders; Hollon, DeRubeis, Shelton, et al., Prevention of relapse following cognitive therapy vs. medications in moderate to severe depression; Rush, Trivedi, Wisniewski, et al., Acute and longer-term outcomes in depressed outpatients; Teasdale, Segal, Williams, Ridgeway, Soulsby, and Lau, Prevention of relapse/recurrence in major depression by mindfulness-based cognitive therapy.

p. 176 sidebar, *Exercise and the Brain:* There has been an explosive growth of research on the effects of exercise and brain plasticity, both in mice and rats studied in the research laboratory and in humans.

Convit, Wolf, Tarshish, and de Leon, Reduced glucose tolerance is associated with poor memory performance and hippocampal atrophy among normal elderly; Dunn, Trivedi, Kampert, Clark, and Chambliss, DOSE study; Erickson and Kramer, Aerobic exercise effects on cognitive and neural plasticity in older adults; Mather, Rodriguez, Guthrie, McHarg, Reid, and McMurdo, Effects of exercise on depressive symptoms in older adults; Pereira, Huddleston, Brickman, et al.,

In vivo correlate of exercise-induced neurogenesis in the adult dentate gyrus; Russo-Neustadt, Beardy, Huang, and Cotman, Physical activity and antidepressant treatment potentiate the expression of specific brain-derived neurotrophic factor transcripts in the rat hippocampus; Trivedi, Greer, Grannemann, Chambliss, and Jordan, Exercise as an augmentation strategy for treatment of major depression; van Praag, Shubert, Zhao, and Gage, Exercise enhances learning and hippocampal neurogenesis in aged mice.

p. 177, *We now see the brain as a dynamic organ that is continually being remodeled in response to its environment:* Dias-Ferreira et al. described how chronic stress remodels the brain in rats and leads to behavior becoming more routine and compulsive. With rest, this process is reversed. See also Angier, Brain is a co-conspirator in a vicious stress loop.
Dias-Ferreira, Sousa, Melo, et al., Chronic stress causes frontostriatal reorganization and affects decision-making.

p. 178, *learning clearly is associated with neurogenesis and plasticity in the brain:* Maguire's studies clearly show this phenomenon. Also, Draganski and colleagues cleverly showed this in a study of people who learned to juggle.
Burgess, Maguire, and O'Keefe, Human hippocampus and spatial and episodic memory; Draganski, Gaser, Busch, Schuierer, Bogdahn, and May, Neuroplasticity; Maguire, Burgess, Donnett, et al., Knowing where and getting there; Maguire, Gadian, Johnsrude, et al., Structural change in the hippocampi of taxi drivers.

p. 179, *Adjusting Medication to Stay in Remission:* Lam and Kennedy, Evidence-based strategies for achieving and sustaining full remission in depression; Rush, Trivedi, Wisniewski, et al., Acute and longer-term outcomes in depressed outpatients.

p. 180 sidebar, *Sexuality, Disorder, and Recovery:* Pfaus, Neurobiology of sexual behavior; Crenshaw and Goldberg, *Sexual Pharmacology;* Rosen, Lane, and Menza, Effects of SSRIs on sexual function.

p. 184 sidebar, *Pregnancy, Childbirth, and After:* Blier, Pregnancy, depression, antidepressants and breast-feeding; Donahue Jennings, Ross, Popper, and Elmore, Thoughts of harming infants in depressed and nondepressed mothers; Freeman, Antenatal depression; Hallberg and Sjoblom, Use of selective serotonin reuptake inhibitors during pregnancy and breastfeeding; Wisner, Parry, and Piontek, Postpartum depression; Yonkers, Treatment of women suffering from depression who are either pregnant or breastfeeding.
Useful Web sites include the Canadian www.motherisk.org and the Harvard University (Massachusetts General Hospital) site www.womensmentalhealth.org.

p. 187, *Panic disorder, for instance, often runs in families:* Hettema, Neale, and Kendler, A review and meta-analysis of the genetic epidemiology of anxiety disorders.

p. 189, *development of children exposed in utero to SSRI medications:* Einarson and Einarson, Newer antidepressants in pregnancy and rates of major malformations.

p. 193, *the neurobiological changes of becoming parents, and whether this too may facilitate brain recovery:* Insel and Young, Neurobiology of attachment; Pfaus, Neurobiology of sexual behavior.

Chapter 7. Mapping the Route

p. 196, *perhaps one-third of patients are now treatment resistant:* Fagiolini and Kupfer, Is treatment-resistant depression a unique subtype of depression?; Fava, Diagnosis and definition of treatment-resistant depression. See also p. X below for the sidebar on Treatment-Resistant Depression.

p. 200 sidebar, *Options in Treatment-Resistant Depression:* Many different approaches have been shown to be effective for treatment-resistant depression, including medication combinations and the use of psychotherapy. The Texas Medication Algorithm Project, available online, offers guidance when remission is not achieved, in the form of a series of treatment choices. Psychopharmacologist Stephen Stahl described a number of medication combinations for treatment-resistant depression, including what is called "California rocket fuel," a combination of two potent antidepressants, venlafaxine and mirtazapine. Alternative therapies, such as omega-3 fatty acids, and behavioral approaches, such as mindfulness meditation, have also been shown to be helpful.

Mayo Clinic staff, Treatment-resistant depression; Peet and Stokes, Omega-3 fatty acids in the treatment of psychiatric disorders; Rush, Crismon, Kashner, et al. The Texas Medication Algorithm Project for major depression, Phase 3; Severus, Littman, and Stoll, Omega-3 fatty acids, homocysteine, and the increased risk of cardiovascular mortality in major depressive disorder; Shelton, Treatment-resistant depression; Stahl and Muntner, *Stahl's Essential Psychopharmacology*, 655-56; Suehs, Argo, Bendele, Crimson, Trivedi, and Kurian, *Texas Medication Algorithm Project: Procedural Manual.*

p. 204 sidebar, *Possible Genetic Reasons for Lack of Response to Treatment:* These can include a wide range of possibilities, such as those resulting from genetic differences, such as how one's body absorbs or metabolizes a drug (Lohoff) or how one's brain deals with life stresses (Anguelova, Benkelfat, and Turecki; Caspi et al.). On a more prosaic level, the most common reason depression does not respond to medication treatment is that the medication is not being taken as prescribed. Misdiagnosis must also be considered, particularly in the case of bipolar II disorder (see chapter 4, p. 19, above*).* Though genetics offers much long-term promise and though companies are now promoting genetic testing packages, it is doubtful that they currently provide much benefit, as Roy-Byrne notes.

Anguelova, Benkelfat, and Turecki, Systematic review of association studies investigating genes coding for serotonin receptors and the serotonin transporter; Caspi, Sugden, Moffitt, et al., Influence of life stress on depression; Lohoff, Pharmacogenetics of major depressive disorder; Roy-Byrne, Predictive power of genes.

p. 209, *poor treatment response of patients who have anxious depression:* Fava, Rush, Alpert, et al., Difference in treatment outcome in outpatients with anxious versus nonanxious depression.

p. 211, *Mindfulness is a meditation-based form of stress reduction:* Brantley and Kabat-Zinn, *Calming Your Anxious Mind;* Grossman, Niemann, Schmidt, and Walach, Mindfulness-based stress reduction and health benefits; Kabat-Zinn, *Full Catastrophe Living;* Stein, Ives-Deliperi, and Thomas, Psychobiology of mindfulness.

p. 212 sidebar, *Increasing Resilience:* Charney, Nemeroff, and Braun, *Peace of Mind Prescription;* Stein, Psychobiology of resilience.

p. 217, *Patricia clearly had borderline personality disorder:* People who have this condition (see the DSM-IV definition) generally have unstable personal relationships and impulsive behavior (including self-injury and suicide attempts) and make frantic efforts to avoid real or imagined abandonment. They often have chronic feelings of emptiness, have difficulty in controlling anger, and act impulsively in sexual relationships or in using drugs or alcohol. Interesting brain imaging studies have shown that people who have borderline personality disorder often have abnormal connections between the brain's frontal lobe and the anxiety centers of the amygdala, suggesting that this condition may be as "biological" as many other psychiatric disorders, such as bipolar illness or schizophrenia.

American Psychiatric Association, *Diagnostic and Statistical Manual of Mental Disorders,* 4th edition; Lis, Greenfield, Henry, Guile, and Doughtery, Neuroimaging and genetics of borderline personality disorder; New and Hazlett, Amygdala–prefrontal disconnection in borderline personality disorder.

p. 218, *DBT is a prime example of New Neuropsychiatry therapies:* DBT, or dialectical behavioral therapy, was developed by Marsha Linehan, PhD. In addition to DBT, other treatment approaches have been developed for the treatment of borderline personality disorder. A recent study (Clarkin et al.) compared three different treatments for this disorder: DBT, transference-focused psychotherapy, and brief supportive psychotherapy. Patients treated with all three of these approaches improved over the course of treatment, with significant relief of depression and core symptoms of BPD and improvement of social functioning.

Clarkin, Levy, Lenzenweger, and Kernberg, Evaluating three treatments for borderline personality disorder; Linehan, *Skills Training Manual for Treating Borderline Personality Disorder;* Palmer, Dialectical behavior therapy for borderline personality disorder.

p. 220, *Neuropsychiatry theorist Dr. Daniel Siegel talks about how "complexity theory" applies to the personality:* Siegel, *The Developing Mind,* p. 215.

p. 223. *In "A Life on the Decline, and Then the 'Why?'"* Winerip, *New York Times,* September 18, 2009.

Chapter 8. Returning Home

p. 226 sidebar, *The Safety Center:* Rogan, Leon, Perez, and Kandel, Distinct neural signatures for safety and danger in the amygdala and striatum of the mouse.

p. 227 sidebar, *Recently, Daniela Pollak, PhD, another Columbia researcher:* Pollak, Monje, Zuckerman, Denny, Drew, and Kandel, Animal model of a behavioral intervention for depression.

p. 234 sidebar, *Do I Need to Keep Taking Medicine?* Geddes, Carney, Davies, et al., Relapse prevention with antidepressant drug treatment in depressive disorders; Kupfer, Frank, Perel, et al., Five-year outcome for maintenance therapies in recurrent depression; Nierenberg, Petersen, and Alpert, Prevention of relapse and recurrence in depression.

p. 234 sidebar, *In the late 1980s, Ellen Frank and David Kupfer:* Kupfer, Frank, Perel, et al., Five-year outcome for maintenance therapies in recurrent depression.

p. 235 sidebar, *We have numerous other studies as well:* Otto, Smits, and Reese, Cognitive-behavioral therapy for the treatment of anxiety disorders.

p. 240 sidebar, *Gradually taper off medicine:* Haddad, Antidepressant discontinuation syndromes; Viguera, Baldessarini, and Friedberg, Discontinuing antidepressant treatment in major depression.

p. 240 sidebar, *social rhythms therapy:* This approach has been studied in bipolar disorder, in which it has been shown to help people remain stable and avoid the return of disorder, but has not yet been reported in major depression. Frank, Hlastala, Ritenour, et al., Inducing lifestyle regularity in recovering bipolar disorder patients.

p. 241 sidebar, *Psychotherapy may be a way to make tapering off medicine go more smoothly:* Bockting, Schene, Spinhoven, et al., Preventing relapse/recurrence in recurrent depression with cognitive therapy; Fava, Rafanelli, Grandi, Conti, and Belluardo, et al., Prevention of recurrent depression with cognitive behavioral therapy; Fava, Ruini, Rafanelli, et al., Six-year outcome of cognitive behavioral therapy for prevention of recurrent depression; Frank, Kupfer, Wagner, et al., Efficacy of interpersonal psychotherapy as a maintenance treatment of recurrent depression; Hollon, DeRubeis, Shelton, et al., Prevention of relapse following cognitive therapy vs. medications in moderate to severe depression.

Bibliography

Addis, M.E., and Martell, C.R. *Overcoming Depression One Step at a Time: The New Behavioral Activation Approach to Getting Your Life Back*. Oakland, CA: New Harbinger Publications, 2004.

Albers, L.J., Hahn, R.K., and Reist, C., eds. *Handbook of Psychiatric Drugs*. Mission Viejo, CA: Current Clinical Strategies Publishing, 2007.

American Psychiatric Association. *Diagnostic and Statistical Manual of Mental Disorders*, 3rd edition. Washington, DC: American Psychiatric Association, 1980.

_____. *Diagnostic and Statistical Manual of Mental Disorders*, 4th edition. Washington, DC: American Psychiatric Association, 1994.

_____. *Diagnostic and Statistical Manual of Mental Disorders*, 4th edition, text revision. Washington, DC: American Psychiatric Association, 2000.

Amsterdam, J.D., Williams, D., Michelson, D., et al. Tachyphylaxis after repeated antidepressant drug exposure in patients with recurrent major depressive disorder. *Neuropsychobiology* 2009;59:227-33.

Andrade, L., Caraveo-Anduaga, J.J., Berglund, P., et al. The epidemiology of major depressive episodes: results from the International Consortium of Psychiatric Epidemiology (ICPE) surveys. *International Journal of Methods in Psychiatric Research* 2003;12:3-21.

Angier, N. Brain is a co-conspirator in a vicious stress loop. *The New York Times*, Aug. 18, 2009.

Anguelova, M., Benkelfat, C., and Turecki, G. A systematic review of association studies investigating genes coding for serotonin receptors and the serotonin transporter: I. Affective disorders. *Molecular Psychiatry* 2003;8:574-91.

Azmitia, E.C., and Whitaker-Azmitia, P.M. Cell biology and maturation of the seroto-
    nergic system: neurotrophic implications for the actions of psychotropic drugs. In
    Bloom, F.E., and Kupfer, D.J., eds., *Neuropsychopharmacology: The Fourth Generation
    of Progress*. Nashville, TN: American College of Neuropsychopharmacology, 2000.
Baer, L. *The Imp of the Mind: Exploring the Silent Epidemic of Obsessive Bad Thoughts*. New
    York: Dutton, 2001.
Barlow, D.H. *Clinical Handbook of Psychological Disorders*, 4th edition. New York: Guilford
    Press, 2007.
Barlow, D.H., and Cerny, J. *Psychological Treatment of Panic*. New York: Guilford Press,
    1988.
Barlow, D.H., and Craske, M.G. *Mastery of Your Anxiety and Panic: Workbook*, 4th edition.
    New York: Oxford University Press, 2007.
Bauer, M., Whybrow, P.C., Angst, J., et al. World Federation of Societies of Biological
    Psychiatry (WFSBP) guidelines for biological treatment of unipolar depressive
    disorders. I: acute and continuation treatment of major depressive disorder. *World
    Journal of Biological Psychiatry* 2002;3:5-43.
Beck, A.T., Emery, G., and Greenberg, R.L. *Anxiety Disorders and Phobias: A Cognitive
    Perspective*. New York: Basic Books, 1985.
Beck, A.T., Rush, A.J., Shaw, B.I., and Emery, G. *Cognitive Therapy of Depression*. New
    York: Guilford Press, 1987.
Beck, A.T., Ward, C.H., Mendelson, M, Mock, J., Erbaugh, J. An inventory for measuring
    depression. *Archives of General Psychiatry* 1961;4:561-571.
Belmaker, R.H., and Agam, G. Major depressive disorder. *New England Journal of
    Medicine* 2008;358:55-68.
Black, K.J., and Sheline, Y.I. Personality disorder scores improve with effective pharmaco-
    therapy of depression. *Journal of Affective Disorders* 1997;43:11-18.
Blier, P. Pregnancy, depression, antidepressants and breast-feeding. *Journal of Psychiatry &
    Neuroscience* 2006;31:226-28.
Bockting, C.L., Schene, A.H., Spinhoven, P., et al. Preventing relapse/recurrence in
    recurrent depression with cognitive therapy: a randomized controlled trial. *Journal
    of Consulting and Clinical Psychology* 2005;73:647-57.
Borkovec, T.D., and Costello, E. Efficacy of applied relaxation and cognitive-behavioral
    therapy in the treatment of generalized anxiety disorder. *Journal of Clinical and
    Consulting Psychology* 1993;61:611-19.
Bourne, C. *The Anxiety and Phobia Workbook*, 4th edition. Oakland, CA: New Harbinger,
    2005.
Bowden, C.L. Strategies to reduce misdiagnosis of bipolar depression. *Psychiatric Services*
    2001;52:51-55.
Brantley, J., and Kabat-Zinn, J. *Calming Your Anxious Mind: How Mindfulness and
    Compassion Can Free You from Anxiety, Fear and Panic*. Oakland, CA: New
    Harbinger, 2003.
Burgess, N., Maguire, E.A., and O'Keefe, J. The human hippocampus and spatial and
    episodic memory. *Neuron* 2002;35:625-41.

Carlson, P.J., Singh, J.B., Zarate, C.A., Jr., Drevets, W.C., Manji, H.K. Neural circuitry and neuroplasticity in mood disorders: insights for novel therapeutic targets. *NeuroRx* 2006;3:22-41.

Caspi, A., Sugden, K., Moffitt, T.E., et al. Influence of life stress on depression: moderation by a polymorphism in the 5-HTT gene. *Science* 2003;301:386-89.

Charney, D.S., and Drevets, W.C. Neurobiological basis of anxiety disorders. In Davis, K.L., Charney, D., Coyle, J.T., and Nemeroff, C., eds., *Neuropsychopharmacology: The Fifth Generation of Progress.* New York: Lippincott Williams & Wilkins, 2002:901-30.

Charney, D.S., Nemeroff, C.B., and Braun, S. *The Peace of Mind Prescription.* Boston: Houghton Mifflin, 2004.

Cipriani, A., Geddes, J., Furukawa, T., and Barbui, C. Metareview on short-term effectiveness and safety of antidepressants for depression: an evidence-based approach to inform clinical practice. *Canadian Journal of Psychiatry* 2007;52:553-62.

Clarkin, J.F., Levy, K.N., Lenzenweger, M.F., and Kernberg, O.F. Evaluating three treatments for borderline personality disorder: a multiwave study. *American Journal of Psychiatry* 2007;164:922-28.

Cloninger, C.R. *The Tridimensional Personality Questionnaire*, version IV. St. Louis, MO: Department of Psychiatry, Washington University School of Medicine, 1987.

Cloninger, C.R., Svrakic, D.M., and Przybeck, T.R. A psychobiological model of temperament and character. *Archives of General Psychiatry* 1993;50:975–90.

Conrad, A., and Roth, W.T. Muscle relaxation therapy for anxiety disorders: it works, but how? *Journal of Anxiety Disorders* 2007;21:243-64.

Convit, A., Wolf, O.T., Tarshish, C., and de Leon, M.J. Reduced glucose tolerance is associated with poor memory performance and hippocampal atrophy among normal elderly. *Proceedings of the National Academy of Sciences of the USA* 2003;100:2019-22.

Crenshaw, T.L., and Goldberg, J.P. *Sexual Pharmacology: Drugs That Affect Sexual Function.* New York: Norton, 1996.

Cross-National Collaborative Group. The changing rate of major depression. *JAMA* 1992;268:3098-3105.

Davidson, R.J., Jackson, D.C., and Kalin, N.H. Emotion, plasticity, context and recognition: perspectives from affective neuroscience. *Psychological Bulletin* 2000;126:890-909.

Davidson, J.R.T., Stein, D.J., Shalev, A.Y., and Yehuda, R. Posttraumatic stress disorder: acquisition, recognition, course and treatment. *Journal of Neuropsychiatry and Clinical Neurosciences* 2004;16:135-37.

Davis, M. Neural circuitry of anxiety and stress disorders. In Davis, K.L., Charney, D., Coyle, J.T., and Nemeroff, C., eds., *Neuropsychopharmacology: The Fifth Generation of Progress.* New York: Lippincott, Williams & Wilkins, 2000:931-52.

———. Neurobiology of fear responses: the role of the amygdala. *Journal of Neuropsychiatry and Clinical Neurosciences* 1997;9:382-402.

Dias-Ferreira, E., Sousa, J.C., Melo, I., et al. Chronic stress causes frontostriatal reorganization and affects decision-making. *Science* 2009;325:621-25.

Dixon, J.F., and Hokin, L.E. Lithium acutely inhibits and chronically upregulates and stabilizes glutamate uptake by presynaptic nerve endings in mouse cerebral cortex. *Proceedings of the National Academy of Sciences* 1998;95:8363-68.

Donahue Jennings, K., Ross, S., Popper, S., and Elmore, M. Thoughts of harming infants in depressed and nondepressed mothers. *Journal of Affective Disorders* 1999;54:21-28.

Donaldson, C., and Lam, D. Rumination, mood and social problem-solving in major depression. *Psychological Medicine* 2004;34:1309-18.

Downey, G., Feldman, S.I. Implications of rejection sensitivity for intimate relationships. *Journal of Personality and Social Psychology* 1996;70:1327-43.

Draganski, B., Gaser, C., Busch, V., Schuierer, G., Bogdahn, U., and May, A. Neuroplasticity: changes in grey matter induced by training. *Nature* 2004;427:311-12.

Draganski, B., Gaser, C., Kempermann, G., et al. Temporal and spatial dynamics of brain structure changes during extensive learning. *Journal of Neuroscience* 2006;26:6314-17.

Dranovsky, A., and Hen, R. Hippocampal neurogenesis: regulation by stress and antidepressants. *Biological Psychiatry* 2006;59:1136-43.

Drevets, W.C., Price, J.L., Simpson, J.R., Todd, R.D., et al. Subgenual prefrontal cortex abnormalities in mood disorders. *Nature* 1997;386:824-27.

Driessen, M., Beblo, T., Mertens, M., et al. Posttraumatic stress disorder and fMRI activation patterns of traumatic memory in patients with borderline personality disorder. *Biological Psychiatry* 2004;55:603-11.

Dunn, A.L., Trivedi, M.H., Kampert, J.B., Clark, C.G., and Chambliss, A.O. The DOSE study: a clinical trial to examine efficacy and dose response of exercise as treatment for depression. *Controlled Clinical Trials* 2002;23:584-603.

Einarson, T.R., and Einarson, A. Newer antidepressants in pregnancy and rates of major malformations: A meta-analysis of prospective comparative studies. *Pharmacoepidemiology and Drug Safety* 2005;14:823-27.

Ellis, A., and Dryden, W. *The Practice of Rational Emotive Behavior Therapy*, 2nd edition. New York: Springer Publishing Co., 2007.

Ellis, A., and Harper, R.A. *A Guide to Rational Living*, 3rd revised edition. Chatsworth, CA: Wilshire Book Co., 1975.

Erickson, K.I., and Kramer, A.F. Aerobic exercise effects on cognitive and neural plasticity in older adults. *British Journal of Sports Medicine* 2009;43:22-24.

Erlangsen, A., Canudas-Romo, V., and Conwell, Y. Increased use of antidepressants and decreasing suicide rates: a population-based study using Danish register data. *Journal of Epidemiology and Community Health* 2008;62:448-54.

Fagiolini, A., and Kupfer, D.J. Is treatment-resistant depression a unique subtype of depression? *Biological Psychiatry* 2003;53:640–48.

Fava, G.A., Rafanelli, C., Grandi, S., Conti, S., and Belluardo, P. Prevention of recurrent depression with cognitive behavioral therapy: preliminary findings. *Archives of General Psychiatry* 1998;55:816-20.

Fava, G.A., Ruini, C., Rafanelli, C., et al. Six-year outcome of cognitive behavioral therapy for prevention of recurrent depression. *American Journal of Psychiatry* 2004;161:1872-76.

Fava, M. Diagnosis and definition of treatment-resistant depression. *Biological Psychiatry* 2003;53:649-59.

Fava, M., Rush, A.J., Alpert, J.E., et al. Difference in treatment outcome in outpatients with anxious versus nonanxious depression: a STAR*D report. *American Journal of Psychiatry* 2008;165:342-51.

Frank, E., Hlastala, S., Ritenour, A., et al. Inducing lifestyle regularity in recovering bipolar disorder patients: results from the maintenance therapies in bipolar disorder protocol. *Biological Psychiatry* 1997;41:1165-73.

Frank, E., Kupfer, D.J., Wagner, E.F., et al. Efficacy of interpersonal psychotherapy as a maintenance treatment of recurrent depression: contributing factors. *Archives of General Psychiatry* 1991;48:1053-59.

Freedman, R. Long-term effects of early genetic influence on behavior. *New England Journal of Medicine* 2002;347:213-15.

Freeman, M.P. Antenatal depression: navigating the treatment dilemmas. *American Journal of Psychiatry* 2007;164:1162-65.

Freud, S. Mourning and melancholia. In Strachey, J., ed. and trans, *The Standard Edition of the Complete Psychological Works of Sigmund Freud*, vol. 14 (1914-1916): *On the History of the Psycho-Analytic Movement*, Papers on Metapsychology and Other Works. London: Hogarth Press, 1917:237-58.

Frodl, T.S., Koutsouleris, N., Bottlender, R., et al. Depression-related variation in brain morphology over 3 years: effects of stress? *Archives of General Psychiatry* 2008;65:1156-65.

Gage, F.H. Brain, repair yourself. *Scientific American* 2003;289 (3):46-53.

Geddes, J.R., Carney, S.M., Davies, C., Furukawa, T.A., Kupfer, D.J., Frank, E., and Goodwin, G.M. Relapse prevention with antidepressant drug treatment in depressive disorders: a systematic review. *Lancet* 2003;361:653-61.

Gervasoni, N., Aubry, J.-M., Bondolfi, G., et al. Partial normalization of serum brain-derived neurotrophic factor in remitted patients after a major depressive episode. *Neuropsychobiology* 2005;51:234-38.

Ghaemi, S.N., Boiman, E.E., and Goodwin, F.K. Diagnosing bipolar disorder and the effect of antidepressants: a naturalistic study. *Journal of Clinical Psychiatry* 2000;61:804-8.

Gillespie, C.F., and Nemeroff, C.B. Early life stress and depression. *Current Psychiatry* 2005;4(10):15-30.

Goldapple, K., Segal, Z., Garson, C., Lau, M., Bieling, P., Kennedy, S., and Mayberg, H. Modulation of cortical-limbic pathways in major depression: treatment-specific effects of cognitive behavior therapy. *Archives of General Psychiatry* 2004;61:34-41.

Gorman, J. *The New Psychiatry*. New York: St. Martin's Press, 1996.

Gorman, J.M. *The Essential Guide to Psychiatric Drugs*, Revised and Updated, 4th edition. New York: St. Martin's Press, 2007.

Gould, E., Reeves, A.J., Graziano, M.S., and Gross, C.G. Neurogenesis in the neocortex of adult primates. *Science* 1999;286:548-52.

Grawe, K. *Neuropsychotherapy: How the Neurosciences Inform Effective Psychotherapy.* New York: Routledge Press, 2006.

Greene, K. The latest in mental health: working out at the "brain gym." *Wall Street Journal,* March 28, 2009.

Grilo, C.A., Shea, T.M., Skodol, A.E., et al. Two-year prospective naturalistic study of remission from major depressive disorder as a function of personality disorder comorbidity. *Journal of Consulting and Clinical Psychology* 2005;73:78-85.

Grossman, P., Niemann, L., Schmidt, S., and Walach, H. Mindfulness-based stress reduction and health benefits: a meta-analysis. *Journal of Psychosomatic Research* 2004;57:35-43.

Grove, G., Coplan, J.D., and Hollander, E. The neuroanatomy of 5-HT dysregulation and panic disorder. *Journal of Neuropsychiatry* 1997;9:198-207.

Gunnell, D., Saperia, J., and Ashby, D. Selective serotonin reuptake inhibitors (SSRIs) and suicide in adults: meta-analysis of drug company data from placebo controlled, randomized controlled trials submitted to the MHRA's safety review. *British Medical Journal* 2005;330:385-89.

Gurling, H., Smyth, C., Kalsi, G., et al. Linkage findings in bipolar disorder. *Nature Genetics* 1995;10:8-9.

Habermas, T., and Bluck, S. Getting a life: the emergence of the life story in adolescence. *Psychological Bulletin* 2000;126:748-69.

Haddad, P.M. Antidepressant discontinuation syndromes: clinical relevance, prevention and management. *Drug Safety* 2001;24:183-97.

Hales, R.E., and Yudofsky, S.C. *Essentials of Clinical Psychiatry,* 2nd edition. Washington, DC: American Psychiatric Press, 2004.

Hallberg, P., and Sjoblom, V. The use of selective serotonin reuptake inhibitors during pregnancy and breastfeeding: a review and clinical aspects. *Journal of Clinical Psychopharmacology* 2005;25:59-73.

Hamilton, M. A rating scale for depression. *Journal of Neurology, Neurosurgery and Psychiatry* 1960;23:56-62.

Hellerstein, D.J., Kocsis, J.H., Chapman, D., Stewart, J.W., and Harrison, W. Double-blind comparison of sertraline, imipramine, and placebo in the treatment of dysthymia: effects on personality. *American Journal of Psychiatry* 2000;157:1436-44.

Hellerstein, H.K., with Snyder, A. *A Matter of Heart.* Caldwell, ID: Griffith Publishing, 1994.

Hendrie, H.C., Albert, M.S., Butters, M.A., et al. The NIH cognitive and emotional health project: report of the critical evaluation study committee. *Alzheimer's and Dementia* 2006;2:12-32.

Hettema, J.M., Neale, M.C., and Kendler, K.S. A review and meta-analysis of the genetic epidemiology of anxiety disorders. *American Journal of Psychiatry* 2001;158:1568-78.

Higgins, E.S. Is depression neurochemical or neurodegenerative? *Current Psychiatry* 2004;3 (9):39-40.

Hiller, J. Speculations on the links between feelings, emotions and sexual behaviour: are vasopressin and oxytocin involved? *Sexual and Relationship Therapy* 2004;19:393-412.

Hirschfeld, R.M.A., Lewis, L., and Vornik, L.A. Perceptions and impact of bipolar disorder: how far have we really come? Results of the National Depressive and Manic-Depressive Association 2000 survey of individuals with bipolar disorder. *Journal of Clinical Psychiatry* 2003;64:161-74.

Holden, C. Future brightening for depression treatments. *Science* 2003;302:810-13.

Hollon, S.D., DeRubeis, R.J., Shelton, R.C., et al. Prevention of relapse following cognitive therapy vs. medications in moderate to severe depression. *Archives of General Psychiatry* 2005;62:417-22.

Hull, A.T. Neuroimaging findings in posttraumatic stress disorder: systematic review. *British Journal of Psychiatry* 2002;181:102-10.

Insel, T.R., and Quirion, R. Psychiatry as a clinical neuroscience discipline. *JAMA* 2005;294:2221-24.

Insel, T.R., and Young, L.J. The neurobiology of attachment. *Nature Reviews/Neuroscience* 2001;2:129-36.

Israel, J.A. Remission in depression: definition and initial treatment approaches. *Journal of Psychopharmacology* 2006;20(3):5-10.

Jacobs, B.L., van Praag, H., and Gage, F.H. Adult neurogenesis and psychiatry: a novel theory of depression. *Molecular Psychiatry* 2000;5:262-69.

———. Depression and the birth and death of brain cells. *American Scientist* 2000;88:340-45.

Jacobson, E. *Progressive Relaxation*, 3rd edition. Chicago: University of Chicago Press, 1974.

Jick, H., Kaye, J., and Jick, S. Antidepressants and the risk of suicidal behaviors. *JAMA* 2004;292:338-43.

Jindal, R.D., and Thase, M.E. Integration of care: integrating psychotherapy and pharmacotherapy to improve outcomes among patients with mood disorders. *Psychiatric Services* 2003;54:1484-90.

Johnstone, T., van Reekum, C.M., Urry, H.L., Kalin, N.H., and Davidson, R.J. Failure to regulate: counterproductive recruitment of top-down prefrontal-subcortical circuitry in major depression. *Journal of Neuroscience* 2007;27:8877-84.

Judd, L.L., Akiskal, H.S., Maser, J.D., et al. Major depressive disorder: a prospective study of residual subthreshold depressive symptoms as predictor of rapid relapse. *Journal of Affective Disorders* 1998;50;97–108.

Judd, L.L., Paulus, M.J., Schettler, P.J., et al. Does incomplete recovery from first lifetime major depressive episode herald a chronic course of illness? *American Journal of Psychiatry* 2000;157:1501–4.

Kabat-Zinn, J. *Full Catastrophe Living: Using the Wisdom of Your Body and Mind to Face Stress, Pain and Illness*. New York: Delta, 1990.

Kandel, E.R. The molecular biology of memory storage: a dialog between genes and synapses. *Bioscience Reports* 2004;24:477-522.

Keitner, G.I., and Miller, I.W. Family functioning and major depression: an overview. *American Journal of Psychiatry* 1990;147:1128-37.

Keller, M.B., McCullough, J.P., Klein, et al. A comparison of nefazodone, the cognitive behavioral-analysis system of psychotherapy, and their combination for the treatment of chronic depression. *New England Journal of Medicine* 2000;342:1462-70.

Kessler, R.C., Berglund, P., Olga Demler, M.S., et al. The epidemiology of major depression: results from the National Comorbidity Survey Replication (NCS-R). *JAMA* 2003;289:3095-3105.

Kessler, R.C., DuPont, R.L., Berglund, P., and Wittchen, H.U. Impairment in pure and comorbid generalized anxiety disorder and major depression at 12 months in two national surveys. *American Journal of Psychiatry* 1999;156:1915-23.

Khan, A., Khan, S., Kolts, R., and Brown, W. Suicide rates in clinical trials of SSRIs, other antidepressants, and placebo: analysis of FDA reports. *American Journal of Psychiatry* 2003;160:790-92.

Kim, S.W., Dysken, M.W., and Kuskowski, M. The Yale-Brown Obsessive-Compulsive Scale: a reliability and validity study. *Psychiatry Research* 1990;34:99-106.

Koehl, M., Meerlo, P., Gonzales, D., et al. Exercise-induced hippocampal cell proliferation requires beta endorphin. *FASEB Journal* 2008;22;2253-62.

Kupfer, D.J., Frank, E., Perel, J.M., et al. Five-year outcome for maintenance therapies in recurrent depression. *Archives of General Psychiatry* 1992;49:769-73.

Lam, R.W., and Kennedy, S.H. Evidence-based strategies for achieving and sustaining full remission in depression: focus on meta-analyses. *Canadian Journal of Psychiatry* 2004;49 (suppl 1):17-26.

LeDoux, J. *The Emotional Brain.* New York: Simon & Schuster, 1996.

LeDoux, J. *The Synaptic Self: How Our Brains Become Who We Are.* New York: Penguin Group, 2002.

Li, L., Ma, N., Li, Z., et al. Prefrontal white matter abnormalities in young adult with major depressive disorder: a diffusion tensor imaging study. *Brain Research* 2007;1168:124-28.

Linehan, M.M. *Skills Training Manual for Treating Borderline Personality Disorder.* New York: Guilford Press, 1993.

Lis, E., Greenfield, B., Henry, M., Guile, J.M., and Dougherty, G. Neuroimaging and genetics of borderline personality disorder: a review. *Journal of Psychiatry Neuroscience* 2007;32:162-73.

Lohoff, F.W. Pharmacogenetics of major depressive disorder. *Psychiatric Annals* 2008;36:414-18.

Lydiard, R.B. Break the "fear circuit" in resistant panic disorder. *Current Psychiatry* 2003;11(2):12-22.

Lyubomirsky, S., and Nolen-Hoeksema, S. Effects of self-focused rumination on negative thinking and interpersonal problem solving. *Journal of Personality and Social Psychology* 1995;69:176-90.

MacQueen, G.M., and Young, L.T. Bipolar II disorder: symptoms, courses, and response to treatment. *Psychiatric Services* 2001;52:358-61.

Maguire, E.A., Burgess, N., Donnett, J.G., et al. Knowing where and getting there: a human navigation network. *Science* 1998;280:921-24.

Maguire, E.A., Gadian, D.G., Johnsrude, I.S., et al. Navigation-related structural change in the hippocampi of taxi drivers. *Proceedings of the National Academy of Sciences* 2000;97:4398-4403.

Malberg, J. Implications of adult hippocampus neurogenesis in antidepressant action. *Journal of Psychiatry and Neuroscience* 2004;29:196-205.

Malberg, J.E., Amelia, J.E., Nestler, E.J., and Duman, R.S. Chronic antidepressant treatment increases neurogenesis in adult rat hippocampus. *Journal of Neuroscience* 2000;20:9104-10.

Manji, H.K., Moore, G.J., and Chen, G. Clinical and preclinical evidence for the neurotrophic effects of mood stabilizers: implication for the pathophysiology and treatment of manic-depressive illness. *Biological Psychiatry* 2000;38:740-54.

Manji, H.K., Quiroz, J.A., and Gould, T.D. Cellular resistance and neuroplasticity in mood disorders. *Psychiatric Times*, January 2003:55-59.

Mann, J.J. The medical management of depression. *New England Journal of Medicine* 2005;353:1819-34.

Markowitz, J.C. Psychotherapy of the post-dysthymic patient. *Journal of Psychotherapy Practice and Research* 1993;2:157-63.

Martell, C.R., Addis, M.E., and Jacobson, N.S. *Depression in Context: Strategies for Guided Action*. New York: W.W. Norton, 2001.

Martin, J.B. Integration of neurology, psychiatry and neuroscience in the 21st century. *American Journal of Psychiatry* 2002;159:695-704.

Mather, A.S., Rodriguez, C., Guthrie, M.F., McHarg, A.M., Reid, I.C., and McMurdo, M.E.T. Effects of exercise on depressive symptoms in older adults with poorly responsive depressive disorder. *British Journal of Psychiatry* 2002;180:411-15.

Mayberg, H.S. Defining neurocircuits in depression. *Psychiatric Annals* 2006;36:259-68.

_____. Modulating dysfunctional limbic-cortical circuits in depression: toward development of brain-based algorithms for diagnosis and optimized treatment. *British Medical Bulletin* 2003;65:193-207.

Mayberg, H.S., Brannan, S.K., Tekell, J.L., et al. Regional metabolic effects of fluoxetine in major depression: serial changes and relationship to clinical response. *Biological Psychiatry* 2000;48:830-43.

Mayberg, H.S., Lozano, A.M., Voon, V., et al. Deep brain stimulation for treatment-resistant depression. *Neuron* 2005;45:651-60.

Mayo Clinic staff. Treatment-resistant depression: explore options when depression won't go away. August 29, 2007. www.mayoclinic.com/print/treatment-resistant-depression/DN00016.

McEwen, B.S. The neurobiology of stress: from serendipity to clinical relevance. *Brain Research* 2000;886:172-89.

Montgomery, S.A., Asberg, M. A new depression scale designed to be sensitive to change. *British Journal of Psychiatry* 1979;134:382-89.

Mulder, R.T. Personality pathology and treatment outcome in major depression: a review. *American Journal of Psychiatry* 2002;159:359-71.

Nestler, E.J., Barrot, M., DiLeone, R.J., et al. Neurobiology of depression. *Neuron* 2002;34:13-25.

New, A.S., and Hazlett, E.A. Amygdala–prefrontal disconnection in borderline personality disorder. *Neuropsychopharmacology* 2007;32:1629–40.

Nierenberg, A.A., Petersen, T.J., and Alpert, J.E. Prevention of relapse and recurrence in depression: the role of long-term pharmacotherapy and psychotherapy. *Journal of Clinical Psychiatry* 2003;64 (suppl 15):13-17.

Nierenberg, A., and Wright, E. Evolution of remission as the new standard in treatment of depression. *Journal of Clinical Psychiatry* 1999;60:7–11.

Olfson, M., Marcus, S.C., Druss, B., Elinson, L., Tanielian, T., and Pincus, H.A. National trends in the outpatient treatment of depression. *JAMA* 2002;287:203-9.

Otto, M.W., Smits, J.A.J., and Reese, H.E. Cognitive-behavioral therapy for the treatment of anxiety disorders. *Journal of Clinical Psychiatry* 2004;65 (suppl 5):34-41.

Pakpan, A. Lithium and valproate may provide neurotrophic and neuroprotective effects. *Bipolar Disorder and Impulsive Spectrum Newsletter* August 2001;1-3.

Palmer, R.L. Dialectical behavior therapy for borderline personality disorder. *Advances in Psychiatric Treatment* 2002;8:10-16.

Patoine, B. Move your feet, grow new neurons? Exercise-induced neurogenesis shown in humans. *BrainWork*. Dana Foundation, May 1, 2007.

Peet, M., and Stokes, C. Omega-3 fatty acids in the treatment of psychiatric disorders. *Drugs* 2006;65:1061-69.

Pereira, A.C., Huddleston, D.E., Brickman, A.M., et al. An in vivo correlate of exercise-induced neurogenesis in the adult dentate gyrus. *Proceedings of the National Academy of Sciences* 2007;104:5638-43.

Pfaus, J.G. Neurobiology of sexual behavior. *Current Opinion in Neurobiology* 1999;9:751-58.

Pilkonis, P.A., and Frank, E. Personality pathology in recurrent depression: nature, prevalence, and relationship to treatment response. *American Journal of Psychiatry* 1988;145:435-41.

Pollak, D.D., Monje, F.J., Zuckerman, L., Denny, C.A., Drew, M.R., and Kandel, E.R. An animal model of a behavioral intervention for depression. *Neuron* 2008;60:149-61.

Quitkin, F.M. Depression with atypical features: diagnostic validity, prevalence, and treatment. *Primary Care Companion Journal of Clinical Psychiatry* 2002;4:94-99.

Rizzolatti, G., and Craighero, L. The mirror-neuron system. *Annual Review of Neurosciences* 2004;27:169-92.

Rogan, M.T., Leon, K.M., Perez, D.L., and Kandel, E.R. Distinct neural signatures for safety and danger in the amygdala and striatum of the mouse. *Neuron* 2006;46:309-20.

Rosen, R.C., Lane, R.M., and Menza, M. Effects of SSRIs on sexual function: a critical review. *Journal of Clinical Psychopharm* 1999;19:67-85.

Roy-Byrne, P. Predictive power of genes: stronger but not ready for the clinic. *Journal Watch: Psychiatry* 2009;15(1):7-8.

Rush, A.J., Crismon, M.L., Kashner, T.M., et al. The Texas Medication Algorithm Project for major depression, Phase 3. *Journal of Clinical Psychiatry* 2003;64:357-69.

Rush, A.J., Kraemer, H.C., Sackeim, H.A., et al. Report by the ACNP Task Force on response and remission in major depressive disorder. *Neuropsychopharmacology* 2006;31:1841–53.

Rush, A.J., Trivedi, M.H., Ibrahim, H.M., et al. The 16-Item Quick Inventory of Depressive Symptomatology (QIDS), Clinician Rating (QIDS-C), and Self-report (QIDS-SR): a psychometric evaluation in patients with chronic major depression. *Biological Psychiatry* 2003;54:573–83.

Rush, A.J., Trivedi, M.H., Wisniewski, S.R., et al. Acute and longer-term outcomes in depressed outpatients requiring one or several treatment steps: A STAR*D report. *American Journal of Psychiatry* 2006;163:1905-17.

Russo-Neustadt, A.A., Beardy, R.C., Huang, Y.M., and Cotman, C.W. Physical activity and antidepressant treatment potentiate the expression of specific brain-derived neurotrophic factor transcripts in the rat hippocampus. *Neuroscience* 2000;101:305-12.

Sabshin, M. Turning points in twentieth-century American psychiatry. *American Journal of Psychiatry* 1990;147:1267-74.

Sacks, O. *Awakenings*. New York: Knopf, 1990.

Sadock, B.J., and Sadock, V.A. Clinical manifestations of psychiatric disorders. In Sadock, B.J., and Sadock, V.A., eds., *Kaplan and Sadock's Comprehensive Textbook of Psychiatry*. Philadelphia: Lippincott Williams and Wilkins, 2009;789-823.

———. Diagnosis and psychiatry: examination of the psychiatric patient. In Sadock, B.J., and Sadock, V.A., eds., *Kaplan and Sadock's Comprehensive Textbook of Psychiatry*. Philadelphia: Lippincott Williams and Wilkins, 2009;652-788.

———. Psychological factors affecting medical conditions. In Sadock, B.J., and Sadock, V.A., eds., *Kaplan and Sadock's Comprehensive Textbook of Psychiatry*. Philadelphia: Lippincott Williams and Wilkins, 2009;1765-1887.

Santarelli, L., Saxe, M., Gross, C., et al. Requirement of hippocampal neurogenesis for the behavioral effects of antidepressants. *Science* 2003;301:805-9.

Sapolsky, R.M. Stress is bad for your brain. *Science* 1996;273:749-50.

Schiraldi, G.R. *The Post-Traumatic Stress Disorder Sourcebook: A Guide to Healing, Recovery, and Growth*. New York: McGraw Hill, 2009.

Schore, A.N. Effects of a secure attachment relationship on right brain development, affect regulation, and infant mental health. *Infant Mental Health Journal* 2001;22:7-66.

Schwartz, J.M., and Begley, S. *The Mind and the Brain: Neuroplasticity and the Power of Mental Force*. New York: Harper Collins, 2003.

Sen, S., Duman, R., and Sanacora, G. Serum brain-derived neurotrophic factor, depression and antidepressant medications: meta-analyses and implications. *Biological Psychiatry* 2008;64:527-32.

Severus, W.E., Littman, A.B., and Stoll, A.L. Omega-3 fatty acids, homocysteine, and the increased risk of cardiovascular mortality in major depressive disorder. *Harvard Review of Psychiatry* 2001;9:280-93.

Sheline, Y.I. Neuroimaging studies of mood disorder effects on the brain. *Biological Psychiatry* 2003;54:338-52.

Sheline, Y.I., Wang, P.W., Gado, M.H., et al. Hippocampal atrophy in recurrent major depression. *Proceedings of the National Academy of Sciences* 1996;93:3908-13.

Shelton, R.C. Treatment-resistant depression: therapeutic options. Medscape Psychiatry and Mental Health eJournal 1(6), 1996. www.medscape.com/viewarticle/431515.

Shulman, R.B. Response versus remission in the treatment of depression: understanding residual symptoms. *Primary Psychiatry* 2001;8:28-34.

Siegel, D.J. An interpersonal neurobiology approach to psychotherapy. *Psychiatric Annals* 2006;36:248-56.

_____. *The Developing Mind: Toward a Neurobiology of Interpersonal Experience*. New York: Guilford Press, 1999.

_____. Toward an interpersonal neurobiology of the developing mind: attachment relationships, "mindsight," and neural integration. *Infant Mental Health Journal* 2001;22:67-94.

Silbersweig, D., Clarkin, J.F., Goldstein, M., et al. Failure of frontolimbic inhibitory function in context of negative emotion in borderline personality disorder. *American Journal of Psychiatry* 2007;164:1832-41.

Simon, G.E., Savarino, J., Operskalski, B., and Wang, P.S. Suicide risk during antidepressant treatment. *American Journal of Psychiatry* 2006;163:41-47.

Solomon, D.A., Leon, A.C., Mueller, T.I., et al. Tachyphylaxis in unipolar major depressive disorder. *Journal of Clinical Psychiatry* 2005;66:283-90.

Stahl, S.M., and Muntner, N. *Stahl's Essential Psychopharmacology: Neuroscientific Basis and Practical Applications*. New York: Cambridge University Press, 2006.

Stein, D.J. The neurobiology of panic disorder: toward an integrated model. *CNS Spectrums* 2005;10(suppl 12):12-24.

Stein, D.J., Ives-Deliperi, V., Thomas, K.G.F. Psychobiology of mindfulness. *CNS Spectrums* 2008;13:752-756.

_____. The psychobiology of resilience. *CNS Spectrums* 2009;14(2, suppl 3):41-47.

Storr, A. *Solitude: A Return to the Self*. New York: Free Press, 1988.

Stout, S.C., and Musselman, D.L. Depression and cardiovascular disease. *Depression: Mind and Body* 2005;2(1):2-10.

Suehs, B., Argo, T.R., Bendele, S.D., Crismon, M.L., Trivedi, M.K., and Kurian, B. *Texas Medication Algorithm Project: Procedural Manual*. Texas Department of State Health Services, Austin, Texas, 2008.

Suppes, T., and Dennehy, E.B. Evidence-based long-term treatment of bipolar II disorder. *Journal of Clinical Psychiatry* 2002;63(suppl 10)29-33.

Teasdale, J.D., Segal, Z.V., Williams, G.M.G., Ridgeway, V.A., Soulsby, J.M., and Lau, M.A. Prevention of relapse/recurrence in major depression by mindfulness-based cognitive therapy. *Journal of Consulting and Clinical Psychology* 2000;68:615-23.

Thase, M. Evaluating antidepressant therapies: remission as the optimal outcome. *Journal of Clinical Psychiatry* 2003;64(suppl 13):18-25.

_____. When are psychotherapy and pharmacotherapy combinations the treatment of choice for major depressive disorder? *Psychiatric Quarterly* 1999;70:333-46.

Trivedi, M.H., Greer, T.L., Grannemann, B.D., Chambliss, H.O., and Jordan, A.N. Exercise as an augmentation strategy for treatment of major depression. *Journal of Psychiatric Practice* 2006;12:205-13.

van Praag, H., Shubert, T., Zhao, C., and Gage, F.H. Exercise enhances learning and hippocampal neurogenessis in aged mice. *Journal of Neuroscience* 2006;25:8680-85.

Van Rhoads, R., and Gelenberg, A.J. Treating depression to remission: target recovery, and give patients back their lives. *Current Psychiatry* 2005;4(9):15-28.

Viamontes, G.I., and Beitman, B.D. Neural substrates of psychotherapeutic change. I: The default brain. *Psychiatric Annals* 2006;36:225-237.

Viamontes, G.I., and Beitman, B.D. Neural substrates of psychotherapeutic change. II: Beyond default mode. *Psychiatric Annals* 2006;36:238-47.

Videbech, P., and Ravnkilde, B. Hippocampal volume and depression: a meta-analysis of MRI studies. *American Journal of Psychiatry* 2004;161:1957-66.

Viguera, A.C., Baldessarini, R.J., and Friedberg, J. Discontinuing antidepressant treatment in major depression. *Harvard Review of Psychiatry* 1998;5(6),293-306.

Watkins, E., and Baracaia, S. Rumination and social problem-solving in depression. *Behavior Research and Therapy* 2002;40:1179-89.

Weissman, M.M., Bland, R.C., Canino, G.J., et al. Cross-national epidemiology of major depression and bipolar disorder. *JAMA* 1996;276:293-99.

Williams, J.M.G., Barnhofer, T., Crane, C., et al. Autobiographical memory specificity and emotional disorder. *Psychological Bulletin* 2007;133:123-48.

Winerip, M. A life on the decline, and then the "Why?" *New York Times*, September 18, 2009.

Winslow, J.T., Hastings, N., Carter, C.S., Harbaugh, C.R., and Insel, T.R. A role for central vasopressin in pair bonding in monogamous prairie voles. *Nature* 1993;365:545-48.

Wisner, K.L., Parry, B.L., and Piontek, C.M. Postpartum depression. *New England Journal of Medicine* 2002;347:194-99.

Yatham, L.N. Diagnosis and management of patients with bipolar II disorder. *Journal of Clinical Psychiatry* 2005;66 (suppl 1):13-17.

Yonkers, K.A. The treatment of women suffering from depression who are either pregnant or breastfeeding. *American Journal of Psychiatry* 2007;164:1457-59.

Yudofsky, S.C., and Hales, R.E. Neuropsychiatry and the future of psychiatry and neurology. *American Journal of Psychiatry* 2002;159:1261-64.

Zimmerman, M., Posternak, M.A., and Chelminski, I. Implications of using different cutoffs on symptom severity scales to define remission from depression. *International Clinical Psychopharmacology* 2004;19:215–20.

Index

adjustment reaction, 59, 83

adrenal glands, 24, 57, 113, 139, 198

adrenaline, 96, 100

agitation, 19, 92, 107, 109, 143, 195, 210

alcohol, 24, 186, 195, 199; and depression, 89; effects of, 51; and evaluation, 66; and medication, 120, 240; and neurogenesis, 122; and resilience, 212; and serotonin system, 59; and treatment, 88

alcoholism, 16, 46, 56

amygdala, 71, 111, 114, 162, 207, 208, 209; blocking false alarms of, 44; and borderline personality disorder, 217–18; changes in, 128, 141, 142, 148; and cognitive-behavioral therapy, 152; and depression, 22, 23, 31, 128; effect of medication on, 98; evaluation of, 42, 43; and fear, 9, 23, 37, 75, 112, 116, 230; and hippocampus, 100, 148; and hyperventi-lation, 72–73; and panic disorder, 64; and recovery, 166, 177; and remission, 139; and safety, 227; and sexual behavior, 167; and stress hormones, 24; and treatment resistance, 198. *See also* brain, parts of

antidepressant medication, 52, 92; choice of, 86; and cognitive-behavioral therapy, 152; combinations of, 200; and dentate gyrus, 113; and exercise, 176, 214; high-side-effect, 8; and metabolism, 204; and neurogenesis, 122; and pregnancy, 184, 186; response to, 58, 127; and serotonin system, 58; and sexuality, 180; and side effects, 86; tricyclic (TCAs), 58, 84, 87. *See also* medication, specific

anxiety, 35–36, 63, 110, 137, 146, 161–62, 208, 210; as ally vs. enemy, 118; and amygdala, 23; anticipatory, 71, 73–74; and brain function, 115; and depression, 16; and evaluation, 42; management of, 71–74, 102, 116; and New Neuropsychiatry, 5; and panic attacks, 17; recovery from, 166; and relaxation exercises, 72–73; and serotonin system, 54, 55; toleration of, 77; as useful, 135

anxiety disorder, 54–58; and avoidance, 153; biological vulnerability for, 74; and brain changes, 140, 141; brain damage from, 7; and brain physiology, 23;

medial prefrontal cortex, 139, 198; mirror neurons, 114; orbitofrontal cortex, 111, 114, 148; pineal gland, 114; premotor cortex, 114; putamen, 111, 113, 230; pyramidal cells, 118; raphe/raphe nuclei, 54, 114; reticular activating system of, 42, 115; reticular formation, 115; right frontal area, 22; right prefrontal cortex, 22; right temporal-parietal cortex, 22; rostral cingulate, 142; subcortical areas, 115; subgenual anterior cingulate, 2, 115; subgenual prefrontal cortex, 151; synaptic cleft, 18; temporal lobes, 113; thalamus, 43, 115; ventral tegmental area, 198. *See also* amygdala; hippocampus; prefrontal cortex

brain imaging, 67. *See also* MRI (magnetic resonance imaging) scan; PET (positron emission tomography) scan

brain-derived neurotrophic factor (BDNF), 57, 90, 177, 178, 198. *See also* neurotrophic factors

breathing exercises, 71, 116, 122, 157, 211, 242; and bottom-up control, 104; and medication, 241; method of, 72–73; and present moment, 121; and remission, 158; and treatment, 74, 80, 90. *See also* exercise; meditation; mindfulness exercises

case studies: Adrienne, 50; Ahmad, 150; Alexandra, 150, 159; Amelia, 50; Becca, 52, 53; Betty, 53; Bob, 180; Britta, 149; Cecil, 96; George, 50; Herb, 151; Ilene, 51; Ivan, 149; Joan, 85; Julius, 51; Kenneth, 214–16, 220, 224, 237; Kevin, 135, 136; Luanne, 180; Marianne, 87; Marsha, 83; Marvin, 151; Nell, 50, 51–52, 53; Alexandra O'Connor, 132–33, 134, 145; Patricia, 216–20, 224, 237; Paul, 181; Ricardo, 53; Rob, 52, 53; Robert, 50; Ryan, 153–54; Steven Schnipper, 223; Stella, 53; Timothy, 52, 53; Toby, 135,

136; Tony, 149; Warner, 242–43. *See also* Johnson, Allen (case study); Linden, Lynette (case study); Maple, Mark (case study); Marietta (case study); Prince, Cindy (case study); Ramos, Hannah Wrenn (case study)

case synthesis: defined, 62, 65–69; and panic disorder, 63–65; and treatment, 73–74, 91–93. *See also individual case studies*

Celexa (citalopram), 18, 96, 154, 182, 184; and breast-feeding, 191; dose of, 200; maintenance of, 232; off-label use of, 87; and pregnancy, 184, 187, 188, 189, 243, 244; and treatment resistance, 200

children, 172; decision to have, 168–69, 170, 183–93, 195; relationship with, 16, 31, 45–46, 48–49, 215, 216. *See also* postpartum depression; pregnancy and childbirth

Cognitive Behavioral Analysis System of Psychotherapy (CBASP), 88

cognitive therapy, 70, 78, 88, 149, 243

cognitive-behavioral therapy (CBT), 29, 155, 156, 211, 242, 244; choice of, 81; and ending medication, 241; medicine-like effects of, 84; and negative thoughts, 151; and New Neuropsychiatry, 157; and panic disorder, 9, 70, 83, 116–18; principles of, 152

concentration: causes for lack of, 59; improvements in, 97, 102, 139, 160, 174, 211, 215, 221; problems with, 14, 19, 40, 48, 50, 197, 209, 210; as residual symptom, 130; and serotonin system disorders, 55

cortisol, 23, 24, 57, 100, 212, 221

couples therapy, 21, 159–60

crisis, 33, 36, 41, 101–9, 106

cure, possibility of, 29, 49, 170

cytokines, 24, 96, 166

depression, 53, 60, 75, 168, 197, 207, 208; acute, 36; and age, 15; and amygdala, 112;

medication, specific (*cont.*)
Luvox, 18, 52, 135, 184; mirtazapine, 181; modafinil, 200; Nardil, 8; Paxil (paroxetine), 18, 77, 87, 135, 180, 186, 209, 215; Pristiq, 182; Remeron, 18–19, 84, 180, 200, 220; Restoril, 53, 209, 210, 221; Risperdal, 107, 109, 179, 241; risperidone, 184; Seroquel, 200; Serzone, 18; Synthroid, 50; Thorazine, 50; Topamax, 208; topiramate, 132; trazodone, 92–93, 99, 238; Valium, 107, 186, 242; Viagra, 181, 182, 201; Xanax, 184, 186, 209, 210, 211, 221; yohimbine, 181; Zithromax, 30; Zyprexa, 63, 200. *See also* Celexa (citalopram); Prozac (fluoxetine); Wellbutrin (bupropion); Zoloft

meditation, 156, 157, 211; and control, 104; and end of medication, 241; and neurogenesis, 7; and remission, 149, 158; and self-calming, 121; use of, 5. *See also* breathing exercises; mindfulness exercises

melatonin, 24, 25, 114, 202

memory, 2, 40, 59, 221; autobiographical, 4, 113; and brain function, 112, 114; consolidation of, 6, 122; declarative, 113; and depression, 22; and exercise, 176; and hippocampus, 5, 6, 22–23, 24, 113, 115, 122, 128–29; and Old Psychiatry, 120; of positive experiences, 157; and PTSD, 75; and remission, 139; working, 31, 129, 139

mind-body connection, 21, 24–25, 89

mindfulness exercises, 5, 70, 121, 149, 157, 211, 220, 241. *See also* breathing exercises; meditation

mood: and borderline personality disorder, 217; and brain function, 115; cycling of, 107, 109, 143, 144; depressed, 19; and disorders, 17; diurnal variation in, 40; evaluation of, 42; improvements in, 102; and omega-3 fatty acids, 201; regulation of, 75, 106; and serotonin system, 54,

55; stabilization of, 107. *See also* mood disorder

mood disorder, 39–40, 54–58, 201, 219; and avoidance, 153; and brain changes, 140; escape from, 7; and genetic vulnerability, 40; ongoing treatment of, 235; personality traits worsened by, 215; and pregnancy, 190; recovery from, 133–34; and relationships, 169; as responsive to SSRIs, 55; and treatment resistance, 196. *See also* mood

MRI (magnetic resonance imaging) scan, 2–3, 4, 10, 22, 55, 112, 127; and borderline personality disorder, 217; and brain connections, 168; and cognitive-behavioral therapy, 152; and jugglers, 178

muscle relaxation, 73, 80, 90, 116, 122, 158, 242. *See also* exercise

neurotrophic factors, 2, 90, 139, 166, 177, 178, 221. *See also* brain-derived neurotrophic factor (BDNF)

New Neuropsychiatry, 1, 2; and brain imaging, 10; and evaluations, 21; focus on present in, 120–21; as interrupting damage to brain, 7; and life story, 47; and narrative, 41; and neuroscience, 4–5; personal challenges of, 27; and stories, 8; treatment goal of, 119

norepinephrine, 18, 19, 55–56, 182, 210, 221, 227

obsessive-compulsive disorder (OCD), 37, 40, 52, 60, 75, 135; and anterior cingulate cortex, 112; and brain changes, 141; and depression, 39–40, 58; and dopamine, 58; evaluation of, 42; and genetics, 187; improvement in, 95; and libido, 165; medication for, 58, 87; ongoing treatment of, 235, 236; rise in, 56; self-education about, 77; and serotonin, 58; and SSRI medication, 55, 74; symptoms of, 17, 28

suicide (*cont.*)

58; and pregnancy, 186; preoccupation with, 17; rates of, 16, 56; and serotonin, 56; and SSRIs, 8, 9; thoughts of, 19, 108, 217, 222

symptoms, 29, 40, 90, 98, 105–6, 128, 171; breathing to cope with, 73; control of, 5, 106, 203, 224; and daily life, 25, 53; decrease of, 95, 96, 97, 108, 119, 127; and diagnosis, 49; and emotion, 149; evaluation of, 100; frequency of, 234; and loss of motivation, 104; and medication, 70, 88–89, 107; as motivating therapy, 128; and Old Psychiatry, 103–4; and physical ailment, 21; and psychoanalysis, 128–29; reappearance of, 135; residual, 130, 171; review of physical, 66; and self-care, 172; significant and persistent, 16, 19; and therapy, 83, 115

therapist, 19, 20, 21, 67, 80–82

therapy, 5, 102, 103, 108, 109, 169; and achievement of control, 103–4; break from, 98, 110; and catharsis, 102, 103; continuance of, 224; end of, 231–32; evaluation for, 20–21; evidence-based, 81; and hyperactive stress, 115; with initially effective medication, 96; for life problems, 88, 89; and medication, 31, 32, 79, 88–89, 184; and ongoing treatment, 237; previous experiences of, 66; process of, 82; and recovery, 175, 177; during remission, 131; and split treatment, 80; symptoms as motivating, 128; time frame for, 82, 84. *See also* behavioral therapy; cognitive therapy; cognitive-behavioral therapy (CBT); couples therapy; dialectical behavioral therapy (DBT); exposure therapy; interpersonal therapy (IPT); psychotherapy

thought(s), 113; change of negative, 150, 151–53, 154–55, 157, 210; intrusive, 110, 121,

122, 153, 210; negative, 2, 121–22, 130, 147, 210

trauma, 40, 57, 74, 90, 207, 208; and brain changes, 140, 236; experience of, 17; and medical history, 66; memories of, 221; and posttraumatic stress, 17. *See also* posttraumatic stress disorder (PTSD)

treatment, 62–92; after remission, 136; avoidance of, 17–18; beginning of, 94–124; benefits of continuing, 234–35; and case synthesis, 62, 63, 65–69, 73–74, 91–93; changing of, 85; and choice points, 69–74; choices for, 79; collaboration on, 20, 61, 63, 68, 193, 206; completion of, 203, 224; desire for former life through, 26; different responses to, 118–20; effect on brain, 4; end of, 228, 231–45; expectations for, 70; explanation of, 62–63; goal of, 95–96; and history of present illness, 66; and initial treatment package, 62, 69, 70, 79; insight in, 120–24; lifetime, 235; map of, 117, 118; and medication, 84–85; necessity of, 16; obstacles derailing, 96–97; options for, 79, 82; planning of, 5, 70; reevaluation of, 69, 70; refusal to continue, 110; and remission, 119; reregulation of life through, 68–69; response to, 79, 127; return to the normal rhythms and patterns with, 96; and self-healing, 24–25; serial, 79; and series of treatment packages (STP), 69, 79; for several coexisting problems, 88; strategy for, 78; time frame for, 70, 77–78, 79, 234; and treatment package, 71; variety of, 70. *See also* medication; therapy

treatment resistance, 195–224; and anxious depression, 209–10; and brain, 198–99; and complexity, 220; and genetics, 203–5; medication options for, 200–202; and ongoing treatment, 237; and personality style, 214–20; and resilience exercises, 212; and treatment and life-map flowcharts, 206, 207, 209

Wellbutrin (bupropion), 58, 84, 86, 181, 182, 196; function of, 19; and pregnancy, 184; side effects of, 95, 180, 181; and treatment resistance, 200

work, 16, 27, 28, 66, 145, 172

Zoloft, 18, 69, 132, 182; and panic disorder, 58; and pregnancy, 170, 184, 186, 189, 191, 192; and Cindy Prince, 30, 31, 32, 93, 99, 106, 109; side effects of, 77, 182

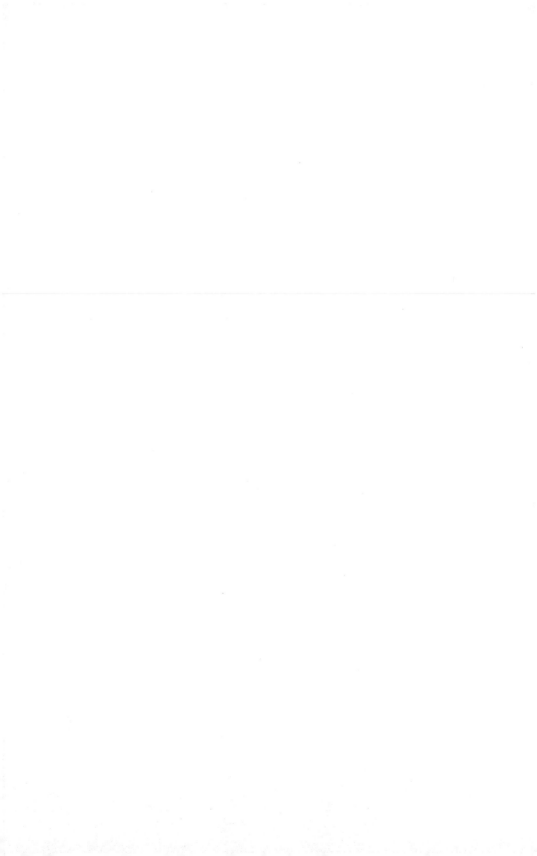